Ovarian Cancer Biomarkers

Khalid El Bairi
Editor

Ovarian Cancer Biomarkers

Mapping to Improve Outcomes

Springer

Editor
Khalid El Bairi
Cancer Biomarkers Working Group
Oujda, Morocco

ISBN 978-981-16-1872-7 ISBN 978-981-16-1873-4 (eBook)
https://doi.org/10.1007/978-981-16-1873-4

This Springer imprint is published by the registered company Springer Nature Singapore Pte Ltd.
The registered company address is: 152 Beach Road, #21-01/04 Gateway East, Singapore 189721, Singapore

We wrote this book with love for oncology and cancer research
Khalid El Bairi

To my parents (Mohammed and Fatima) and
my family for always supporting me
To my friends young oncologists and
researchers on ovarian cancer worldwide
And, particularly to cancer patients

Foreword

Ovarian cancer is often referred to as a silent killer. In the Western world, it is the most lethal gynecological disease, and the fifth most common cancer-related death in women. One reason for the high mortality is a lack of specific symptoms in postmenopausal women and accurate diagnostic testing for detection of the disease at early stages as well as the inevitable development of treatment resistance. Although the 5-year death rate has slightly decreased in the last decade, the overall prognosis and quality of life has not improved substantially. That said, there are major advances being made in ovarian cancer research that have improved the understanding of the disease and might ultimately lead to the development of new therapeutic options. Since the discovery of ovarian cancer, a long road of research has been explored. Ovarian carcinoma is actually no longer considered to be one disease but a spectrum of pathologies with subtype-specific molecular and clinical features. In this book edited by my friend *Khalid El Bairi* from Morocco, Chap. 1 presents the etiology of tubo-ovarian carcinoma and the involvement of several tissues of origin. A better knowledge of the molecular mechanisms and genomic profiles of this cancer has revealed a very complex disease. Chapters 2 and 3 offer a comprehensive summary of the molecular hallmarks of ovarian carcinoma. It is understood that a reduction in the death rate will inevitably be achieved through a better screening of patients. The search for biomarkers for early detection has been relatively unsuccessful in the past. In this regard, major progress has recently been made, with deeper knowledge in the proteomics and genetics of ovarian carcinoma. The most promising biomarkers and guiding treatment options are presented in Chap. 4. In addition, Chap. 5 presents how genomic profiling of ovarian carcinoma could translate into better patient management, in using newer types of circulating biomarkers to measure treatment response. Other novel biomarkers for early diagnosis of tubo-ovarian carcinoma are presented in Chap. 6. Finally, Chap. 7 presents how recent innovative technologies applied to the development of precision medicine, guided by tumor phenotype, can be optimized for the identification of actionable molecular targets. Recent advances in the field continue to push the boundaries of our understanding of this disease and help the evolution of treatments to manage ovarian cancer so that it is no longer the silent killer we know today. I hope that this book will be valuable in offering up-to-date knowledge on this topic for a broad range of ovarian cancer specialists worldwide.

McGill University Health Centre
Montréal, QC, Canada

Cecile Le Page, PhD

Acknowledgments

This book is a part of the annual scientific activities of the *Cancer Biomarkers Working Group* and OVANORDEST studies.

Funding: No funding was received for writing this book.

Contents

About the Editor

Khalid El Bairi is the principal investigator of OVANORDEST studies and the founder of *The Cancer Biomarkers Working Group*, and he is currently pursuing clinical and translational research in medical oncology. He has published many peer-reviewed articles in the field of predictive and prognostic cancer biomarkers to improve survival outcomes in several WoS and Medline-indexed journals. His research focuses particularly on biomarkers for digestive and gynecological cancers such as ovarian and colorectal malignancies. He is currently a member of the board of various international scientific societies such as the International Gynecologic Cancer Society (IGCS), European Society for Medical Oncology (ESMO), American Society of Clinical Oncology (ASCO), European Society of Gynaecological Oncology (ESGO), and the American Association for Cancer Research (AACR). He is also an editor and reviewer for more than 40 academic journals and a guest editor for several special issues on emerging topics in gynecological cancers such as platinum-resistant ovarian cancer. He is also highly interested in teaching evidence-based medicine, clinical research methods, and publishing ethics to medical and PhD students and was selected for the 70th Lindau Nobel Laureate Meeting as a young scientist.

Origins and Pathology of Epithelial Ovarian Cancer: A Brief Overview

1

Sara Nasser, Khalid El Bairi, Dario Trapani, and Boubacar Efared

Abstract

Since the emergence of data about the natural history of ovarian cancer (OC) approximately 150 years ago, tremendous advances have been made in the area of the molecular pathology of this aggressive cancer. However, OC remains one of the most lethal gynecological cancers worldwide, with no adequate screening and prevention program available yet to avoid diagnosis in advanced stages. Despite OC still being the silent killer, it has seen dynamic shifts in its classification, staging, and theories regarding its origins in the last years. In fact, the term OC has experienced a shift to include primary peritoneal and tubal cancer, as these tumors behave identically. The prognosis and treatment of OC are dependent on multiple factors, including tumor biology and extent of tumor spread, which has recently been reclassified in a new FIGO staging system. In the literature throughout the years, attempts to identify the origins of these heterogeneous tumor entities have better guided our diagnostic strategies and therapeutic arsenal. This chapter aims to give a general overview of the epidemiology, the natural history as well as the pathology of epithelial OC.

S. Nasser
Charite Comprehensive Cancer Center, Department of Gynecologic Oncology and Center for Tumor Surgery, Charite Campus Virchow Clinic, Berlin, Germany

K. El Bairi (✉)
Cancer Biomarkers Working Group, Oujda, Morocco
e-mail: k.elbairi@ump.ac.ma

D. Trapani
European Institute of Oncology, IRCCS, Milan, Italy

B. Efared
Laboratory of Pathology, Faculty of Medicine, Abdou Moumouni University, Niamey, Niger

K. El Bairi (ed.), *Ovarian Cancer Biomarkers*,
https://doi.org/10.1007/978-981-16-1873-4_1

Keywords

Ovarian cancer · Epidemiology · Pathology · FIGO classification

1.1 Introduction

Epithelial ovarian cancer (OC) is a leading cause of morbidity, mortality, and disability for women worldwide (Sung et al. 2021). With the advances of clinical and molecular knowledge, OC has been dissected in a heterogeneous group of malignancies, characterized by reproducible specific prognostic and predictive features (Haunschild and Tewari 2021; Govindarajan et al. 2020; Lheureux et al. 2019a). To date, OC is viewed more as a spectrum of diseases, and not a single tumor entity, with different trajectories of ontogenesis, pathogenesis, and carcinogenesis (Shih et al. 2021; Wu et al. 2019). The identification of diversified drivers of the tumorigenesis in the different pathology subtypes of OC has enhanced the pathology-molecular biology continuum and facilitated the clinical implementation of therapeutic interventions per histology and molecular subtypes (Lheureux et al. 2019b). This chapter will briefly address ovarian carcinogenesis, portraying a pathology landscape with key elements of molecular pathogenesis. Useful elements in the clarification of the pathology-molecular biology continuum will be highlighted, and key points on the pathology diagnosis and staging will be presented to outline the essential knowledge on this aggressive women's cancer.

1.2 Epidemiology of Ovarian Cancer

OC is one of the most commonly diagnosed gynecological cancers, associated with the highest mortality rates among women (Bray et al. 2018). For instance, although it has a lower prevalence than breast cancer, it is three times more lethal (Bray et al. 2018; Yoneda et al. 2012; Momenimovahed et al. 2019). OC has been named "*The Silent Killer,*" for the indolent initial progression and the onset of non-specific symptoms only in advanced stages of the disease. Despite significant advances that have been made over the last decades in the diagnosis and treatment of OC, more than 75% of patients still presents in advanced stages (Bray et al. 2018; Bereck et al. 2015, 2018) due to lack of evidence-based and effective screening interventions, along with the delayed onset of symptoms and initial asymptomatic tumor growth (Ahmed et al. 2012; Wu et al. 2018). For the vague associated symptoms, initial OC can be misdiagnosed with other conditions, including gastro-intestinal and other pelvic disorders (Ahmed et al. 2012; Wu et al. 2018). OC is highly diverse in its epidemiological and geographical distribution. Approximately, one-third of OC cases are registered from European countries (Bray et al. 2018; Momenimovahed et al. 2019). Within Europe, OC has a North-to-South distribution gradient with the highest incidence rates in the Scandinavian Region (i.e., Denmark, Finland, and Sweden) and the lowest rates in southern Europe (i.e., Portugal, Greece,

Spain, Italy) (Sehouli and Fotopoulou 2006). This gradient in the incidence rates is also reflected in the worldwide distribution of OC, as it has a higher incidence in high-income countries and a lower incidence in low- and middle-income countries. According to the International Agency for the Research on Cancer (IARC) global cancer registry (GLOBOCAN), OC has an age-standardized incidence rate (ASR) of 8.5 per 100,000 women per year in countries with a very high Human development index (HDI) as compared to an ASR of almost half (4.7 per 100,000 women per year) in countries with a low HDI (Bray et al. 2018; Momenimovahed et al. 2019), based on 2018 estimates. The differences between high and low HDI countries have remained unchanged since 1973, as evaluated by Zhang et al. (2019a). In general, age-adjusted incidence rates for cancer has been increasing in the last decades, as a result of lifestyle changes and enhanced healthcare, with more longevous populations (Bray et al. 2018); however, still, the highest rates for OC are observed in high HDI countries, especially Central Europe, and Central and South America (Zhang et al. 2019a). These differences in the incidence are most likely attributable to the various risk factors associated with OC. It can be argued that factors such as obesity rates, smoking, use of the contraceptive pill, number of pregnancies, nutritional, and lifestyle factors do vary significantly between high HDI and low HDI countries and hence may influence the incidence rates of OC in these regions (Bray et al. 2018). Furthermore, in low HDI countries, quality registration of health conditions may be only partially implemented, and the lower incidence rates may mirror low population coverage of cancer registration and overall under diagnosis of cancer (Bray et al. 2018). Hence, this could be a confounding factor in representing the true incidence rates in these regions. In contrast to the above, the mortality rate for OC is inversely distributed to the incidence rates, with higher mortality rates in low HDI compared to high HDI countries. According to GLOBOCAN 2018 data, 184,799 deaths were registered due to OC in 2018, of which only one-third in countries at very-high HDI (Bray et al. 2018). This represents 4.4% of the mortality rate of all cancers in women (Bray et al. 2018; Momenimovahed et al. 2019). The highest mortality rates are seen in Asia (specifically in India) (Bray et al. 2018). The global disparities in cancer mortality can be attributed to the lack of resilient health systems and sufficient healthcare resources to deliver quality, timely, accessible, available, and affordable cancer care (Bray et al. 2018). For OC, the disparities in cancer mortality are mostly related to the delayed access to surgical treatments and to affordable chemotherapy (Bray et al. 2018). OC remains one of the deadly gynecological cancers worldwide until to date. Mortality varies greatly according to geographical distribution and mirrors the environmental, lifestyle, health system, socioeconomic, and reproductive risk factors around the world.

1.3 Origins of Ovarian Cancer

The exact origin of OC has remained controversial throughout the 150-year known natural history of the disease. The earliest theory was the development from the ovarian surface epithelium (OSE) (Desai et al. 2014). In the earliest study by Cheng et al., mouse ovarian surface epithelial cells (MOSEC) with ectopic expression of *HOXA9*, *HOXA10* and *HOXA11* genes were injected into mice (Cheng et al. 2005). This resulted in the development of serous, endometrioid, and mucinous cancers, supporting the theory that OC can indeed originate from malignant transformation of OSE. Additionally, the OSE can also be vulnerable to malignant transformation due to repeated injury (such as the following ovulation or due to hormonal factors) (Eisen and Weber 1998). Ovarian inclusion can arise following ovulation and the invagination of the OSE into the ovarian stroma. The OSE was then postulated to undergo malignant transformation (Zheng and Fadare 2012). This is further supported by observational studies that suggest that factors suppressing ovulation (such as pregnancy, birth-control pill or breast-feeding) can reduce the occurrence of OC (Eisen and Weber 1998; Zheng and Fadare 2012; Purdie et al. 2003), whereas a higher number of lifetime ovulations increase the risk of OC (Zheng and Fadare 2012; Purdie et al. 2003; Risch 1998). However, the OSE theory was then reshaped in 1999 by Dubeau et al. (Dubeau 1999). The author argued that epithelial OCs do not resemble mesothelial tumors, though OSE cells are identical to the mesothelial cells lining the peritoneum. Moreover, the authors highlighted that precancerous lesions are most often not found in the OSE of ovarian inclusion cysts but in the adjacent organs. In 2001, Piek et al. then firstly proposed the fallopian tube as the origin from which epithelial OCs arise and implant on the peritoneum and the ovarian surface (Piek et al. 2001). Consequently, over the last decades, we have seen increasing evidence in the literature that, in fact, epithelial OCs are not a single entity and indeed develop from distinct binary pathways. These pathways result in type I tumors (low-grade serous cancers, low-grade endometrioid, clear cell, mucinous and Brenner tumors) and type II tumors (high-grade serous cancers) (Desai et al. 2014; Bowtell 2010). High-grade serous OC (HGSOC) typically shows *TP53* mutations and frequently occurs in the distal end of the fallopian tubes (Shih et al. 2021). This has been shown in prophylactic salpingectomy specimens obtained from patients with *BRCA1* or *BRCA2* mutation carriers (Shih et al. 2021). Studies have shown that serous tubal intraepithelial carcinomas (STICs) in the distal fimbriated end of the tube are the most likely precursors for the development of HGSOC. The STICs theory is further supported by the following findings:

- Fifty percent of pelvic HGSOCs show the presence of intraepithelial cancers in the fallopian fimbriae (Stanciu et al. 2019; Kindelberger et al. 2007).
- STICs have been found in 10–15% of fallopian tubes that have been prophylactically removed from women with *BRCA* mutations (Finch et al. 2006; Medeiros et al. 2006).
- Ninety-two percent of STICs have shown *TP53* mutations like those found in HGSOCs samples (Stanciu et al. 2019; Ahmed et al. 2010; Cancer Genome Atlas Research Network 2011).
- STICs-related oncogene products (e.g., cyclin E1, Rsf-1, and fatty acid synthase) are also overexpressed in HGSOCs (Stanciu et al. 2019).

Table 1.1 Clinical, histological, and molecular characteristics of type I and type II ovarian cancer

Type I tumors	Type II tumors
Mutated *RAS*	Wild-type *RAS*
Progress from LMP	De novo
Usually LGSC	Usually HGSC
Wild-type *BRCA*	*BRCA* mutations
Generally wild-type *TP53*	*TP53* mutations
Platinum resistant	Platinum sensitive

Abbreviations: *LMP* low malignant potential, *LGSC* low-grade serous cancer, *HGSC* high-grade serous cancer, *BRCA* breast cancer gene, *TP53* tumor protein 53

- STICs have also been found to be present in prophylactic salpingectomy samples without the presence of ovarian carcinomas, and hence, are unlikely it had been formed due to metastasis from an adjacent HGSOC (Desai et al. 2014).

The above observations support the theory that STICs are the origin of HGSOC in either women harboring or not a germline *BRCA* mutation. Compared with high-grade carcinomas, the low-grade serous OC (LGSOC) has a much lower expression of *TP53* mutations and higher expression of estrogen and progesterone receptors and PAX2 (Bowtell 2010). They typically display mutations related to specific signaling pathways which are not present in HGSOC, for example, *KRAS* and *BRAF*, and rarely *TP53* (Kyo et al. 2020). Cystadenomas and borderline tumors represent early stages in the carcinogenesis of LGSOCs (Ho et al. 2004). This is supported by several findings showing that both LGSOCs and borderline tumors express *KRAS* and *BRAF* mutations in about 30–35% of cases (Singer et al. 2003; Kyo et al. 2020). Interestingly, *KRAS* and *BRAF* mutations have even been detected in benign cystadenomas.

LGSOCs initiate their tumorigenesis from tubal epithelial cells invaginating into the ovarian surface epithelium and forming ovarian inclusion cysts or serous cystadenomas (Kyo et al. 2020; Bowtell 2010). These develop into borderline tumors and subsequently into carcinomas. In this process, molecular mutations in *KRAS*, *BRAF*, and *ERBB2* are increased. In contrast, HGSOCs are believed to develop from a different pathway. They start from the tubal epithelium, develop into latent pre-cancer (p53 signature), precancerous lesion (tubal dysplasia), early cancer (STICs) and ultimately into HGSOCs. In this process, the earliest change is the p53 mutation which is currently considered as a hallmark of OC initiation. Table 1.1 summarizes type I and type II pathways for the development of HGSOC and LGSOC (Kyo et al. 2020).

In summary, two distinct trajectories of ovarian carcinogenesis have been reported, associated with specific clinical conditions (e.g., hyperestrinism, endometriosis), pathology and molecular landscapes, resulting in a spectrum of ovarian epithelial malignancies with peculiar treatment-response patterns and prognosis. While the ontogenetic theories of OC seem to diverge substantially, it cannot be excluded that the different theories apply to different experimental and clinical scenarios and may be characteristic of specific OC types. To date, the better definition of the ontogenesis of the high-grade tumors has resulted in a new perspective for cancer staging (i.e., 2014 FIGO system) and in the identification of precursor lesions in the fallopian fimbriae, and not exclusively in the ovaries—suggesting new options for the fertility-preserving risk-reducing surgical interventions for women carrying germline mutations at higher risk of OC (e.g., prophylactic fimbriectomy).

1.4 Ovarian Cancer Histotypes and Staging

1.4.1 Pathology of Epithelial Ovarian Cancer

OC encompasses a spectrum of diverse histology entities (Scully et al. 1998; Vargas 2014), with peculiar carcinogenesis, clinical and molecular patterns, and prognostic significance. Most of the OC arises from the malignant epithelial transformation, and only 10% origins from non-epithelial tissues, including germ cells, sex cord or stroma cells and mesenchymal tumors of the ovary. The majority of ovarian epithelial tumors present with a serous histology (around 80% of all) (Scully et al. 1998). However, a multitude of histology types has been reported, such as mucinous, endometrioid, clear cell, transitional and undifferentiated types, as shown in Table 1.2 (Vargas 2014; Scully et al. 1998). Two-thirds of the deaths from OC are related to high-grade serous adenocarcinomas that are associated with the poorest prognosis. Serous carcinomas are further classified into LGSOCs and HGSOCs. HGSOCs have a peculiar intrinsic biological aggressiveness, with local invasiveness and early peritoneal spread (Bell 2005). In fact, these tumors are more commonly diagnosed as bilateral or locally advanced with conspicuous spread into the peritoneum. HGSOC seems to originate from the coelomic Mullerian epithelium of the

Table 1.2 Overview of epithelial ovarian tumors

	Adenoma	Borderline	Carcinoma
Serous	Serous cystadenoma	Serous borderline tumor (BOT)	Serous ovarian carcinoma
Mucinous	Mucinous cystadenoma	Mucinous BOT of either intestinal type or endocervical type	Mucinous ovarian carcinoma
Endometrioid	Endometrioid cystadenoma	Endometrioid BOT	Endometrioid ovarian carcinoma
Clear cell	Clear cell cystadenoma	Clear cell BOT	Clear cell ovarian carcinoma
Transitional	Brenner tumor	Brenner BOT	Malignant Brenner tumor or transitional cell carcinoma
Undifferentiated	–	–	Undifferentiated ovarian carcinoma
Mixed	Cystadenoma	BOT	Carcinoma

ovarian surface, as well as from the tubo-ovarian fallopian fimbriae and the peritoneum (Zhang et al. 2019b). High-grade serous neoplasms are enriched in mutations of the breast cancer associated genes 1 and 2 (*BRCA1/2*), resulting in a deficiency in the DNA repair machinery and a high burden of DNA mutations, that is a key characteristic of serous tumors (i.e., higher tumor mutational burden) (Zweemer et al. 2000). Of note, the presence of these specific stigmata of the homologous recombination DNA repair mechanism is also associated with enhanced sensitivity to some DNA-targeting agents, including platinum compounds and targeted agents against Poly-ADP-ribose polymerase (PARP) (Alkema et al. 2016). Also, another distinguishing feature of HGSOCs is the presence of *TP53* mutations (with non-synonymous mutations more common than frameshift mutations or deletions) (Zhang et al. 2016; Singh et al. 2017; Ruba et al. 2020). The macroscopic aspects of HGSOCs are not specific; most patients present with advanced stages, with abdominopelvic extension, fallopian tubes are usually embedded in the tumor bulk (WHO 2020). HGSOCs are described at the gross pathology as variably-sized, exophytic tumors with solid or papillary growth patterns and solid areas with necrotic and hemorrhagic parts or bloody fluid-filled cysts (Kaku et al. 2003). Histologically, HGSOCs present with serous differentiation, high mitotic count (>5 mitoses/mm^2 equivalent to >12 mitosis/10 HPF of 0.55 mm in diameter and 0.24 mm^2 in the area) and marked cellular atypia associated sometimes with necrosis. The tumors may have a solid, cribriform papillary or glandular architecture with infiltrative borders (WHO 2020; Singh et al. 2017). At immunohistochemistry, HGSOCs particularly show abnormal p53 oncoprotein immunostaining, reflecting the *TP53* mutation (defined as diffuse and strong p53 nuclear expression (≥80%) or complete absence of immunohistochemical staining with retained internal control staining); rarely, HGSOCs show aberrant cytoplasmic p53 expression (McCluggage 2012; Singh et al. 2017). Also, p16 is diffusely positive ("block-type" staining) in most cases of HGSOCs (McCluggage et al. 2015). Other non-distinctive immunohistochemical staining of HGSOCs (as well as other serous tumors) include the cancer-associated antigen Wilms tumor 1 (WT1) and the paired box 8 transcription factor (PAX8) positivity. Also, they can variously express estrogen and progesterone receptors; the pattern of cytokeratin (CK) staining is also quite peculiar, with CK7-positivity and CK20-negativity (Lee et al. 2002). The above-mentioned immunohistochemical features of HGSOCs may be particularly important in the differential diagnosis with other ovarian carcinomas or metastatic tumors to the ovaries.

LGSOC is a rarer entity of serous carcinomas, representing 1–3% of all epithelial OCs (Gadducci and Cosio 2020). These tumors present mostly in younger patients (i.e., 20–40 years), with an initial more indolent biological behavior. Though less sensitive to chemotherapy, their intrinsic, more indolent nature has been associated with better prognosis, especially in the earlier stages (Gershenson et al. 2006). Grossly, LGSOCs present as unilateral or bilateral solid-cystic tumors with ovarian surface involvement. Histologically, LGSOCs appear as cuboidal, columnar cells, with monotonous proliferation patterns, without high-grade cellular atypia and lower mitotic count (≤12 mitoses/10 HPF), with usually papillary or micropapillary architecture, destructive stromal invasion and frequent calcifications (psamommas)

(WHO 2020). The key IHC finding of this serous variant is the low proliferation index, with Ki-67 staining usually less than 10%. LGSOCs often express estrogen and progesterone receptors, with a normal p53 pattern of immunoexpression (Slomovitz et al. 2020).Notably, the carcinogenesis of a half of low-grade serous proliferation can be peculiarly driven by molecular alterations of the mitogen-activated protein kinases (MAPKs), like *KRAS* and *BRAF*. Eventually, *BRCA* alterations are uncommon.

Mucinous OC (MOC) encompasses up to 5% of all epithelial OCs (Köbel et al. 2010). The clinical and pathology of mucinous malignancies in the ovaries is commonly challenging, as three-quarter of mucinous tumors in ovaries are secondary tumors (i.e., Krukenberg tumors, generally bilateral), and only one-third is a primitive MOC (generally unilateral) (McCluggage 2012). In addition, only a minority of MOC in the ovaries are primary malignant proliferation (i.e., pure MOC), as 90–95% can present in the context of benign or borderline proliferation (Rodríguez and Prat 2002). Younger women are mostly affected. MOC often appears as unilateral solid-cystic neoplasms with a smooth external surface filled with a large amount of gelatinous secretions. Two patterns of tissue invasion have been reported, expansive, and infiltrative (i.e., destructive stromal growth), respectively; the presence of an infiltrative pattern has been associated independently with an adverse prognosis, including in early-stage MOC (Lee and Scully 2000). The immunohistochemical feature of MOC includes positive staining with CK20, CK7, carcinoembryonic antigen (CEA), CA19-9 and CDX2 (McCluggage 2012). MOC stains negative to PAX8, WT1, and hormone receptors (estrogen and progesterone), in contrast with serous OC (McCluggage 2012). This immunostaining profile lacks unfortunately any specificity as many metastatic tumors to ovaries may have these immunohistochemical staining patterns, especially tumors from the digestive tract. Distinguishing primitive MOC from metastases is a challenging issue that requires histopathological, clinical, and imaging correlations (McCluggage 2012; Simons et al. 2019). For their intrinsic chemoresistance, MOC has a better prognosis when diagnosed early and dismal in advanced stages (Kelemen and Köbel 2011).

Endometrioid OC accounts for 10–25% of all epithelial OCs; in 10–15% of the cases, a diagnosis of endometrioid OC is contextual to pre-existing endometriosis, with or without synchronous endometrial hyperplasia or carcinoma (Oswald and Gourley 2015). Endometrioid OC presents mostly as unilateral and as solid hemorrhagic masses without papillae. Squamous metaplasia and adeno-fibroma components are reported in half of the specimens (Gilks and Prat 2009). Endometrioid OC is histologically, graded as its uterine counterpart according to the extent of glandular component and cellular atypia: <5% solid growth (grade 1); 5–50% solid growth (grade 2); >50% solid growth (grade 3) (WHO 2020; Fadare and Parkash 2019). At immunohistochemistry, typically, endometrioid OC stains positive with CK7, PAX8, hormone receptors, and stains negative with WT1, CK20, CDX2, with wild-type p53 staining (normal staining) (Fadare and Parkash 2019). Loss of *PTEN* is a hallmark of carcinogenesis in these tumors, described in 20–25%; also, in 10–20%, patients may have a Lynch syndrome, with a family history of multiple tumors—therefore presenting a hyper-mutating DNA phenotype, recorded as microsatellite instability (MSI) (Pierson et al. 2020).

Clear cell OC are rarer variants, diagnosed in 5–10% of the patients; in women from Japan, this tumor type can encompass up to 25% of the epithelial OCs (Iida et al. 2020). Clear cell OC is associated with endometriosis in up to 70% of the cases (Iida et al. 2020). The prognosis of this tumor is stage-dependent: in the earlier setting, these tumors can have an excellent prognosis (Fujiwara et al. 2016). However, for their intrinsic platinum resistance, patients with advanced disease have a poor prognosis (Sugiyama et al. 2000). At the gross pathology, clear cell OC appears as unilateral cystic mass with solid components, mostly a single and marginated one (Sugiyama et al. 2000). Microscopically, this tumor exhibits tubule-cystic, papillary, or solid architecture, cells with clear to eosinophilic cytoplasm and dense eosinophilic intracytoplasmic secretions (Fadare and Parkash 2019). Cells with a hobnail appearance are typically found in tumors with tubule-cystic architecture. The typical immunohistochemical characteristics of clear cell OC are positive staining with Napsin A, HNF-1β (hepatocyte nuclear factor 1β), PAX8, CK7, and negative staining with hormone receptors (estrogen and progesterone), CK20, and WT1 (McCluggage et al. 2015; Fadare and Parkash 2019). An association with Lynch syndrome has been reported; however, the most characteristic genomic stigmata of these tumors are the presence of *ARID1A* alterations in a half of cases, resulting in a hyper-mutating DNA phenotype (Berns et al. 2018).

Other malignant ovarian epithelial tumors include malignant Brenner tumor, mixed ovarian carcinomas, and undifferentiated carcinomas. These are very rare cancers, and their molecular and histopathological features are not yet well established (WHO 2020; Bennett and Olivia 2020; Tafe et al. 2010). Malignant Brenner tumors resemble histologically invasive urothelial carcinoma but are associated with foci of benign or borderline Brenner tumors (Cuatrecasas et al. 2009). They are usually unilateral and express urothelial markers at immunohistochemistry (p63, GATA3 mainly) (Cuatrecasas et al. 2009). Mixed ovarian carcinomas show two or more histological differentiation (serous, mucinous, endometrioid, clear cell, etc.) (Mackenzie et al. 2015). These tumors seem to be monoclonal, suggesting a common precursor cell of all of the mixed histological components (WHO 2020). Undifferentiated carcinomas are defined as malignant carcinoma with no obvious morphological differentiation. Some are associated with foci of differentiated ovarian carcinomas (especially low-grade endometrioid carcinomas), suggesting progression or dedifferentiation from these tumors (WHO 2020; Tafe et al. 2010).

1.4.2 Staging of Ovarian Cancer

The surgical and pathological staging of epithelial OC is crucial and is a major determinant of the treatment choices and of the prognosis. A standardized international staging system aids in determining the following (Binder et al. 2015):

1. Extent of tumor spread
2. Individual prognosis
3. Treatment efficacy
4. Overall, disease-free and progression-free survival rates

There has been increasing molecular, histological, and genetic evidence in the literature that serous carcinomas of the ovary or peritoneum may have actually originated from the fimbrial end of the fallopian tube (Berek et al. 2018; Prat 2014; Callahan et al. 2007). The theory of the STICs as a precursor of HGSOC has been largely validated and accepted. Some epithelial OCs, in fact, present with extensive pelvic-peritoneal involvement, with no apparent origin in the ovaries (Berek et al. 2018; Callahan et al. 2007; Prat 2014). Therefore, STICs may originate in the fallopian fimbriae and rapidly grow on the ovarian surfaces and implant on the peritoneum, as commonly reported for HGSOC (Kurman and Shih 2010). Hence, the Gynecologic Oncology Committee of the International Federation of Gynecology and Obstetrics (FIGO) revised the staging system in 2014 to incorporate ovarian, fallopian tube, and peritoneal cancer as a single entity (Prat 2014) (Fig. 1.1). The updated staging system enforces the efforts to retrieve the primitive tumor whenever possible; however, when the primary site cannot be successfully identified, the pathologist should label it as "undesigned," more than "unknown primary," as a peritoneal or fallopian origin can still be possible, namely a pelvic origin. In fact, international recommendations are now established for site assignment of the primary tumor in extra-uterine high-grade serous carcinomas of the ovary and distinguish them from fallopian tubes and peritoneal primaries (McCluggage et al. 2015; Singh et al. 2016). For this, the fallopian tubes, or at least their fimbrial ends, should be totally sampled in all the cases of high-grade serous carcinoma (Table 1.3 summarizes diagnostic criteria for assigning primary site in extra-uterine high-grade serous carcinoma according to the latest World Health Organization classification of female genital tumors).

The FIGO staging system includes four stages for OC, based on the peritoneal spread and metastatic pattern (Fig. 1.1). An important addition in the 2014 classification is the subdivision of Stage IC into three risk categories according to the spontaneous or iatrogenic rupture of the tumor capsule and the presence of malignant ascites (Berek et al. 2015). Stage III is now defined according to spread to the retroperitoneal lymph nodes, regardless of the intraperitoneal dissemination (i.e., stage IIIA1 and stage IIIA2, see Fig. 1.1) (Prat 2014). This is based on a study indicating that patients with positive retroperitoneal lymph nodes alone have significantly better survival than those who have intraperitoneal dissemination (Berek 2009). Stage IVB now also includes inguinal lymph nodes metastases (Prat 2014). The FIGO staging system must be considered as a surgical and pathological system. While imaging like computed tomography scan can detect the pelvic and abdominal involvement of epithelial OC, all tumors arising from ovaries, fallopian tubes and primary peritoneal malignancies require a precise surgical staging approach. The findings from operative surgical staging are critical to inform on the prognosis and the optimal treatment choices. In patients with no extra-pelvic symptoms, there is no

Primary tumor (T)		
TNM	FIGO	
TX		Primary tumor cannot be assessed
T0		No evidence of primary tumor
T1	I	Tumor limited to the ovaries (one or both)
T1a	IA	Tumor limited to one ovary; capsule intact, no tumor on ovarian surface; no malignant cells in ascites or peritoneal washings
T1b	IB	Tumor limited to both ovaries; capsules intact, no tumor on ovarian surface; no malignant cells in ascites or peritoneal washings
T1c	IC	Tumor limited to one or both ovaries with any of the subcategories below (IC1-3)
T1c1	IC1	Surgical spill
T1c2	IC2	Capsule ruptured before surgery or tumor on ovarian or fallopian tube surface
T1c3	IC3	Malignant cells in ascites or peritoneal washings
T2	II	Tumor involves one or both ovaries with pelvic extension below pelvic brim
T2a	IIA	Extension and/or implants on the uterus and/or tube(s)
T2b	IIB	Extension to and/or implants in other pelvic tissues
T3	III	Tumor involves one or both ovaries with microscopically confirmed peritoneal metastasis outside the pelvis and/or retroperitoneal lymph node involvement
T3a	IIIA2	Microscopic peritoneal metastasis beyond the pelvis with or without positive retroperitoneal lymph nodes
T3b	IIIB	Macroscopic peritoneal metastasis beyond the pelvis 2 cm or less in greatest dimension with or without positive retroperitoneal lymph nodes
T3c	IIIC	Macroscopic peritoneal metastasis beyond the pelvis >2 cm in greatest dimension including extension to liver capsule or spleen without parenchymal involvement of those organs and with or without positive retroperitoneal lymph nodes
Regional lymph nodes (N)		
TNM	FIGO	
NX		Regional lymph nodes cannot be assessed
N0		No regional lymph node metastasis
N0(i+)		Isolated tumor cells in regional lymph node(s) ≤0.2 mm
N1	IIIA1	Positive (histologically confirmed) retroperitoneal lymph nodes
N1a	IIIAi	Metastasis ≤10 mm in greatest dimension
N1b	IIIAii	Metastasis more than 10 mm in greatest dimension
Distant metastasis (M)		
TNM	FIGO	
M0		No distant metastasis
M1	IV	Distant metastasis including cytology-positive pleural effusion; liver or splenic parenchymal involvement; extra-abdominal organ involvement including inguinal lymph nodes; transmural intestinal involvement
M1a	IVA	Pleural effusion with positive cytology
M1b	IVB	Liver or splenic parenchymal metastases; metastases to extra-abdominal organs (including inguinal lymph nodes and lymph nodes outside the abdominal cavity); transmural involvement of intestine

Fig. 1.1 The current FIGO classification

Table 1.3 Assigning tumor primary site in extra-uterine high-grade serous carcinomas

Primary site	Diagnostic criteria
Fallopian tube	– Presence of STIC, or – Presence of mucosal HGSC, or – Part or the entire length of the fallopian tube in separable from the tumor mass
Ovary	– Both fallopian tubes separate from ovarian mass, and – No STIC or mucosal HGSC in either tubes
Tubo-ovarian	– Fallopian tubes and ovaries not available for complete examination, and – Pathological findings consistent with extra-uterine HGSC
Peritoneal	– Both tubes and both ovaries fully examined, and – No gross or microscopic evidence of STIC or HGSC in tubes or ovaries

Abbreviations: *STIC* serous intraepithelial carcinoma, *HGSC* high-grade serous carcinoma

common need to provide a systemic staging, as the distant metastases are uncommon (Berek et al. 2018). In selected patients with advanced disease at presentation, in which the surgical staging is deemed not appropriate and/or unsafe, a diagnostic biopsy may be considered to provide histologically and molecularly appropriate treatments (Berek et al. 2018).

1.5 Conclusion

The carcinomas of ovarian, tubal, and peritoneal origin remain highly heterogeneous entities. Accumulating epidemiological and molecular evidence shows that the origin for serous high-grade carcinomas is indeed the fallopian tube secretory cells. Additionally, comprehensive molecular analyses have uncovered the key driver events for serous carcinogenesis. This has provided us with novel molecular targets and consequently vast opportunities for new therapies (for additional reading, see Box 1.1).

Box 1.1 Recommended reading of particular interest

Citation	DOI
Iida Y, et al. *Clear cell carcinoma of the ovary: a clinical and molecular perspective*. Int J Gynecol Cancer. 2020: ijgc-2020-001656.	https://doi.org/10.1136/ijgc-2020-001656
Mills AM, Shanes ED. *Mucinous Ovarian Tumors*. Surg Pathol Clin. 2019;12(2):565–585.	https://doi.org/10.1016/j.path.2019.01.008
El Bairi K, et al. *Does the "Devil" originate from the fallopian tubes?* Semin Cancer Biol. 2021:S1044-579X(21)00068-7.	https://doi.org/10.1016/j.semcancer.2021.03.018
Prat J, et al. *Ovarian carcinomas: at least five different diseases with distinct histological features and molecular genetics*. Hum Pathol. 2018;80:11–27.	https://doi.org/10.1016/j.humpath.2018.06.018

(continued)

Box 1.1 (continued)

Kommoss F, Gilks CB. *Pathology of Ovarian Cancer: Recent Insights Unveiling Opportunities in Prevention.* Clin Obstet Gynecol. 2017;60(4):686–696.	https://doi.org/10.1097/GRF.0000000000000314
Jones MR, et al. *Genetic epidemiology of ovarian cancer and prospects for polygenic risk prediction.* Gynecol Oncol. 2017;147(3):705–713.	https://doi.org/10.1016/j.ygyno.2017.10.001
Pietragalla A, et al. *Ovarian cancer predisposition beyond BRCA1 and BRCA2 genes.* Int J Gynecol Cancer. 2020;30(11):1803–1810.	https://doi.org/10.1136/ijgc-2020-001556
Voutsadakis IA. *Low-grade serous ovarian carcinoma: an evolution toward targeted therapy.* Int J Gynecol Cancer. 2020;30(10):1619–1626.	https://doi.org/10.1136/ijgc-2019-000832
Kyo S, et al. *The fallopian tube as origin of ovarian cancer: Change of diagnostic and preventive strategies.* Cancer Med. 2020;9(2):421–431.	https://doi.org/10.1002/cam4.2725

Acknowledgment and Conflicts of Interest KE is an editor in Springer Nature Journals and a previous editor for a Springer Book (https://link.springer.com/book/10.1007/978-3-030-53821-7). Other authors: none.

Authors' Contribution SN and DT wrote the first draft of the chapter and shared a preliminary content discussion. KE coordinated the development of the chapter and revised the manuscript. BE revised and validated the pathology data of the manuscript. The final draft was reviewed and approved by all the authors. The contents of the chapter reflect the authors' perspectives and not of their institutions of affiliation.

References

Ahmed AA, Etemadmoghadam D, Temple J, Lynch AG, Riad M, Sharma R, Stewart C, Fereday S, Caldas C, Defazio A, Bowtell D, Brenton JD (2010) Driver mutations in TP53 are ubiquitous in high grade serous carcinoma of the ovary. J Pathol 221(1):49–56. https://doi.org/10.1002/path.2696

Ahmed AA, Becker CM, Bast RC Jr (2012) The origin of ovarian cancer. BJOG 119(2):134–136. https://doi.org/10.1111/j.1471-0528.2011.03149.x

Alkema NG, Wisman GB, van der Zee AG, van Vugt MA, de Jong S (2016) Studying platinum sensitivity and resistance in high-grade serous ovarian cancer: different models for different questions. Drug Resist Updat 24:55–69. https://doi.org/10.1016/j.drup.2015.11.005

Bell DA (2005) Origins and molecular pathology of ovarian cancer. Mod Pathol 18(Suppl 2):S19–S32. https://doi.org/10.1038/modpathol.3800306

Bennett JA, Oliva E (2020) Undifferentiated and dedifferentiated neoplasms of the female genital tract. Semin Diagn Pathol. S0740-2570(20)30099-X. https://doi.org/10.1053/j.semdp.2020.11.002

Berek JS (2009) Lymph node-positive stage IIIC ovarian cancer: a separate entity? Int J Gynecol Cancer 19(Suppl 2):S18–S20. https://doi.org/10.1111/IGC.0b013e3181bf8111

Berek JS, Friedlander M, Hacker NF (2015) Epithelial ovarian, fallopian tube, and peritoneal cancer. In: Berek JS, Hacker NF (eds) Berek and Hacker's gynecologic oncology, 6th edn. Lippincott Williams and Wilkins, Philadelphia, PA, pp 464–529

Berek JS, Kehoe ST, Kumar L, Friedlander M (2018) Cancer of the ovary, fallopian tube, and peritoneum. Int J Gynaecol Obstet 143(Suppl 2):59–78. https://doi.org/10.1002/ijgo.12614

Berns K, Caumanns JJ, Hijmans EM, Gennissen AMC, Severson TM, Evers B, Wisman GBA, Jan Meersma G, Lieftink C, Beijersbergen RL, Itamochi H, van der Zee AGJ, de Jong S, Bernards R (2018) ARID1A mutation sensitizes most ovarian clear cell carcinomas to BET inhibitors. Oncogene 37(33):4611–4625. https://doi.org/10.1038/s41388-018-0300-6

Binder PS, Prat J, Mutch DG (2015) The future role of molecular staging in gynecologic cancer. Int J Gynaecol Obstet 131(Suppl 2):S127–S131

Bowtell DD (2010) The genesis and evolution of high-grade serous ovarian cancer. Nat Rev Cancer 10(11):803–808. https://doi.org/10.1038/nrc2946

Bray F, Ferlay J, Soerjomataram I, Siegel RL, Torre LA, Jemal A (2018) Global cancer statistics 2018: GLOBOCAN estimates of incidence and mortality worldwide for 36 cancers in 185 countries. CA Cancer J Clin 68(6):394–424

Callahan MJ, Crum CP, Medeiros F, Kindelberger DW, Elvin JA, Garber JE, Feltmate CM, Berkowitz RS, Muto MG (2007) Primary fallopian tube malignancies in BRCA-positive women undergoing surgery for ovarian cancer risk reduction. J Clin Oncol 25 (25):3985–3990. https://doi.org/10.1200/JCO.2007.12.2622

Cancer Genome Atlas Research Network (2011) Integrated genomic analyses of ovarian carcinoma. Nature 474(7353):609–615. https://doi.org/10.1038/nature10166. Erratum in: Nature 2012;490 (7419):298

Cheng W, Liu J, Yoshida H, Rosen D, Naora H (2005) Lineage infidelity of epithelial ovarian cancers is controlled by HOX genes that specify regional identity in the reproductive tract. Nat Med 11(5):531–537. https://doi.org/10.1038/nm1230

Cuatrecasas M, Catasus L, Palacios J, Prat J (2009) Transitional cell tumors of the ovary: a comparative clinicopathologic, immunohistochemical, and molecular genetic analysis of Brenner tumors and transitional cell carcinomas. Am J Surg Pathol 33(4):556–567. https://doi.org/10.1097/PAS.0b013e318188b84c

Desai A, Xu J, Aysola K, Qin Y, Okoli C, Hariprasad R, Chinemerem U, Gates C, Reddy A, Danner O, Franklin G, Ngozi A, Cantuaria G, Singh K, Grizzle W, Landen C, Partridge EE, Rice VM, Reddy ES, Rao VN (2014) Epithelial ovarian cancer: an overview. World J Transl Med 3(1):1–8. https://doi.org/10.5528/wjtm.v3.i1.1

Dubeau L (1999) The cell of origin of ovarian epithelial tumors and the ovarian surface epithelium dogma: does the emperor have no clothes? Gynecol Oncol 72(3):437–442. https://doi.org/10.1006/gyno.1998.5275

Eisen A, Weber BL (1998) Primary peritoneal carcinoma can have multifocal origins: implications for prophylactic oophorectomy. J Natl Cancer Inst 90(11):797–799. https://doi.org/10.1093/jnci/90.11.797

Fadare O, Parkash V (2019) Pathology of endometrioid and clear cell carcinoma of the ovary. Surg Pathol Clin 12(2):529–564. https://doi.org/10.1016/j.path.2019.01.009

Finch A, Shaw P, Rosen B, Murphy J, Narod SA, Colgan TJ (2006) Clinical and pathologic findings of prophylactic salpingo-oophorectomies in 159 BRCA1 and BRCA2 carriers. Gynecol Oncol 100(1):58–64. https://doi.org/10.1016/j.ygyno.2005.06.065

Fujiwara K, Shintani D, Nishikawa T (2016) Clear-cell carcinoma of the ovary. Ann Oncol 27 (Suppl 1):i50–i52. https://doi.org/10.1093/annonc/mdw086

Gadducci A, Cosio S (2020) Therapeutic approach to low-grade serous ovarian carcinoma: state of art and perspectives of clinical research. Cancers (Basel) 12(5):1336. https://doi.org/10.3390/cancers12051336

Gershenson DM, Sun CC, Lu KH, Coleman RL, Sood AK, Malpica A, Deavers MT, Silva EG, Bodurka DC (2006) Clinical behavior of stage II-IV low-grade serous carcinoma of the ovary. Obstet Gynecol 108(2):361–368

Gilks CB, Prat J (2009) Ovarian carcinoma pathology and genetics: recent advances. Hum Pathol 40(9):1213–1223. https://doi.org/10.1016/j.humpath.2009.04.017

Govindarajan M, Wohlmuth C, Waas M, Bernardini MQ, Kislinger T (2020) High-throughput approaches for precision medicine in high-grade serous ovarian cancer. J Hematol Oncol 13 (1):134. https://doi.org/10.1186/s13045-020-00971-6

Haunschild CE, Tewari KS (2021) The current landscape of molecular profiling in the treatment of epithelial ovarian cancer. Gynecol Oncol 160(1):333–345. https://doi.org/10.1016/j.ygyno.2020.09.043

Ho CL, Kurman RJ, Dehari R, Wang TL, Shih IM (2004) Mutations of BRAF and KRAS precede the development of ovarian serous borderline tumors. Cancer Res 64(19):6915–6918. https://doi.org/10.1158/0008-5472.CAN-04-2067

Iida Y, Okamoto A, Hollis RL, Gourley C, Herrington CS (2020) Clear cell carcinoma of the ovary: a clinical and molecular perspective. Int J Gynecol Cancer. https://doi.org/10.1136/ijgc-2020-001656

Kaku T, Ogawa S, Kawano Y, Ohishi Y, Kobayashi H, Hirakawa T, Nakano H (2003) Histological classification of ovarian cancer. Med Electron Microsc 36(1):9–17. https://doi.org/10.1007/s007950300002

Kelemen LE, Köbel M (2011) Mucinous carcinomas of the ovary and colorectum: different organ, same dilemma. Lancet Oncol 12(11):1071–1080. https://doi.org/10.1016/S1470-2045(11)70058-4

Kindelberger DW, Lee Y, Miron A, Hirsch MS, Feltmate C, Medeiros F, Callahan MJ, Garner EO, Gordon RW, Birch C, Berkowitz RS, Muto MG, Crum CP (2007) Intraepithelial carcinoma of the fimbria and pelvic serous carcinoma: evidence for a causal relationship. Am J Surg Pathol 31 (2):161–169. https://doi.org/10.1097/01.pas.0000213335.40358.47

Köbel M, Kalloger SE, Huntsman DG, Santos JL, Swenerton KD, Seidman JD, Gilks CB, Cheryl Brown Ovarian Cancer Outcomes Unit of the British Columbia Cancer Agency, Vancouver BC (2010) Differences in tumor type in low-stage versus high-stage ovarian carcinomas. Int J Gynecol Pathol 29(3):203–211. https://doi.org/10.1097/PGP.0b013e3181c042b6

Kurman RJ, Shih IM (2010) The origin and pathogenesis of epithelial ovarian cancer: a proposed unifying theory. Am J Surg Pathol 34:433–443

Kyo S, Ishikawa N, Nakamura K, Nakayama K (2020) The fallopian tube as origin of ovarian cancer: change of diagnostic and preventive strategies. Cancer Med 9(2):421–431. https://doi.org/10.1002/cam4.2725

Lee KR, Scully RE (2000) Mucinous tumors of the ovary: a clinicopathologic study of 196 borderline tumors (of intestinal type) and carcinomas, including an evaluation of 11 cases with 'pseudomyxoma peritonei'. Am J Surg Pathol 24(11):1447–1464. https://doi.org/10.1097/00000478-200011000-00001

Lee BH, Hecht JL, Pinkus JL, Pinkus GS (2002) WT1, estrogen receptor, and progesterone receptor as markers for breast or ovarian primary sites in metastatic adenocarcinoma to body fluids. Am J Clin Pathol 117(5):745–750. https://doi.org/10.1309/QLV6-HH0H-UCTF-WEF6

Lheureux S, Braunstein M, Oza AM (2019a) Epithelial ovarian cancer: evolution of management in the era of precision medicine. CA Cancer J Clin 69(4):280–304. https://doi.org/10.3322/caac.21559

Lheureux S, Gourley C, Vergote I, Oza AM (2019b) Epithelial ovarian cancer. Lancet 393 (10177):1240–1253. https://doi.org/10.1016/S0140-6736(18)32552-2

Mackenzie R, Talhouk A, Eshragh S, Lau S, Cheung D, Chow C, Le N, Cook LS, Wilkinson N, McDermott J, Singh N, Kommoss F, Pfisterer J, Huntsman DG, Köbel M, Kommoss S, Gilks CB, Anglesio MS (2015) Morphologic and molecular characteristics of mixed epithelial ovarian cancers. Am J Surg Pathol 39(11):1548–1557. https://doi.org/10.1097/PAS.0000000000000476

McCluggage WG (2012) Immunohistochemistry in the distinction between primary and metastatic ovarian mucinous neoplasms. J Clin Pathol 65(7):596–600. https://doi.org/10.1136/jcp.2010.085688

McCluggage WG, Judge MJ, Clarke BA, Davidson B, Gilks CB, Hollema H, Ledermann JA, Matias-Guiu X, Mikami Y, Stewart CJ, Vang R, Hirschowitz L, International Collaboration on Cancer Reporting (2015) Data set for reporting of ovary, fallopian tube and primary peritoneal carcinoma: recommendations from the International Collaboration on Cancer Reporting (ICCR). Mod Pathol 28(8):1101–1122. https://doi.org/10.1038/modpathol.2015.77

Medeiros F, Muto MG, Lee Y, Elvin JA, Callahan MJ, Feltmate C, Garber JE, Cramer DW, Crum CP (2006) The tubal fimbria is a preferred site for early adenocarcinoma in women with familial ovarian cancer syndrome. Am J SurgPathol 30(2):230–236. https://doi.org/10.1097/01.pas.0000180854.28831.77

Momenimovahed Z, Tiznobaik A, Taheri S, Salehiniya H (2019) Ovarian cancer in the world: epidemiology and risk factors. Int J Womens Health 11:287–299. https://doi.org/10.2147/IJWH.S197604

Oswald AJ, Gourley C (2015) Low-grade epithelial ovarian cancer: a number of distinct clinical entities? Curr Opin Oncol 27(5):412–419. https://doi.org/10.1097/CCO.0000000000000216

Piek JM, van Diest PJ, Zweemer RP, Kenemans P, Verheijen RH (2001) Tubal ligation and risk of ovarian cancer. Lancet 358(9284):844. https://doi.org/10.1016/S0140-6736(01)05992-X

Pierson WE, Peters PN, Chang MT, Chen LM, Quigley DA, Ashworth A, Chapman JS (2020) An integrated molecular profile of endometrioid ovarian cancer. Gynecol Oncol 157(1):55–61. https://doi.org/10.1016/j.ygyno.2020.02.011

Prat J (2014) FIGO Committee on Gynecologic Oncology. Staging classification for cancer of the ovary, fallopian tube, and peritoneum. Int J Gynecol Obstet 124:1–5

Purdie DM, Bain CJ, Siskind V, Webb PM, Green AC (2003) Ovulation and risk of epithelial ovarian cancer. Int J Cancer 104(2):228–232. https://doi.org/10.1002/ijc.10927

Risch HA (1998) Hormonal etiology of epithelial ovarian cancer, with a hypothesis concerning the role of androgens and progesterone. J Natl Cancer Inst 90(23):1774–1786. https://doi.org/10.1093/jnci/90.23.1774

Rodríguez IM, Prat J (2002) Mucinous tumors of the ovary: a clinicopathologic analysis of 75 borderline tumors (of intestinal type) and carcinomas. Am J Surg Pathol 26(2):139–152. https://doi.org/10.1097/00000478-200202000-00001

Ruba S, Doherty D, Stewart CJR (2020) A detailed morphological and immunohistochemical comparison of primary endometrial and tubo-ovarian high-grade serous carcinomas and their corresponding omental metastases. Pathology 52(2):197–205. https://doi.org/10.1016/j.pathol.2019.10.007

Scully RE, Young RH, Clement PB (1998) Tumors of the ovary, maldeveloped gonads, fallopian tube, and broad ligament, vol Fascicle 23, 3rd series. Atlas Tumor Pathol. Armed Forces Institute of Pathology, Washington, DC, pp 1–168

Sehouli J, Fotopoulou C (2006) Multimodales Management des Ovarialkarzinoms. Uni-Med Verlag AG, D-28323men

Shih IM, Wang Y, Wang TL (2021) The origin of ovarian cancer species and precancerous landscape. Am J Pathol 191(1):26–39. https://doi.org/10.1016/j.ajpath.2020.09.006

Simons M, Bolhuis T, De Haan AF, Bruggink AH, Bulten J, Massuger LF, Nagtegaal ID (2019) A novel algorithm for better distinction of primary mucinous ovarian carcinomas and mucinous carcinomas metastatic to the ovary. Virchows Arch 474(3):289–296. https://doi.org/10.1007/s00428-018-2504-0

Singer G, Oldt R III, Cohen Y, Wang BG, Sidransky D, Kurman RJ, Shih IM (2003) Mutations in BRAF and KRAS characterize the development of low-grade ovarian serous carcinoma. J Natl Cancer Inst 95(6):484–486. https://doi.org/10.1093/jnci/95.6.484

Singh N, Gilks CB, Hirschowitz L, Kehoe S, McNeish IA, Miller D, Naik R, Wilkinson N, McCluggage WG (2016) Primary site assignment in tubo-ovarian high-grade serous carcinoma: consensus statement on unifying practice worldwide. Gynecol Oncol 141(2):195–198. https://doi.org/10.1016/j.ygyno.2015.10.022

Singh N, McCluggage WG, Gilks CB (2017) High-grade serous carcinoma of tubo-ovarian origin: recent developments. Histopathology 71(3):339–356. https://doi.org/10.1111/his.13248

Slomovitz B, Gourley C, Carey MS, Malpica A, Shih IM, Huntsman D, Fader AN, Grisham RN, Schlumbrecht M, Sun CC, Ludemann J, Cooney GA, Coleman R, Sood AK, Mahdi H, Wong KK, Covens A, O'Malley DM, Lecuru F, Cobb LP, Caputo TA, May T, Huang M, Siemon J, Fernández ML, Ray-Coquard I, Gershenson DM (2020) Low-grade serous ovarian cancer: state of the science. Gynecol Oncol 156(3):715–725. https://doi.org/10.1016/j.ygyno.2019.12.033

Stanciu PI, Ind TEJ, Barton DPJ, Butler JB, Vroobel KM, Attygalle AD, Nobbenhuis MAE (2019) Development of Peritoneal Carcinoma in women diagnosed with Serous Tubal Intraepithelial Carcinoma (STIC) following Risk-Reducing Salpingo-Oophorectomy (RRSO). J Ovarian Res 12(1):50

Sugiyama T, Kamura T, Kigawa J et al (2000) Clinical characteristics of clear cell carcinoma of the ovary: a distinct histologic type with poor prognosis and resistance to platinum-based chemotherapy. Cancer 88(11):2584–2589

Sung H, Ferlay J, Siegel RL, Laversanne M, Soerjomataram I, Jemal A, Bray F (2021) Global cancer statistics 2020: GLOBOCAN estimates of incidence and mortality worldwide for 36 cancers in 185 countries. CA Cancer J Clin. https://doi.org/10.3322/caac.21660

Tafe LJ, Garg K, Chew I, Tornos C, Soslow RA (2010) Endometrial and ovarian carcinomas with undifferentiated components: clinically aggressive and frequently under recognized neoplasms. Mod Pathol 23(6):781–789. https://doi.org/10.1038/modpathol.2010.41

Vargas AN (2014) Natural history of ovarian cancer. Ecancermedicalscience 8:465. https://doi.org/10.3332/ecancer.2014.465

WHO (2020) WHO classification of female genital tumours. IARC Press, Lyon

Wu J, Sun H, Yang L et al (2018) Improved survival in ovarian cancer, with widening survival gaps of races and socioeconomic status: a period analysis, 1983-2012. J Cancer 9(19):3548–3556. https://doi.org/10.7150/jca.26300

Wu RC, Wang P, Lin SF, Zhang M, Song Q, Chu T, Wang BG, Kurman RJ, Vang R, Kinzler K, Tomasetti C, Jiao Y, Shih IM, Wang TL (2019) Genomic landscape and evolutionary trajectories of ovarian cancer precursor lesions. J Pathol 248(1):41–50. https://doi.org/10.1002/path.5219

Yoneda A, Lendorf ME, Couchman JR, Multhaupt HA (2012) Breast and ovarian cancers: a survey and possible roles for the cell surface heparansulfate proteoglycans. J Histochem Cytochem 60 (1):9–21. https://doi.org/10.1369/0022155411428469

Zhang Y, Cao L, Nguyen D, Lu H (2016) TP53 mutations in epithelial ovarian cancer. Transl Cancer Res 5(6):650–663. https://doi.org/10.21037/tcr.2016.08.40

Zhang Y, Luo G, Li M, Guo P, Xiao Y, Ji H, Hao Y (2019a) Global patterns and trends in ovarian cancer incidence: age, period and birth cohort analysis. BMC Cancer 19(1):984. https://doi.org/10.1186/s12885-019-6139-6

Zhang S, Dolgalev I, Zhang T, Ran H, Levine DA, Neel BG (2019b) Both fallopian tube and ovarian surface epithelium are cells-of-origin for high-grade serous ovarian carcinoma. Nat Commun 10(1):5367. https://doi.org/10.1038/s41467-019-13116-2

Zheng W, Fadare O (2012) Fallopian tube as main source for ovarian and pelvic (non-endometrial) serous carcinomas. Int J Clin Exp Pathol 5(3):182–186

Zweemer RP, van Diest PJ, Verheijen RH, Ryan A, Gille JJ, Sijmons RH, Jacobs IJ, Menko FH, Kenemans P (2000) Molecular evidence linking primary cancer of the fallopian tube to BRCA1 germline mutations. Gynecol Oncol 76(1):45–50. https://doi.org/10.1006/gyno.1999.5623

An Introduction to the Current Management of Ovarian Cancer in the Era of Precision Oncology

2

Emilio Francesco Giunta, Annalisa Pappalardo, Dario Trapani, and Angelica Petrillo

Abstract

Ovarian cancer (OC) is a leading cause of premature mortality worldwide, mainly because of its advanced stage at diagnosis and poor outcomes in metastatic phase. Quality and timely surgery is the key intervention for both the curative and the palliative setting, providing one of the largest benefits on the survival outcomes. However, patients with OC, at all stages, benefit of a number of pharmacological treatments, both chemotherapy and targeted agents. Therapeutic advances in OC reflect a better knowledge of the biology and the critical pathogenetic mechanisms of tumorigenesis. For instance, the discovery of homologous recombination deficiency, particularly *BRCA* gene mutations, and the implementation of anti-(Poly ADP-ribose polymerase) PARP treatments have been largely considered to be milestones in cancer treatment. PARP inhibitors are now approved as maintenance therapy in platinum-sensitive OC. Antiangiogenic agents can play an important role in the advanced disease. Immunotherapy has been tested in OC with less impactful results, suggesting the need of more efforts to identify predictive factors to refine the patient selection. Despite the progresses in treatment discovery, the prognosis of patients with more advanced diseases or exhibiting treatment resistance still remains dismal. The personalization of

E. F. Giunta · A. Pappalardo
Medical Oncology Unit, Department of Precision Medicine, School of Medicine, University of Campania "Luigi Vanvitelli", Naples, Italy

Medical Oncology Unit, Ospedale del Mare, Naples, Italy

D. Trapani
European Institute of Oncology (IEO), IRCCS, Milan, Italy

A. Petrillo (✉)
Medical Oncology Unit, Ospedale del Mare, Naples, Italy

K. El Bairi (ed.), *Ovarian Cancer Biomarkers*,
https://doi.org/10.1007/978-981-16-1873-4_2

treatment, together with the developing of new drugs, will improve the prognosis of this disease, addressing an unmet area of the cancer treatment.

Keywords

Ovarian cancer · Therapy · Biomarkers · Precision medicine · PARP inhibition

2.1 Introduction

Ovarian cancer (OC) is the third most common gynecologic malignancy diagnosed, after cervical and endometrial cancer and the most lethal gynecological tumor: 295,414 new cases and 184,799 deaths were estimated in 2018, worldwide (Bray et al. 2018; Momenimovahed et al. 2019). The highest age-standardized incidence of OC is observed in Europe; however, an increasing trend has been observed over the last years in Central and South America and Asia (Zhang et al. 2019). One of the greatest challenges in the field of OC remains the lack of an effective screening, resulting in common late stage tumors at diagnosis, leading to a dismal prognosis. Despite the attempts to introduce early diagnostic tools, such as transvaginal ultrasound and/or tumor markers (e.g., CA-125, HE4), the high rates of false-positive screening test results and the poor screening performance led the authorities to advise against screening in non-selected population (i.e., asymptomatic women, not selected per cancer risk) (Grossman et al. 2018; Aust and Seebacher-Shariat 2020).

Regarding the histology, the current classification of OC comprises a spectrum of ovarian neoplasms according to the tissues of origin: surface epithelial (65%), germ cell (15%), sex cord-stromal (10%), and miscellaneous tumors. Among surface epithelial tumors, five major histology variants can be distinguished (*for more details see below*), each of them further divided into benign, borderline, and malignant (https://www.pathologyoutlines.com/topic/ovarytumorwhoclassif.html. Accessed August 6, 2020).The pathogenesis of the epithelial OC (EOC) is mostly unclear. The "incessant ovulation" theory has been claimed as one of the strongest biological hypotheses, related to the retainment of inclusion cysts and subsequent epithelial metaplasia driving the carcinogenetic mechanisms (Fleming et al. 2006). Additionally, researchers have suggested the "hormonal" and "inflammation hypothesis," mostly due to the gonadotropin stimulation for the ovulation dynamics. However, the current perspectives seem to conclude for apathogenesis based on a multifactorial process, involving different biological events and multi-step mechanisms (Hunn and Rodriguez 2012).

Regarding the risk factors for EOC, the most critical is the family history for OC. In fact, 10–20% of women diagnosed with EOC harbors germline mutations in *BRCA* (Breast cancer susceptibility gene) 1 or 2, accounting for nearly 80% of hereditary EOCs. Other mutated genes are *TP53* (responsible for Li-Fraumeni syndrome), mismatch repair genes (responsible for Lynch syndrome), *CHEK2*,

RAD51, *BRIP1*, and *PALB2* (all of them involved in double-strand break repair pathway, some presenting in *BRCA*-like syndromes) (Toss et al. 2015).

The discovery in the mid-1990s of the *BRCA* genes and the identification of their key role in the oncogenesis of ovarian and breast carcinomas is considered the most important turning point to inform the identification of high-risk patients, the evaluation of prophylactic interventions, and the development of therapeutics for personalized treatments (Walsh 2015). *BRCA*-mutant EOC patients show a better survival, probably due to better response to platinum chemotherapy (Cass et al. 2003), becoming object of study for new therapeutic strategies. Poly-(ADP-ribose)-polymerase (PARP) inhibitors, whose development started in the 1980s, have been investigated in several types of human cancers, since they could increase sensitivity to chemotherapy (mainly DNA-alkylating agents and topoisomerase inhibitors) and ionizing radiation (Curtin 2005). The discovery, *as better outlined below,* of a "synergism" between *BRCA* mutations and PARP inhibitors is a milestone in EOC therapeutic research, opening the door to new scenarios of tailored treatments for EOC. In this chapter, the current advances in the therapeutic management of OC in the era of precision medicine are discussed.

2.2 Epithelial Ovarian Cancer Histotypes

EOC comprises the majority of ovarian neoplasms. They can be classified according to the cell of origin in five major histopathological subgroups: high- and low-grade serous OC (HGSOC and LGSOC, respectively), endometrioid, clear cell (CCO), and mucinous (MOC) carcinomas. Each subtype shows peculiar characteristics of epidemiology, risks factors, immunohistochemistry (IHC) patterns, biological behavior, and response to treatment (Table 2.1). HGSOCs are the most common EOC subtype (80%). They are usually diagnosed as bilateral disease or in advanced stage due to the lack of specific symptoms prompting early detection. The detection of occult OCs in the fimbrial portion of the fallopian tubes in *BRCA1* and *2* carriers who underwent risk-reduction salpingo-oophorectomy led to the proposal of physio-pathological model of HGSOC precursor cells arising from fallopian tube and secondarily involving the ovary (Hirst et al. 2009; Yates et al. 2011).The IHC profile of HGSOC typically reports p53, WT1 staining, harboring more commonly *BRCA1* and *2* and *TP53* mutations; additionally, they express estrogen and progesterone receptors (ER and PgR, respectively). Recently, the TCGA has distinguished four molecular subtypes among the HGSOC subgroup: immunoreactive, proliferative, differentiated, and mesenchymal; each TCGA subgroup is characterized by peculiar genes alterations and different outcome (TCGA 2011).

LGSOC represents a subgroup of rare serous cancers, the recognition of which is relatively recent (Kurman et al. 2014). Due to that, still today there is a lack of consistent data in this field on large samples of patients. In general, LGSOCs cover the 4.7% of serous histotypes and almost 2% of all EOC (Matsuo et al. 2018). They are diagnosed mostly in women in their 40s, younger than those in the HGSOC group; the association with higher risk of relapse and death in case of former

Table 2.1 Epithelial ovarian cancer histotypes

Histotype	Frequency	Molecular alterations	Clinical features
High-grade serous ovarian cancer	70–80%	*BRCA1/2, Tp53, WT1*	Bilateral disease, advanced stage at diagnosis
Low-grade serous ovarian cancer	4%	*KRAS, NRAS, BRAF, HER2*	Younger age, indolent disease
Endometrioid	10–15%	*ARID1A, KRAS, PTEN, MSI*	Perimenopause, associated with endometriosis and endometrial carcinoma
Clear cell	10%	*AKT, PI3KCA*	Early stage at diagnosis, chemoresistant
Mucinous	3–5%	*KRAS, BRAF, PI3KCA, cMET*	Large cystic mass, early stage at diagnosis, chemoresistant

Abbreviations: *BRCA* Breast Related Cancer Antigens, *TP53* tumor protein P53, *WT1* Wilms' tumor 1, *KRAS* Kirsten RAt Sarcoma virus, *NRAS* neuroblastoma RAS viral oncogene homolog, *BRAF* v-Raf murine sarcoma viral oncogene homolog B, *HER2* receptor tyrosine-protein kinase erbB-2, *ARID1A* AT-rich interactive domain-containing protein 1A, *PTEN* phosphatase and tensin homolog, *MSI* microsatellite instability, *AKT* protein kinase, *PI3KCA* phosphatidylinositol-4,5-bisphosphate 3-kinase-catalytic subunit alpha, *cMET* hepatocyte growth factor receptor

smokers and high BMI has been reported. Additionally, LGSOC is characterized by lower CA-125 levels at diagnosis (Fader et al. 2014) and a more indolent behavior with a better outcome if compared with HGSOC (i.e., overall survival (OS): 102.9 vs 72.8 months; progression free survival (PFS): 31.2 vs 17.8 months, respectively) (Gershenson 2016; Della Pepa et al. 2015). From a molecular point of view, LGSOC is characterized by a peculiar pattern of alterations, which distinguish this group from HGSOC. The IHC analysis show that they stain positive to WT-1, ER and PgR expression with a proliferative index (Ki-67) $\leq$10% and wild-type *TP53* status in the majority of cases. In few cases, LGSOC can be positive to Her-2 (28%) or c-kit (4.5%) (O'Neill et al. 2005; Wong et al. 2007). However, the definition of its molecular profile is one of the most important research topics in this field. The MAPK pathways play a key role in the process of LGSOC's carcinogenesis and the activating mutations in *KRAS*, *BRAF*, *NRAS*, *HER-2* genes represent the most frequent alterations detected by next generation sequencing (NGS) assays. In particular, *KRAS* mutations were present in a range between 35% and 54% of LGSOC, depending on the samples analyzed (Singer et al. 2003a, b), while a wild-type status was reported in the entire HGSOC population. Like *KRAS*, also *BRAF* mutation was reported in a range between 2% and 33% in different series of LGSOC with no cases in HGSOC. This mutation, mostly V600E, is mutually exclusive with *RAS* mutations like in other tumor types, such as colorectal cancer and melanoma (Singer et al. 2003a, b; Hunter et al. 2015). Additionally, these tumors rarely show alterations in *BRCA* genes, even if their determination is recommended still today in the context of serous OCs (Vineyard et al. 2011). Therefore, the discrepancy in the gene profile between HGSOC and LGSOC seems to suggest a divergent tumorigenesis, in which peculiar molecular alterations can be recognized at each step of the process (Kurman and Shih 2016). In particular, some analyses reported the appearance of *KRAS* activating mutation in a very early stage of development from the ovarian epithelium to the LGSOC, which is not present in the HGSOC carcinogenesis. Thus, several analyses defined and confirmed the hypothesis of two distinct pathways of carcinogenesis: RAS (or MAPK) related for LGSOC and RAS (MAPK) independent for HGSOC (Della Pepa et al. 2015).

Endometrioid cancers represent approximately 10–15% of EOC. They are usually detected in perimenopausal women, with a better prognosis, potentially associated with the high percentage of low-grade tumors and early diagnoses (Storey et al. 2008). Additionally, endometrioid cancers are frequently associated with endometriosis as well as synchronous endometrial carcinoma (15–20% of cases). They typically have a WT1 positivity, so the distinction with HGSOC—which expresses WT1 as well—is crucial. The pathways leading to the carcinogenesis are not entirely understood and the ARID1A is one of the most investigated genes in this EOC subgroup. In fact, almost 30% of endometrioid OC is *ARID1A* positive (Guan et al. 2011), showing better survival (5-years OS rate: 84.9% vs 60.2% in *ARID1A* positive and negative, respectively) (Heckl et al. 2018). Additionally, endometrioid cancer harbors *KRAS*, *CTNNB1* (beta-catenin), and *PTEN* mutations (Prat et al. 2018) as well as microsatellite instability (MSI) in 12–19% of cases, mostly related to Lynch syndrome (Gras et al. 2001).

CCO (almost 10% of EOC) is frequently diagnosed at early stages, if compared with the other histology types of OC; the prognosis in the early stage of OCC is favorable. However, when CCO is diagnosed as an advanced disease, it is associated with poor prognosis and lack of response to chemotherapy. One of the most important pathways investigated in this subgroup is the AKT/mTOR signaling. This pathway is activated in up to 70% of EOC (Itamochi et al. 2017); in particular, in CCO the *PI3KCA* gain functions mutations are present in a third of the tumors (Gasparri et al. 2017). Additionally, CCO shows *ARID1A* alterations in 50% of cases, loss of *PTEN* in 33%, and MSI in <10% of cases and they are linked to spectrum of tumors of the Lynch syndrome.

MOCs represent the 3–5% of all EOC (Shimada et al. 2009). They are typically diagnosed in young women (median age 20–40 years old) who presented large cystic masses, mostly at early stage (80%) with a good prognosis. Otherwise, they show worse outcome in case of metastatic disease due to the chemoresistance. Over the last decades, the research has investigated on the origin of MOCs, questioning about the primary site of those tumors: OCs or metastasis from tumors arose in the gastrointestinal tract. In this context, Cheasley et al. recently perform a genetic analysis on 500 specimens of MOC, including all histological grades, such as benign and borderline tumors, and comparing those with mucinous neoplasms from other extra-ovarian sites of origin. The authors showed that MOCs express some molecular alterations, such as *CDKN2A*, *KRAS*, and *TP53* (76%, 64%, and 64%, respectively) as well as *HER-2* (26%, mutually exclusive with *KRAS*), *BRAF* and *PI3KCA* (8–12%), which clearly identify the ovarian origin of MOCs and their distinction from metastasis and from the HGSOCs (Cheasley et al. 2019). Therefore, the diagnosis of MOCs requires a careful evaluation of the specimen from dedicated pathologists by using firstly IHC and then the molecular assessment. In this light, Friedlander et al. did a comprehensive evaluation of 304 cases of MOCs reporting a very heterogeneous landscape: alterations in *KRAS* (49%), *BRAF* (3.5%), *PIK3CA* (12%), cMET overexpression (33%, no gene amplification), *TP53* mutation (37%), *HER-2* amplification (11%), programmed death 1 (PD-1) positivity in tumor-infiltrating lymphocytes (TILs) (43%), and programmed death ligand 1 (PD-L1) positivity (14%) (Friedlander et al. 2015). However, up to date no data about prognostic and predictive biomarkers for these tumor types are available in literature. Therefore, like in the LGSOC, still today the most important prognostic factor in MOCs remains the presence of residual disease after curative surgery (Kajiyama et al. 2019).

2.3 The Personalized Era of Advanced Ovarian Cancer Care: The Intersection of Histology and Molecular Paradigms

The treatment of EOC has been dictated traditionally by the response to the platinum compounds, informing on the prognosis of the patients and orienting on the best therapeutic approaches (NCCN guidelines 2020). The choice of treatments for recurrent EOC is essentially based on the so-called platinum-free interval (PFI). PFI is defined as the interval between the completion of the last platinum-based treatment and the clinical and/or radiological evidence of relapse or progression (Colombo et al. 2019). Tumors are classified according to the platinum response, based on the PFI. Platinum-refractory ovarian tumors recur during therapy or within 4 weeks after the last dose; platinum-resistant tumors show PFI less of 6 months, platinum-intermediate sensitive progress between 6 and 12 months, and platinum-sensitive has a PFI superior to 12 months (Stuart et al. 2011).

The current knowledge on platinum sensitivity seems to suggest unique molecular mechanisms underlying the response to treatments. In fact, the acquisition of a platinum-resistant phenotype has been related to several mechanisms, for example, with the increase of the function of the efflux pumps for chemotherapeutics and the alteration of binding proteins in the intracellular milieu of cancer cells, capable to inactivate the platinum reactive properties (Ishida et al. 2010; Okuno et al. 2003). However, the principal mechanism commonly recalled for the platinum resistance is in the alteration of the DNA repair mechanisms of the tumor cells (Darzynkiewicz et al. 2009). When cellular mechanisms of response to the DNA damage are impaired, the tumor can be more susceptible to the platinum-adduct related damage, with an enhanced platinum sensitivity: that is the case of tumors presenting alterations of the homologous recombination DNA damage repair (HRR), for germinal stigmata or acquired somatic genomic events. In fact, it has been estimated that 50% of HGSOC exhibits an inactivation of the homologous recombination mechanism (HRD) related to mutations or promoter methylation of *BRCA1* and *2* genes, as well as of other molecules involved in this process, classified under the protein family called "Fanconi Anemia." These molecules have a prominent role in the preservation of genome integrity (Dai et al. 2015; Ledermann et al. 2016; Arts-de Jong et al. 2016).

The further development of specific compounds capable to result in synthetic lethality is closely related to the molecular definition of platinum sensitivity, on the comprehension of the mechanisms of tumor susceptibility and how to manipulate the delivery of pharmacological interventions. Nowadays, the high-throughput research methodologies of the molecular biology like NGS have generated multiple genetic characterizations of the ovarian neoplasms, in the attempt to identify possible driver genetic alterations of pharmacological interest and define reproducible trajectories of carcinogenesis. Large-scale genomics reported *TP53* mutations in all high-grade tumors, along with conspicuous copy number alterations (Bodelon et al. 2019). However, when other tumor types are taken into consideration, the mutational landscape seems to diverge quite consistently.

Endometrioid, CCO, LGSOC, and MOC present a spectrum of peculiar alterations of *BRAF*, *KRAS*, *PTEN,* and beta-catenin, *as stated above*. Specifically, LGSOC is enriched in ER and PgR, though the role of hormone manipulations is still controversial for therapeutic intentions (Gershenson et al. 2017). In addition, this subtype seems to depend upon pathogenetic alterations of MAPK signaling pathway, including *KRAS*, *BRAF,* and *NRAS* (Slomovitz et al. 2020). However, the effective and safe targetability of the MAPK components in LGSOC is still controversial: in fact, one randomized trial using a MEK inhibitor (selumetinib) versus physician's choice of chemotherapy resulted in premature withdrawn, for futility at the interim analysis (Farley et al. 2013). Endometrioid cancer, on the other hand, presents a unique molecular profile, that includes alterations in beta-catenin and *PTEN* along with a more common occurrence of MSI. This specific alteration has been associated with the co-existence of germline mutations of the DNA mismatch repairing mechanisms, capable to enhance formation of effective tumor-associated neoantigens to arm an antineoplastic immune response. In general, MSI tumors are deemed immunogenic. When an endometrioid tumor is detected in a woman, especially if presenting MSI, a diagnosis of Lynch syndrome should be ruled out (Ryan et al. 2017). Of interest, the presence of MSI, and in general of a defect in the mismatch repair of the DNA, has been associated with an enhanced response to immunotherapy agents, representing one appealing strategy for patients with advanced disease, for example, non-responsive to standard treatments (Sidaway 2020). On the other hand, though not commonly associated with Lynch syndrome, CCO seems to be also capable of effective immune-modulatory properties, related to unique genetic alterations and a hypermutator phenotype. As aforementioned, more than 50% of CCO harbor a mutation of *ARID1A*, a major component of the SWI/SNF remodeling complex of the chromatin (Jones et al. 2010). The mutations in *ARID1A* have been associated with an impairment of the mismatch repair mechanism of the DNA, with increased tumor mutation load and enhanced formation of tumor-associated neoantigens (Shen et al. 2018). This means that CCO converges eventually on a mismatch repair-like phenotype, associated with an increase response to immune-therapeutic agents. Finally, MOC presents a high rate of MSI (Babaier and Ghatage 2020) and HER-2 overexpression, providing a rationale for anti-HER2 or HER2/HER3 blockers such as monoclonal antibodies, small molecules, or their combination (Chung et al. 2019).

The most common enthusiastic declination of precision medicine in ovarian tumors can be related to the successes of the inhibitors of PARP in HGSOC. With the availability of a plethora of different PARP inhibitors now approved, as single agents or in combination either with chemotherapy or with antivascular agents, the paradigm of a molecular approach in the selection of the treatments of EOC patients is largely accepted (Longo 2019). However, the approval of multiple PARP inhibitors, *as more extensively discussed below*, has been accompanied with the broader concept of HRD as a predictive marker useful for therapeutic decisions. Alterations of the DNA damage response in EOC can be several, related to the mutations or epigenetic silencing of the *BRCA* genes. Accordingly, in the attempt to capture the entire mutational landscape of HRD and recapitulate the synthetic lethality observed with PARP inhibition in *BRCA* mutated patients, the concept of HRD has been introduced. Briefly, HRD defines the spectrum of alterations of the homologous recombination machinery, and is intended to test multiple genes (e.g., *ATM*, Fanconi-anemia related, *RAD51*) to define high (deficient) or low (proficient DNA repair machinery) HRD phenotypes (Patel et al. 2018). Together with the BRCA testing, HRD DNA sequencing panels have been introduced in the clinical practice, as companion diagnostics of some PARP inhibitors.

The research in OC has been prolific in some areas of the cancer investigations, providing paradigm of treatment across multiple tumor types, for example, in the clinical use of PARP inhibitors in non-ovarian tumors. Vice versa, OC research is now applying the broader context of the gene sequencing for the discovery of pharmacological targets, to enhance the implementation of effective and safe compounds for cancer care. While multiple studies are ongoing with innovative molecules, more often biomarker-driven, the histology classification still has a major role in the treatment decision of the early stage and platinum response still dictates the treatment sequences in the advanced stage. With the advent of some agnostic indications for drugs, approved on the base of biomarkers regardless the histology-restriction of the drug development, more data will be collected with small molecules, such as the anti-NTRK compounds and antibodies like the anti-PD1 drugs. This could be applied especially in case of tumors with mismatch repair deficiency or high mutational burden—permitting to understand if such innovative paradigms of the oncology will find a place in EOC treatment.

2.3.1 HRD, PARP Inhibitors, and Synthetic Lethality

OC is characterized by a wide variety of genomic alterations, being *TP53* somatic mutation the most frequent (96%) (TCGA 2011). Among EOC subtypes, HGSOCs show a peculiar biological behavior, with alterations in HRR pathway in almost half of cases (*for more details, see Sect.* 2). HRR is an important DNA repair mechanism: its main role consists in protecting chromosomal integrity through reparation of double-strand breaks (DSBs) (Prakash et al. 2015). DSBs are the most dangerous

DNA damages that could occur in mammalian cells, although they can play a role in biologic diversity and adaptability in some physiological conditions such as meiotic recombination between homologous chromosomes, V(D)J recombination to generate a diverse repertoire of antibodies and T cell receptors and immunoglobulin class-switching (Khanna and Jackson 2001). DSBs could be caused by both endogenous insults, such as oxidative damage, and exogenous insults, such as chemotherapeutic drugs and ionizing radiations (Mehta and Haber 2014). During HRR, the undamaged homologous DNA double helix is recruited to allow the restoration of the disrupted DNA strands, with an extremely low rate of errors. However, another mechanism of DSBs repair has been described in human cells, called non-homologous end joining (NHEJ). NHEJ differs from HRR in a substantial way: in fact, it consists of direct ligation of the DSB ends without the use of undamaged partner, resulting in an error-prone process, with frequent insertions, deletions, and translocations (Chapman et al. 2012).

HRR is carried out by proteins functioning, in concert to prevent genomic instability and, consequently, apoptosis or tumorigenic alterations. *RAD51* plays a central role in recombination, coordinating factors involved in DNA repair, transcription, replication, and cell cycle progression. *RAD51* interacts directly with *TP53* but also with *BRCA 1* and *2* (Baumann and West 1998). *BRCA 1* and *2* are two tumor suppressor proteins involved in HRR mechanisms, which genes are located on chromosome 17 and 13, respectively. BRCA1 binds directly to DSBs and, after being phosphorylated by CHK2, it is required for RAD51 recruitment to the sites of DNA damage through its interactions with PALB2 and BRCA2; conversely, BRCA2 contains a DNA-binding domain (DBD) and a binding domain for RAD51, being the direct link between BRCA1-PALB2-BRCA2 complex and RAD51 itself (Roy et al. 2012). Other genes involved in HRR are *ATM, BARD1,* and BRIP1, which play different roles at different levels of the pathway. HRD is a well-established pathogenetic mechanism involved in EOC. The most common alterations in HGSOCs are germline (~20%) and somatic (<10%) mutations in *BRCA1* and/or 2 genes, being *BRCA1* mutations more frequent than *BRCA2* ones (Konstantinopoulos et al. 2015).

BRCA germline pathogenic mutations, also called "deleterious" mutations, determine the inactivation of BRCA1 and/or BRCA2 proteins ("loss of function"), thus causing hereditary breast–OC syndromes (HBOC). These genetic alterations consist of nonsense mutations, small insertion or deletions, but also larger gene rearrangements.However, not all mutations are pathogenic: the so-called neutral or not pathogenic mutations could be both common single nucleotide polymorphisms and rare variants, but not associated with ovarian and breast cancer risk, most likely because they do not affect protein structure and function. A "grey zone" is characterized by variants of unknown significance, which have undefined/unreported risk of ovarian and breast cancer: subjects harboring them should be assessed for risk in the light of personal and family history (Lindor et al. 2012). Despite playing similar roles in HRR pathway, it is well known that *BRCA1* and *BRCA2* germline mutation carriers have different cumulative risk of breast and OC (47–66% and 35–46% for *BRCA1* and 40–57% and 13–23% for *BRCA2* carriers, respectively)

(Chen and Parmigiani 2007). Furthermore, there are different types of breast cancer in the two groups, being triple negative tumors more frequent in *BRCA1*, suggesting divergent pathogenetic pathways, affecting different cell types and/or cellular differentiation potentials, underlining a non-superimposable role of the two proteins (Roy et al. 2012). Germline mutations in other genes involved in HRR pathway, such as *BARD1*, *BRIP1*, *CHEK1/2*, *PALB2,* and *RAD51*, have been reported, altogether accounting for about 25% of all germline mutations discovered to date (Pennington et al. 2014). Somatic mutations in *BRCA* genes are less frequent than germline ones and it is not clear if they should be considered comparable on the prognostic point of view (Moschetta et al. 2016). Somatic alterations in other genes, such as *CHEK2, ATM,* and *BRIP-1*, are also responsible for HRD in OC (Pennington et al. 2014). HRD causes "genomic scar signatures," which are epiphenomenon of DSBs: loss of heterozygosity, telomeric allelic imbalance, and large-scale state transitions; all these alterations could be identified and classified through ad hoc HRD scores (Telli et al. 2016). HRR pathway became quickly an interesting target for drug development; however, unexpectedly, a different class of therapeutic molecules showed activity in HRD cell lines: PARP inhibitors (Drew 2015). PARPs belong to a family of enzymes that transfer poly(ADP-ribose) from nicotinamide-adenine dinucleotide on a variety of target proteins; this activity is also known as PARylation. PARP-1, the most important in eukaryotes, plays a central role in DNA damage response signaling (Eustermann et al. 2015). However, differently from HR pathway, PARP-1 is involved in DNA single-strand breaks (SSBs) repair: it is a sensor of SSBs by direct binding of damaged DNA sites and it activates (through PARylation) repairing enzymes such as DNA topoisomerases, DNA helicases, and base-excision repair factors (Schreiber et al. 2006).

PARP inhibitors have been developed in order to facilitate the accumulation of SSBs, thus killing tumoral cells. Intriguingly, *BRCA* mutated cell lines showed an extremely high sensitivity to PARP inhibitors if compared to *BRCA* wild-type ones, unveiling a new combination strategy in OC (Javle and Curtin 2011). This mechanism is called "synthetic lethality," which means that two genes are lethal when both are mutated/inactivated while the alteration of only one of them is compatible with cell viability (Kaelin 2005). In the case of PARP inhibitor and *BRCA* mutation, the synthetic lethality takes place by the sum of SSBs, due to the trapping of PARP-1 by the inhibitor that hesitates in the stalled replication forks and DSBs. These last ones cannot be repaired due to loss of function of BRCA; therefore, PARP inhibition results in chromosomal instability, cell cycle arrest and, lastly, cell death (Farmer et al. 2005). Several PARP inhibitors have reached human testing: olaparib, niraparib, veliparib, rucaparib, and talazoparib; they are all small molecules administered orally, but differ in target affinity, with talazoparib showing the highest PARP trapping potency, and also in pharmacokinetics, such as half-life and metabolism (Murthy and Muggia 2019).

2.3.2 The Emerging Role of Immunotherapy in Ovarian Cancer

EOCs have been classically regarded as poorly immunogenic tumors, in the past. However, a subset of EOC seems to exhibit molecular features of some kind of immune-regulation, with higher mutational load and brisk tumor-infiltrating lymphocytes (TILs) (Goodell et al. 2006). HGSOC is a genomically unstable disease, particularly when presenting deficits of the DNA repair system—mainly *BRCA1/2* disruptions and other HRD (Strickland et al. 2016). For patients presenting with tumors enriched of tumor infiltrating immune-competent cells or TILs, a better prognosis has been demonstrated (Zhang et al. 2003); however, when the immune response is set on the immunosuppressive phenotype, the resulting milieu seems to favor the tumor progression, and impair the overall prognosis of patients (Gabrilovich and Nagaraj 2009). Multiple attempts of immunotherapy agents to treat EOC have been provided, mainly in early clinical trials, to study the role and impact of immune-checkpoint inhibitors in various settings of care. The use of the anti-PD1 immune-therapeutics in unselected patients has resulted in poor disease control, with 10–15% objective response (ORR) and short PFS survival rates (between 1 and 3 months) (Brahmer et al. 2012; Matulonis et al. 2019; Varga et al. 2019). Only a trend for improved outcome survival has been so far reported with the use of PD-L1 as a predictive biomarker, in the KEYNOTE-100 trial (Matulonis et al. 2019). This phase 2 clinical trial enrolled patients with OC in two distinct cohorts to receive pembrolizumab: one pre-treated with $\leq$3 lines of therapy, and the second with heavily pretreated patients. The ORR did not significantly differ between the two cohorts, ranging between 7.4% and 9.9%, with PFS of 2.1 months. The patients were stratified for the PD-L1 expression, using the combined positive score (CPS) assessment. CPS is calculated by counting the number of PD-L1-positive cells (immune-competent plus tumor cells) divided by the total number of viable tumor cells and multiplied by 100, aiming to capture the relative staining density of immune-competent cells—namely the effectors of the response. Patients with a PD-L1 CPS < 1.5 experienced an ORR of 4.1% and patients with CPS ≥ 10 reported 10% ORR. Concretely, the CPS seems to poorly skim the population deriving the greatest benefit from immunotherapy, in this setting. A similar result has been observed with the use of the anti-PDL1 avelumab in the OC cohort of the JAVELIN master protocol (Mazzarella et al. 2020). In this clinical trial, the use of the monoclonal antibody avelumab resulted in an ORR of 9.7%: in the PD-L1 positive tumors, the response rates resulted slightly increased against the PD-L1 negative tumors, 12.3% vs 5.9%, respectively (Disis et al. 2019). The PD-L1 staining was reported in JAVELIN by assessing the percentage of tumor cell positive to PD-L1. In the attempt to potentiate the benefit with immunotherapy, combination strategies have been implemented. The escalation of chemotherapy regimens with immunotherapy has been explored in the study JAVELIN 200, a phase 3 trial enrolling patients with platinum-resistant OC, randomized to receive the standard treatment with chemotherapy (pegylated liposomal doxorubicin), avelumab, or their combination (Pujade-Lauraine et al. 2019). The study did not show an improvement in responses and survival outcomes with the combination regimen. However, analysis of enrichment of the population by using the PD-L1 biomarker (as CPS) showed an improvement of the ORR: 18.5% and 3.4% in the positive and negative subgroups, respectively, with slight improvement in PFS (3.7 vs 3.0 months, Hazard Ratio (HR): 0.65) and OS (17.7 vs 13.1 months, HR: 0.72).

The experience with immunotherapy in OC, across diverse settings and platinum sensitivity, seems to be overall disappointing. Accordingly, the identification of biomarkers has been identified as a priority area in the research for OC, as the several declinations of PD-L1 positivity (e.g., proportional scores or absolute scores for positive staining) seem to reveal an imperfect predictive potential to identify the patients deriving large benefits from immunotherapy. Histology can also function as a biomarker per se. Some histological variants of EOC seem to retain an intrinsic immunogenicity, as observed for the CCO. As described above, CCO present with an immune-enhancing MSI-like phenotype related to the *ARID1A* alterations. In KEYNOTE-100 clinical trial, investigators provided a subgroup analysis for patients with clear cell tumors (Matulonis et al. 2019). Authors showed a higher ORR in patients with CCO ($n = 19$ patients), that was 15.8%—including one complete response—suggesting some potentiality of the histology to inform the treatment choice and anticipate the benefits with immunotherapy.

The drug development of immunotherapy for OC should be oriented to the identification of enrichment biomarkers beyond histological types, to storm the intrinsic immunogenic nature of a subgroup of patients and enhance an effective immune-response. Potential biomarkers of clinical utility have been suggested. The positive prognostic role of the TILs and the instrumental role of the T-cells as effectors of the anti-tumor response have suggested using TILs as possible biomarker of treatment response. While the presence of TILs is not expected alone to dictate the immune-response, a detailed characterization of the TILs phenotype and the identification of the milieu—immune-stimulating *vs* immune-suppressive—can aid in the identification of patients at a higher chance to respond to treatment, integrating the information provided by the PD-L1. Additionally, the description of an immunogenic subtype of OC may be critical to understand which patients are more likely to benefit from immunotherapy. In analogy with other tumor types, the use of the neoantigen load or tumor mutational burden and the identification of a hyper-mutating phenotype, like in patients with MSI (e.g., Lynch syndrome) may be critical to refine the patients' selection (Fancello et al. 2019). Even if the research on immunotherapy and OC seems not immediately close to the definition of a new treatment paradigm for patients, the formulation of a multifactorial predictive tool should be prioritized in clinical research, to result in an impact on the patients' outcome.

2.4 Current Clinical Management of Epithelial Ovarian Cancer

2.4.1 Localized Disease

2.4.1.1 Curative Surgery

Unfortunately, more than two-thirds of patients affected by malignant ovarian tumors are diagnosed at an advanced stage (Trimbos 2000). Nevertheless, surgery plays a crucial role in the management of this tumor regardless of the stage of disease, with either diagnostic (i.e., in case of suspicious pelvic mass), staging, and therapeutic aims (Cannistra 2004). According to international guidelines (NCCN guidelines 2020; Ledermann et al. 2013), the standard surgical approach to radically manage EOC is via open surgery, carried out in expert centers by trained gynecologist-oncologists. In the early stages (FIGO I-IIA), which represent almost 20% of EOC at diagnosis, the aim of surgery is to radically remove the tumor and undertake adequate staging, alongside with a macroscopic complete exploration of the abdominal-pelvic peritoneal cavity and the reduction of the risk of the rupture of the primary tumor during its removal. This approach includes hysterectomy with bilateral salpingo-oophorectomy, omentectomy (infracolic or total, if the omentum is or not macroscopically involved), lymph-node dissection of the pelvic and the para-aortic regions up to the left renal vein origin, appendicectomy (in case of mucinous histology), peritoneal washing, and multiple peritoneal biopsies. Up to date, the value of performing a complete abdominal and pelvic lymphadenectomy to all the patients is debated. Patients managed for stage IIB-IV with macroscopically resected tumors and normal intra-abdominal lymph nodes seem to derive no adjunctive benefit from the systematic pelvic and para-aortic lymphadenectomy (LION trial) (Harter et al. 2019). The laparoscopic approach could be considered only in selected patients, to reduce the risk of post-operative complications, exclusively if it allows adequate staging. Additionally, a minimally-invasive surgical approach can increase the risk of rupture of the tumor capsule, with spillage of cancer cells, resulting in an up-staging, based on the FIGO staging system, thus affecting negatively the prognosis (Park et al. 2013). In case of younger patients, wishing to pursue a fertility-sparing strategy, a surgery that preserves the uterus and contralateral ovary can be considered only for low risk ovarian tumors, such as borderline tumors, well differentiated tumors, early stage tumors (IA and some IC tumors, but not IB [bilateral tumor] FIGO stage) and favorable histology (serous, MOC, endometroid subtype) (Bentivegna et al. 2016).

2.4.1.2 Adjuvant Therapy

In the early EOC stages, the prognosis is typically good and the relapse rate is 25–30%. Despite the surgical approach remains the cornerstone in this setting, the addiction of adjuvant platinum-based chemotherapy has demonstrated to prolong long-term OS and PFS in these patients (HR: 0.71 and 0.67, respectively) (Lawrie et al. 2015), especially in those patients who received a suboptimal-staging and in some specific histological subgroups. Multivariate analyses have shown that some clinical (such as age and the presence of ascites) and pathological characteristics (such as grade of differentiation, FIGO substage, histological type, the rupture of the tumor capsule, and the extracapsular tumor growth) are independent prognostic factor (Lawrie et al. 2015). In particular, the tumor grading (well, moderately, and poorly differentiated) has been identified as the most important prognostic factor related of disease-free survival (Vergote et al. 2001).

Therefore, in order to stratify the risk of relapse for each patient and do a better selection of patients who benefit more from adjuvant chemotherapy, we should consider a score including the histology of the tumor (serous versus CCO or endometroid or MOC), the tumor grading, and the FIGO stage. Patients with "low risk" (FIGO stage IA-B G1) and "intermediate risk" (FIGO stage IA-IB G2, IC G1) have an excellent prognosis (surgery is curative in 95% of cases), if well staged; in those patients, adjuvant chemotherapy has not shown a benefit if compared with surgery alone (Collinson et al. 2014). On the other hand, adjuvant chemotherapy should be offered to "high risk" patients (FIGO IC G2, any patient with grade 3 tumor, stage IC clear cell histology, stage IIA) (Trimbos et al. 2003). ACTION (Trimbos et al. 2010) and ICON-1 (Trimbos et al. 2003) studies are the two landmark randomized clinical trials in this setting. They compared the use of platinum-based adjuvant chemotherapy versus observation alone in early EOC.The ACTION trial, after a median follow-up time of 10.1 years, showed that recurrence free survival (RFS) was improved in the group of patients who received chemotherapy versus observation alone (70% vs 62%). However, the difference in OS was not statistically significant and the benefit of adjuvant therapy appeared to be limited to patients who had received suboptimal surgical staging (Trimbos et al. 2010). In a subgroup analysis of ICON-1 trial, a statistically difference in RFS and OS was observed in the group who received chemotherapy, but only in patients with high-risk early stage disease (Colombo et al. 2003). Additionally, combined analysis of both studies showed encouraging results in 5-years OS rate for adjuvant chemotherapy over observation (82% vs 74%) (Colombo and Pecorelli 2003).

Therefore, according to international guidelines (NCCN guidelines 2020), carboplatin monotherapy (six cycles) or the combination of carboplatin/paclitaxel (three–six cycles) is the standard of care for the adjuvant treatment, even if no data suggest that the combination therapy is superior to monotherapy, and there are no clinical trial comparing the two treatments. The optimal duration of adjuvant chemotherapy remains unclear. In GOG 157 trial, 427 patients with stage I–II were randomized to receive three or six cycles of carboplatin/paclitaxel; the six cycles treatment was not associated with significant reduction in recurrence risk, resulting in additional toxicity (Bell et al. 2006). A subsequent unplanned analysis revealed that longer adjuvant therapy was associated with a significant reduction in recurrence risk only for high-grade serous histology (Chan et al. 2010).

Regarding rare EOC subtypes, the role of adjuvant or neoadjuvant platinum-based treatment is controversial, because of the few cases of LGSOC included in the landmark trials (Trimbos et al. 2003, 2010) and the chemoresistance of LGSOC with an ORR of ~4%. Additionally, no dedicated prospective and randomized clinical trials are available in this setting for LGSOC and the majority of the evidences came from retrospective analysis. Regarding MOC, the benefit derived from the adjuvant platinum-based chemotherapy is controversial too for the same reasons. Like adjuvant treatment, also the use of bevacizumab is derived from trials that mostly included HGSOC with a low prevalence of MOCs (Perren et al. 2011). In general, MOCs are considered chemoresistant since they show a range in ORR of 12–35%. In conclusion, the choice of adjuvant chemotherapy should be based on the risk of recurrence assessment. Carboplatin monotherapy (six cycles) or the combination of carboplatin/paclitaxel (three–six cycles) are the possible choice, according to patient's profile.

2.4.2 Advanced Disease: State of the Art

2.4.2.1 Role of Surgery in Advanced Disease

An accurate pre-operative staging of disease is essential in advanced EOC in order to define the best management. Indeed, the standard of care in this setting is the up-front maximal debulking surgery followed by carboplatin/paclitaxel chemotherapy (du Bois et al. 2005). Therefore, patients with good performance status are candidates for up-front debulking surgery in the absence of diffuse infiltration of small bowel mesentery, diffuse carcinomatosis of the small bowel-involving such large parts that resection would lead to a short bowel syndrome-, involvement of stomach, duodenum, or pancreas, non-resectable lymph nodes, multiple unresectable liver or lung metastasis or brain metastasis (Querleu et al. 2017). The main goal of surgery in this setting, indeed, is to achieve a complete cytoreduction, with the resection of all macroscopic disease, being the most important independent prognostic factor for those patients (du Bois et al. 2009). Up to date, according to the ESMO-ESGO consensus conference recommendations, based on retrospective analyses (Colombo et al. 2019), there is no evidence of OS benefit in relation to residual disease (if > or <1 cm). Therefore, the optimal cytoreduction is now defined as no macroscopic visible disease, with no dimensional metric of reference. Another debated question is the role of pelvic and para-aortic lymphadenectomy in advanced disease: in the LION trial, patients with macroscopically resected advanced tumors and normal intrabdominal lymph nodes seemed to derive no adjunctive benefit in OS and PFS from the systematic pelvic and para-aortic lymphadenectomy, with similar quality of life (Harter et al. 2019). Finally, surgical cytoreduction has a role also in recurrence disease. Intraperitoneal relapses represent the majority of cases of recurrence and the aim of surgery in this setting is to achieve a complete secondary cytoreduction (Berek et al. 1983). Several clinical trials have been conducted to identify the best criteria to define the complete cytoreduction and inform on the patients' selection for secondary cytoreduction. The AGO DESKTOP OVAR I trial allowed to identify three predictive factors of complete response: good performance status according to ECOG scale, macroscopically complete resection at first surgery, and absence of ascites greater than 500 ml (i.e., AGO-OVAR score) (Harter et al. 2006). More recently, the AGO DESKTOP III trial prospectively randomized patients with first recurrence of platinum-sensitive OC (PFI $\geq$ 6 months), who have received a complete primary resection and who show an AGO positive score (i.e., resectability is assumed, based on the AGO-OVAR score), to perform secondary cytoreductive surgery followed by chemotherapy or chemotherapy upfront. The trial showed that the secondary cytoreduction was able to improve OS (53.7 vs 46.2 months in the surgical and control arm, respectively; HR: 0.76, *p*: 0.03) and PFS (18.4 vs 14 months in the surgical and control arm, respectively; HR: 0.66; $p < 0.001$) (du Bois et al. 2020). In contrast, the GOG 213 failed to demonstrate a PFS or OS advantage in patients with recurrence platinum-sensitive EOC randomized to receive standard chemotherapy plus bevacizumab with or without surgery. It should be noted that patients in this trial were not systematically selected and the complete resection was lower than AGO DESKTOP III trial (64% vs 72.5%) (Coleman et al. 2018). At least, surgery is also indicated in metastatic disease to control of urinary symptoms and in palliation of malignant bowel obstruction.

2.4.2.2 Neoadjuvant Therapy

The administration of a primary systemic treatment before the radical surgery for patients with EOC has been for long time viewed as controversial, for the contrasting results from clinical trials. The neoadjuvant chemotherapy followed by "interval surgery" in this field has narrow indications, due to the critical role of frontline surgery in curing patients. The quality of surgery and the maximal cytoreduction, in fact, are the most relevant prognostic factors in women with OC (Brand et al. 2017). Accordingly, some gynecology-oncologist have been skeptical on the true impact of a pre-surgical treatment, especially for the fear of a cancer progression resulting in a reduced chance to obtain a radical surgery. Currently, the indication for a neoadjuvant treatment is established after a surgical evaluation, in selected women in whom an optimal cytoreduction is less likely to be reached with the frontline surgery: in such a context, the chemotherapy may shrink the tumor and facilitate the subsequent radical excision (NCCN guidelines 2020). The choice of a neoadjuvant approach commonly regards patients presenting with FIGO III or IV disease. In addition, patients who are poor candidates to surgery may be considered for primary chemotherapy and subsequent surgical re-assessment, for procedural eligibility.

Clinical studies on the neoadjuvant chemotherapy converge on the notion that primary surgery followed by adjuvant treatment and primary neoadjuvant chemotherapy followed by interval surgery can result in similar survival outcomes. The randomized phase III clinical trials CHORUS and EORTC 55971 were designed to respond to this research question (Vergote et al. 2018). Patients presenting with stage IIIA to IV invasive EOC, primary peritoneal, or fallopian tube carcinoma were randomized to receive neoadjuvant or surgery, as initial treatment. The non-inferiority preplanned pooled analysis of these two trials reported a similar outcome with the two alternative initial approaches of treatment. The median OS described is 27.6 months (14.1–51.3 months) vs 26.9 months (12.7–50.1 months), with an HR of 0.97 ($p = 0.586$). PFS was 11.6 months (7.9–17.7 months) and 11.1 months (6.4–17.5 months), respectively, with a HR of 0.98 ($p = 0.688$). The subgroup of patients with stage IV disease seemed to derive the greatest benefit from the primary systemic treatment. In fact, for stage IV patients (i.e., extra-abdominal seeding), PFS was 10.6 (7.9–15.0 months) vs 9.7 months (5.2–13.2

months), HR: 0.77 ($p = 0.049$) and OS was 24.3 months (14.1–47.6 months) vs 21.2 months (10.0–36.4 months), HR: 0.76 ($p = 0.048$), respectively. In addition, one Cochrane meta-analysis investigated the role of neoadjuvant chemotherapy in EOC (Coleridge et al. 2019). The study concluded that patients who are given chemotherapy prior to surgery derive no added benefit, in respect to the OS or PFS. However, the study also suggested speculatively that the chemotherapy-first approach could reduce some surgical complications and possibly improve the quality of life. The controversies around the neoadjuvant therapy in EOC and the critical role of an optimal and timely surgical debulking still limit the broad application of the chemotherapy—first approach in the clinical practice. According to the international guidelines for the treatment of OC (NCCN guidelines 2020), neoadjuvant chemotherapy can be considered when the surgical option is excluded, in patients with poor performance status, high anesthesiologic risk, presenting with abdominal seeding and in any case when the disease is not amenable to optimal primary cytoreduction, based on the surgical assessment.

2.4.2.3 Chemotherapy in the First-Line Setting

According to international guidelines (NCCN guidelines 2020), a first-line chemotherapy with carboplatin area under the curve (AUC) 5 and paclitaxel every 3 weeks for six cycles has been considered the standard of care in case of EOC in advanced stages (II–IV FIGO) for a long time (Piccart et al. 2000). However, despite the treatments, the recurrence rate is high for those patients (70–80% within 2 years). Therefore, over the last decades, the research has focused on different strategies able to overcome this limit, including the evaluation of three-drug chemotherapy regimens, weekly schedules, or by using novel associations. More in detail, the phase III ICON-5 trial, which evaluated paclitaxel and carboplatin versus combinations with gemcitabine, pegylated (PEG)-liposomal doxorubicin or topotecan, failed to show a benefit from the addition of another drug to the doublet carboplatin plus paclitaxel (Bookman et al. 2009). Likewise, the AGO-OVAR trial showed no benefit from the addition of topotecan following carboplatin and paclitaxel (Pfisterer et al. 2006). Regarding the use of new doublets, the MITO-2 trial investigated the efficacy of carboplatin plus PEG-liposomal doxorubicin versus carboplatin plus paclitaxel in 820 patients in this setting (Pignata et al. 2011). However, even if the trial is formally negative, showing no improvement in PFS in the experimental arm (PFS: 19 vs 16.8 months, respectively, p: 0.58; OS: 61.6 vs 53.2 months, $p = 0.32$), the schedule showed manageable toxicities and safety profile. Therefore, it might be considered an alternative treatment option in case of contraindications or non-tolerability to taxanes. The SCOTROC trial evaluated the use of carboplatin plus docetaxel, failing to show a significant improvement of the outcome in this setting along with an adverse safety profile (Vasey et al. 2004).

Regarding the timing, the phase III MITO-7 trial investigated a weekly schedule with carboplatin AUC2 and paclitaxel (60 mg/mq), comparing it to the standard of care schedule, every 3 weeks (Pignata et al. 2014). The trial did not show to improve the PFS in this setting (17.3 months vs 18.3 months, $p = 0.66$); however, the patients in the experimental arm showed a better quality of life if compared with the control arm, suggesting that a weekly regimen can be considered in some cases. Recently, the phase III ICON-8 trial failed to improve the outcome in this setting by using alternative schedules (Clamp et al. 2019). It compared three arms (carboplatin AUC 5 or 6 every 3 weeks plus paclitaxel 80 mg/mq weekly; carboplatin AUC 2 and paclitaxel 80 mg/mq weekly; standard of care) and showed no improvement in PFS (17.7, 21, and 20.8 months, respectively; $p = 0.51$). Interestingly, the ICON-7 and GOG-218 trial (Burger et al. 2011; Perren et al. 2011) were the first phase III trial to demonstrate a benefit by adding a biological agent—the antivascular monoclonal antibody bevacizumab—to the standard carboplatin plus paclitaxel doublet. The findings were especially relevant in patients with high risk of relapse after surgery (stage IV, stage III underwent suboptimal debulking, patients with inoperable disease). Therefore, up to date, the treatment with carboplatin AUC 5 plus paclitaxel and bevacizumab every 3 weeks represents the standard of care in this setting. *For additional details regarding the use of biological agent in EOC, see the Sect. 4.2.2 below.* The treatment of some rare histology subtypes may differ slightly, in the current practice. For instance, in patients with advanced or metastatic LGSOC, the treatment options include the standard platinum-based chemotherapy with bevacizumab or endocrine treatment with aromatase inhibitor until disease progression or toxicity. One way utilized to improve the patients' outcome has been through an alternative delivery of the drugs using intraperitoneal chemotherapy. The GOG 104 (Alberts et al. 1996), GOG 114 (Markman et al. 2001), and GOG 172 (Armstrong et al. 2006) showed a benefit in OS and PFS with the use of intraperitoncal cisplatin-based chemotherapy in this setting, so the FDA approved this approach in patients with stage III EOC who underwent complete resection. However, the high rate of toxicities that lead to discontinuation of treatment is the most important barrier to the diffusion of this approach, along with the procedural complexity not universally available. Finally, the GOG 252 trial compared a standard intravenous chemotherapy (with or without bevacizumab) with the intraperitoneal chemotherapy with bevacizumab, showing no benefit for the experimental arm (Walker et al. 2019). Therefore, its use in EOC is still debated. In conclusion, according to international guidelines (NCCN guidelines 2020), carboplatin plus paclitaxel and bevacizumab should be considered the standard of care treatment in patients with EOC, mainly if presenting high-risk characteristics. In all the other patients, carboplatin AUC5 plus paclitaxel every 3 weeks for six cycles can be considered the first choice; a weekly schedule with carboplatin AUC2 and paclitaxel (60 mg/mq) or 3-weekly carboplatin AUC 5 plus weekly paclitaxel (80 mg/mq) are valid alternatives. In patients with poorer performance status, a first-line chemotherapy with a single agent (carboplatin) or all-weekly (i.e., MITO-7) (Pignata et al. 2014) schedule could be the alternative option. Figure 2.1 summarizes a possible treatment algorithm for advanced epithelial OCs, starting from the first line and according to the "continuum of care."

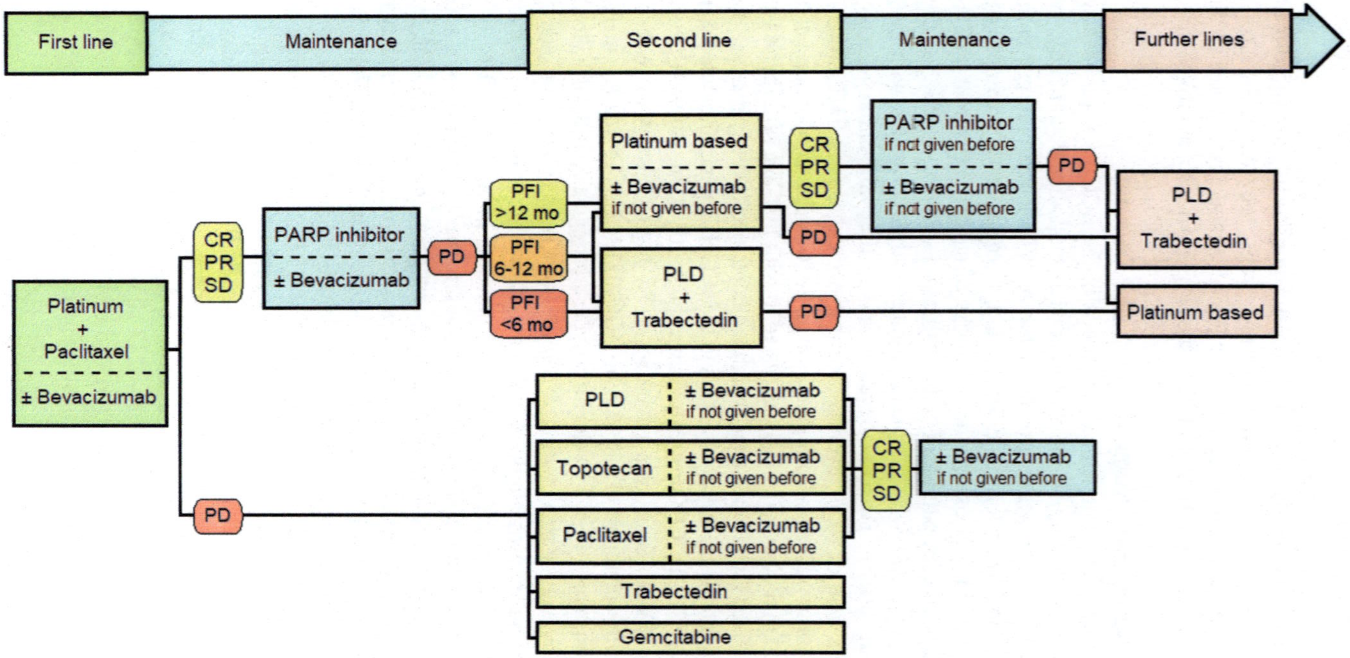

Fig. 2.1 Proposed algorithm for treatment in advanced epithelial ovarian cancer according to the "continuum of care." Abbreviations: *CR* complete response, *PR* partial response, *SD* stable disease, *PD* progression of disease, *PFI* platinum free interval, *mo* months, *PLD* platinum-based chemotherapy, *PLD* pegylated liposomal doxorubicin

2.4.3 The Role of Biological Agents in the Treatment of Epithelial Ovarian Cancer

Biological agents approved by FDA for the treatment of locally advanced/metastatic EOC belong to two classes: antiangiogenic drugs (bevacizumab) and PARP inhibitors (olaparib and niraparib). Other biological agents investigated in the field of EOC are pazopanib and MEK inhibitors; these agents are not approved up to date.

2.4.3.1 Antiangiogenic Drugs

The most important antiangiogenic drugs tested in the EOC field are bevacizumab and pazopanib. Bevacizumab is a humanized monoclonal antibody binding circulating vascular endothelial growth factor A (VEGF-A), thus preventing the activation of its receptor, VEGFR, and, consequently dampening the neoangiogenesis, which is one of the hallmarks of cancer (Ferrara et al. 2004). In OC, VEGF plays a major pathogenetic role, since it is overexpressed virtually in all patients; it is associated with neoplastic ascites and it correlates with prognosis (Colombo et al. 2016). To date, bevacizumab is the only antiangiogenic drug approved in the field of EOC, even if other molecules, namely TKI, are currently under investigation (Ntanasis-Stathopoulos et al. 2016). After encouraging data from phase II clinical trials, bevacizumab was tested in with first-line setting in two phase III clinical trials: the GOG-0218 trial, which included incompletely resected stage III or stage IV patients (Burger et al. 2011), and the ICON-7, which included stage I or IIA grade 3/stage IIB-IV/CCO patients (Perren et al. 2011). In both trials, six cycles of carboplatin (AUC 5–6) and paclitaxel (175 mg/m^2) every 3 weeks were administered. Bevacizumab (15 mg/kg in GOG-0218 and 7.5 mg/Kg in ICON-7 trial) was administered every 3 weeks from cycle 2 (or cycle 1, in ICON-7 trial, only if chemotherapy was started within 4 weeks from surgery) to 6 in addition to chemotherapy and then as single agent maintenance for maximum 22 cycles. A statistically significant increment in PFS was obtained in both trials (HR: 0.72 and 0.81, respectively), but no statistically significant improvement in OS was reported; however, first-line PFS was argued as a better endpoint than OS in EOC, since a prolonged PFS means delayed onset of symptoms and possibly better quality of life. In addition, OS is affected by post-recurrence/progression therapies (Colombo et al. 2016). Bevacizumab was also tested in recurrent EOC, in both platinum-resistant and platinum-sensitive setting. The phase III AURELIA trial showed a modest improvement of PFS in platinum-resistant, bevacizumab-naïve patients treated with chemotherapy (weekly paclitaxel/topotecan or PEG-liposomal doxorubicin) and bevacizumab (15 mg/kg every 3 weeks) versus patients treated with chemotherapy alone (PFS: 6.7 vs 3.4 months) (Pujade-Lauraine et al. 2014). On the other hand, the phase III trials OCEANS and GOG-0213 showed better outcome in platinum-sensitive patients (>6 months of PFI) treated with chemotherapy (carboplatin plus gemcitabine in OCEANS and carboplatin plus paclitaxel in GOG-0213 trial) and bevacizumab (15 mg/kg every 3 weeks) versus chemotherapy alone (12.4 vs 8.4 months and 13.8 vs 10.4 months, respectively). Patients in OCEANS trial were all bevacizumab-naïve, while 10% of GOG213 population had received anti-VEGF in previous treatment lines (Aghajanian et al. 2012; Coleman et al. 2017). The role of bevacizumab beyond progression has been investigated starting from the assumption that resistance to chemotherapy does not affect angiogenesis (Colombo et al. 2016). The MITO 16B trial (NCT01802749) is investigating the role of bevacizumab in platinum-sensitive recurrent EOC previously treated with bevacizumab in the first-line setting (Pignata et al. 2018); it randomized patients to second line chemotherapy (carboplatin plus gemcitabine) alone or in association with bevacizumab. Preliminary results showed a promising increase in PFS from 8.8 to 11.8 months (HR: 0.51, $p < 0.001$); final results are awaited. Likewise, the phase II JGOG3023 trial, evaluating the efficacy and safety of bevacizumab beyond progression, is currently ongoing (Shoji et al. 2018). Therefore, the use of bevacizumab beyond progression appears to be a promising strategy in recurrent EOC. Concerning toxicities, bevacizumab is associated with increased incidence of hypertension, proteinuria, and thromboembolism, and it affects wound healing. No detrimental effect on quality of life has been reported in clinical trials (Colombo et al. 2016). Up to date, FDA currently approved bevacizumab across different therapeutic settings:

1. in combination with carboplatin and paclitaxel followed by single agent maintenance
2. in patients with stage III or IV EOC, fallopian tube, or primary peritoneal cancer following initial surgical resection
3. in combination with carboplatin and paclitaxel or gemcitabine, followed by single agent maintenance, in patients with platinum-sensitive recurrent EOC, fallopian tube, or primary peritoneal cancer and
4. in combination with paclitaxel, PEG-liposomal doxorubicin, or topotecan, in patients with platinum-resistant recurrent EOC, fallopian tube, or primary peritoneal cancer who received no more than two prior chemotherapy regimens (FDA 2018).

Pazopanib is an oral inhibitor of VEGFR-1/2/3, PDGFR-α/β, c-Kit, and FGFR-1/3 kinases, currently approved for advanced soft-tissue sarcoma and renal cell carcinoma (Miyamoto et al. 2018). Pazopanib has been tested in combination with paclitaxel versus paclitaxel single agent in platinum-resistant or refractory patients in the randomized phase II MITO-11 trial, showing a benefit from the addition of pazopanib (PFS: 6.35 vs 3.49 months in the experimental and control arm, respectively) (Pignata et al. 2015). Pazopanib has also been tested as an agent for the maintenance, in EOC patients after receiving and not progressed to first-line platinum-based chemotherapy. The AGO-OVAR16 phase III placebo-controlled randomized clinical trial demonstrated a significant improvement in PFS with the maintenance strategy (Vergote et al. 2019). However, no benefit on the OS was reported. OS was 59.1 months in pazopanib and 64.0 months in placebo arm (HR: 0.960), respectively. Nevertheless, up to date, pazopanib is not approved for the use in EOC patients, in any setting.

2.4.4 PARP Inhibitors

This new class of oral drugs was primarily tested in recurrent EOC and, thereafter, in first-line setting. Table 2.2 shows an overview of the landmark trials in this field. First data about olaparib were published in 2009, with preliminary evidences of activity in *BRCA1/2* mutation carriers EOC patients (Fong et al. 2009). The Study 19 was the phase II, placebo-controlled trial to test olaparib [400 mg bis in die (BID)] as maintenance treatment after first-line. The trial showed a median PFS of 8.4 months in the olaparib arm versus 4.8 months in the placebo arm, reaching 11.2 vs 4.3 months in *BRCA* mutated patients in a preplanned analysis (Ledermann et al. 2012). Another phase II trial—Study 12—tested olaparib (200 or 400 mg BID) versus PEG-liposomal doxorubicin in patients with recurrent germline *BRCA* mutated OC; median PFS was not different among the three arms (Kaye et al. 2012). The phase III SOLO-2 trial evaluated olaparib (300 mg BID tablet) as maintenance treatment in platinum-sensitive relapsed OC patients with *BRCA1/2* mutations; median PFS was 19.1 vs 5.5 months, with an HR of 0.30 (Pujade-Lauraine et al. 2017). The results from SOLO2, together with evidences from Study 19 (Ledermann et al. 2012), led to rapid approval by FDA, in August 2017, of olaparib for the maintenance treatment of adult patients with recurrent HGSOC, fallopian tube, or primary peritoneal cancer, who are in a complete or partial response to platinum-based chemotherapy, regardless of *BRCA* mutation status (FDA 2020a, b). Olaparib was subsequently tested as first-line maintenance therapy in two phase III clinical trials. SOLO1 trial evaluated the efficacy of olaparib (300 mg BID tablet) as maintenance therapy in patients with newly diagnosed advanced HGSOC harboring *BRCA* mutations and experiencing a response to platinum-based chemotherapy, showing a 70% reduction in risk of disease progression/death (HR 0.30, the same value of SOLO2 trial) (Moore et al. 2018). An add-on strategy of olaparib to the standard of care maintenance after chemotherapy with bevacizumab frontline was tested in the PAOLA-1 study. In PAOLA-1 trial, regardless of *BRCA* mutation status, all patients with HGSOC experiencing a response to the first-line platinum- and bevacizumab-containing regimen were randomized (2:1) to receive olaparib tablets (300 mg BID) versus placebo for up to 2 years (Ray-Coquard et al. 2019). Of note, unlike the previous trials conducted in the past, in this study all the patients received bevacizumab as first-line maintenance therapy for up to 15 months. The trial showed valuable results in the overall population, with the median PFS improved of +5.5 months (22.1 vs 16.6 months, HR: 0.59). Additionally, there was a higher benefit in HRD patients (PFS: 37.2 vs 17.7 months, HR: 0.33) as well as in HRD patients excluding *BRCA* mutations (28.1 vs 16.6 months, HR: 0.43). The PAOLA-1 clinical trial did not respond to the clinical question about the added value of olaparib towards bevacizumab, therefore the value of these two agents in the maintenance setting is still debated.

Therefore, in May 2020, FDA approved olaparib plus bevacizumab as maintenance treatment for ovarian, fallopian tube, or primary peritoneal cancers who are in complete or partial response to first-line platinum-based chemotherapy and whose cancer is associated with HRD positive status, defined by either a deleterious or

Table 2.2 PARP inhibitors as maintenance therapy in high-grade serous ovarian cancer

Drug	Trials	Phase	Setting	Control	PFS	References
Olaparib	Study 19	II	Recurrent platinum sensitive	Placebo	– Overall: 8.4 vs 4.8 months ($p < 0.001$) – Mutated *BRCA*: 11.2 vs 4.3 months ($p < 0.0001$)	Ledermann et al. (2012)
	SOLO-2	III	Recurrent platinum sensitive	Placebo	19.1 vs 5.5 months ($p < 0.0001$)	Pujade-Lauraine et al. (2017)
	SOLO-1	III	First-line *BRCA* mutated	Placebo	HR: 0.30 ($p < 0.001$)	Moore et al. (2018)
Olaparib + bevacizumab	PAOLA	III	First-line platinum sensitive	Bevacizumab	– Overall: 22.1 vs 16.6 months (HR: 0.59, $p < 0.001$) – HRD: 37.2 vs 17.7 months (HR: 0.33) – HRD non BRCA mutations: 28.1 vs 16.6 months (HR: 0.43)	Ray-Coquard et al. (2019)
Niraparib	NOVA	III	Recurrentplatinum sensitive	Placebo	– g*BRCA* mut: 21 vs 5.5 months (HR:0.27, $p < 0.001$) – HRD non g*BRCA* mut: 12.9 vs 3.8 months (HR: 0.38, $p < 0.001$) – Non g*BRCA* mut: 9.3 vs 3.9 months (HR: 0.45, $p < 0.001$)	Mirza et al. (2016)
	PRIMA	III	First-line platinum sensitive	Placebo	– Overall: 13.8 vs 8.2 months (HR: 0.62, $p < 0.001$) – HRD: 21.9 vs 10.4 months (HR: 0.43, $p < 0.001$)	González-Martín et al. (2019a, b)
Veliparib	VELIA	III	First-line platinum sensitive	Placebo	– Mutated *BRCA*: 34.7 vs 22 months (HR: 0.44, $p < 0.001$) – HRD: 31.9 vs 20.5 months (HR: 0.57, $p < 0.001$) – Overall: 23.5 vs 17.3 months (HR: 0.68, $p < 0.001$)	Coleman et al. (2019)

Abbreviations: *PFS* progression free survival, *HR* hazard ratio, *HRD* homologous recombination deficiency, *gBRCA mut* germline BRCA mutations, *PLD* pegylated liposomal doxorubicin suspected deleterious *BRCA* mutation, and/or genomic instability (FDA 2020a, b). The FDA also approved Myriad myChoice® CDx (Myriad Genetic Laboratories, Inc.) an NGS-based companion diagnostic for olaparib, for the assessment of the genomic instability on the tumor tissue. The main toxicities of olaparib reported from the trials are nausea (70%) and vomiting (30%), fatigue (61%, G3-4: 5%), anemia (35%, G3-4: 16%), diarrhea (30%), and neutropenia (15%). In general, olaparib could be considered a manageable agent, but toxicities should be optimally managed by clinicians to improve drug compliance (Ricci et al. 2020). It should be noted that, in order to obtain exposure equivalence, olaparib 100 mg tablets and 50 mg capsules have different daily dosing, being 300 mg BID and 400 mg BID, respectively (Mateo et al. 2016). Accordingly, the substitution of capsule and tablets should not be based on the total dose consideration only, but also on the formulation used.

The phase III NOVA trial assessed the efficacy of niraparib versus placebo as maintenance treatment in platinum-sensitive recurrent HGSOC patients; the study population was categorized according to presence or absence of germline *BRCA* mutations. Niraparib (300 mg/die) showed to improve PFS in all three predefined primary efficacy populations. In particular, in the germline-mutated *BRCA* cohort the PFS was prolonged from 5.5 to 21 months (HR: 0.27), in the non-germline-mutated *BRCA* HRD cohort from 3.8 to 12.9 months (HR: 0.38), and in the overall non-germinal mutated *BRCA* cohort from 3.9 to 9.3 months (HR: 0.45) (Mirza et al. 2016). This study led to approval of niraparib as maintenance therapy in recurrent platinum-sensitive HGSOC patients who showed a complete or partial tumor response to platinum-based chemotherapy for recurrence disease, regardless of *BRCA* mutation status (FDA 2020a, b). Niraparib was also tested in newly diagnosed advanced HGSOC patients after a response to first-line platinum-based chemotherapy in the phase III PRIMA trial. In the trial PFS was prolonged from 8.2 to 13.8 months (HR: 0.62) and from 10.4 to 21.9 months (HR: 0.43) in the overall and in HDR population, respectively; data for OS are still immature (González-Martín et al. 2019a, b). In April 2020, FDA approved niraparib for the maintenance treatment of adult patients with advanced EOC, fallopian tube, or primary peritoneal cancer who had a complete or partial response to first-line platinum-based chemotherapy (FDA 2020a, b). Niraparib has a safety profile similar to olaparib, but with a higher incidence of thrombocytopenia.

Another PARP inhibitor, veliparib, was recently tested in the placebo-controlled phase III VELIA trial (Coleman et al. 2019). In this trial, patients with previously untreated stage III/IV HGSOC received veliparib or placebo during chemotherapy with or without a subsequent maintenance phase. A prolonged PFS was observed in the *BRCA* mutated cohort (34.7 vs 22 months in the experimental and control arm, respectively; HR: 0.44), in the HRD cohort (31.9 vs 20.5 months; HR: 0.57) as well as in the overall population (23.5 vs 17.3 months; HR: 0.68). However, the role of veliparib added to chemotherapy (carboplatin was reduced per protocol to minimize additive hematologic toxicities) is still to define and, up to date, veliparib has not been approved yet by FDA.

The evolving landscape of PARP inhibitors in the treatment of HGSOC introduced new treatment options but also new complexities in the treatment-decision making. With multiple companion diagnostics emerging for the single molecules and different predictive biomarkers for response, and their possible overlapping areas, a harmonization process in research is highly warranted. Eventually, the capacity of these agents to improve OS has not yet been reported, deserving precautions in the interpretation of the final data.

2.4.4.1 MEK Inhibitors

MAPK signaling pathway is involved in cell survival and proliferation, and its pathological activation could sustain cancer cell growth (Karin 2001). Among kinases, MEK1/2 (mitogen-activated protein kinase kinase) is considered as principal effector, thus representing a potential bottleneck of the pathway (Zhao and Adjei 2014). Several MEK inhibitors have been developed and subsequently tested in human cancer. Concerning EOC, they have been mainly studied in rare histotypes, such as LGSOC.

The first MEK inhibitor evaluated in an entire LGSOC population after recurrence of disease was the selumetinib. The trial involved 52 patients and showed very promising results, with 80% disease control rate, PFS of 11 months, and good tolerability. However, there was no association between MEK alteration and response to treatment and, therefore, no prognostic or predictive biomarkers were identified (Farley et al. 2013). Then, a phase II trial evaluated the activity of the MEK inhibitor pimasertib with or without a PI3K/mTOR inhibitor (voxtalisib) in 65 patients with serous borderline tumors or LGSOC. Unfortunately, the trial was stopped earlier for futility since it showed similar responses in both arms (12.5% vs 9.4% in the combination and single arm, respectively) (NCT01936363), as well as the phase III trial MILO/ENGOT-OV11 which tested the MEK inhibitor binimetinib in this setting (Grisham et al. 2019). Additionally, a phase II/III trial randomized 260 patients with recurrent LGSOC to receive the MEK inhibitor trametinib or standard chemotherapy. The recently presented preliminary results showed significant improvement in PFS (13 vs 7.2 months, $p < 0.0001$), OS (37 months vs 29.2 months), and responses (26.2% vs 6.2%) for the experimental arm with good tolerability (Gershenson et al. 2019). However, final results as well as the paper in extenso are awaited before introducing trametinib in clinical practice.

2.4.5 Chemotherapy After Recurrence

Unfortunately, the majority of patients show a recurrence after first-line treatments (70–80%). A recurrence is defined as the evidence of relapse of disease, clinical (sign and symptoms of disease) or assessed by scan and evaluated by RECIST 1.1 criteria. The role of cancer antigen 125 (CA-125) in this setting is still debated. In fact, if the increase of CA 125 could precede a radiological recurrence from 2 to 6 months (Lindemann et al. 2016), according to international guidelines (NCCN guidelines 2020) it is not recommended to start a new line of treatment basing only on biochemical progression, since it does not improve the outcome in this setting (Rustin et al. 2010). One of the most important thing to consider in case of relapse is the PFI. In this regard, in fact, we can distinguish patients in two groups, according to the platinum-free interval: patients who show a relapse after 6 months and who can receive again a platinum-based treatment (the "*old*" platinum-sensitive disease); patients who have relapse within 6 months and who cannot receive a platinum-based treatment (the "*old*" platinum-resistant disease). However, the evaluation of *BRCA* status, tumor size, and metastatic sites is important predictive factors that should be take into account in order to choose the most appropriate second line treatments. In patients who can receive a platinum-based treatment, the AGO-OVAR (Pfisterer et al. 2006), CALYPSO (Pujade-Lauraine et al. 2010; Wagner et al. 2012), OCEANS (Aghajanian et al. 2012), and MITO 16B (Pignata et al. 2018) trials showed a benefit with the use of carboplatin plus gemcitabine, carboplatin plus PEG-liposomal doxorubicin, carboplatin plus gemcitabine, in addition to bevacizumab. The last schedule can be used in either patients who previously received bevacizumab [MITO 16B trial (Pignata et al. 2018) or not (OCEANS trial) (Aghajanian et al. 2012)]. More in details, the phase III AGO-OVAR trial (Pfisterer et al. 2006) showed that a doublet chemotherapy (carboplatin plus gemcitabine) was superior in term of PFS in this setting if compared to carboplatin alone (8.6 vs 5.8 months, respectively; HR: 0.72, $p = 0.0031$). Likewise, the phase III CALYPSO trial showed that carboplatin and PEG-liposomal doxorubicin were superior to carboplatin and paclitaxel in PFS (11.3 vs 9.4 months in the experimental and control arm, respectively; HR: 0.821; p: 0.005) (Pujade-Lauraine et al. 2010). However, long-term results did not show benefit in OS, may related to the arm-crossover (Wagner et al. 2012). *For additional details about OCEANS, MITO 16B trial, and the use of PARP inhibitors in these patients, see previous sections.*

In case of patients who experienced intolerance to paclitaxel, some trials with nab-paclitaxel and carboplatin have shown promising preliminary results and are currently ongoing (Benigno et al. 2010). In patients who could receive platinum-based therapy, but with a poorer performance status, a platinum monotherapy could be proposed. Finally, in case of patients in this group who cannot receive platinum-based chemotherapy for other reason, a doublet with trabectedin plus PEG-liposomal doxorubicin showed to be more effective if compared to PEG-liposomal doxorubicin alone (Monk et al. 2012). In these patients, trials regarding the sequence of treatment were conducted, basing on the hypothesis that a first-line non-platinum treatment might improve the responses to follow platinum-based second line and PFI. However, the MITO-8 trial (Pignata et al. 2017) failed to confirm this hypothesis and the sequence "first-line platinum-second-line non-platinum" remains the standard of care up to date. When PFI is 6–12 months, the prolongation of the PFI has been suggested to increase the likelihood of having a response in later lines. To respond to this clinical question, the results of INOVATYON trial (NCT01379989), which use a second line with trabectedin plus PEG-liposomal doxorubicin and a follow platinum line, are awaited in order to clarify this issue in platinum-sensitive EOC patients.

In patients who are not suitable to receive a platinum-based therapy due to a short PFI (resistant or refractory disease), PEG-liposomal doxorubicin, topotecan, gemcitabine, weekly paclitaxel or trabectedin could be alternatives. In particular, the MITO-3 trial showed a benefit in quality of life by using PEG-liposomal doxorubicin versus gemcitabine in this setting, reporting also an improvement in PFS in the platinum-sensitive population (Ferrandina et al. 2008). The AURELIA trial compared weekly paclitaxel/topotecan/PEG-liposomal doxorubicin plus bevacizumab in this setting, showing a benefit in PFS in all arm and in OS in the weekly paclitaxel plus bevacizumab arm (see Sect. 4.2.2 for more details) (Pujade-Lauraine et al. 2014; Poveda et al. 2015). However, today is becoming clear that not all EOC subtypes have the same response to treatment and the same behavior, as previously mentioned. Therefore, if the majority of recommendation are related to HGSOC, those are usually generalized also for the other subtypes, since the pivotal trials have included also those kinds of tumors, not suitable of dedicated studies due to their rarity. Starting from this assumption, the approved treatments are the same for all EOC subtypes, with some peculiarity. In fact, regarding recurrence of LGSOC, secondary resections, endocrine therapy, and chemotherapy with or without target agents or clinical trials are the possible alternatives. In this context, the endocrine therapies showed the higher DCR (~60–70%) (Tang et al. 2019), as well as bevacizumab (~50%) (Dalton et al. 2017). However, clinical trials are currently ongoing and the landscape is quickly evolving especially in these last years in order to depict a personalized landscape also in the field of EOC.

2.5 Current Clinical Management of Non-epithelial Ovarian Cancer

Non-epithelial OCs are a group of rare and heterogeneous tumors that account almost 10% of all OC. They can arise from a variety of ovarian precursor cells and include malignancies of germ cell origin, sex cord-stromal cell origin, and a variety of extremely rare types, such as sarcomas and lipoid cell tumors. The two most common type are sex cord-stromal tumors (SCSTs), that account for approximately in 3–5% of OCs and occur more often in postmenopausal women, and malignant germ cell tumors (GCTs), classified in dysgerminomas and non-dysgerminomas tumors, that occur mainly in young women, with often unilateral presentation (exempt dysgerminomas), representing 5% of all OCs. Instead, small cell carcinoma of the ovary (SCCO) usually affects young women and children with a very low incidence (less than 1% of OCs) (Gatta et al. 2011).

Non-epithelial OC are classified according to the WHO 2014 classification (Kurman et al. 2014) and their staging system is extrapolated from FIGO classification of EOC. They often occur at an early stage (60–70% at stage I, 25–30% at stage III), because of their clinical presentation (abdominal pain, menstrual irregularities, abdominal or pelvic mass). Adverse prognostic factors for GCTs are the stage >I, incomplete surgical resection, age >45 years, and yolk sac histology (Mangili et al. 2011). Instead, intraperitoneal lesion rupture and FIGO stage are the most common prognostic factor for SCSTs, even if also the advanced stage of disease can have a good prognosis because of the response to chemotherapy (Prat and FIGO Committee on Gynecologic Oncology 2014). According to the international guidelines (NCCN guidelines 2020), the standard treatment is surgery; fertility-sparing surgery should be proposed, considering the young age of patients, even in advanced stage, due to the tumor sensitivity to chemotherapy. Patients with stage IA dysgerminoma can be treated with surgery alone, showing a recurrence rate relatively low (15–20%) and a good response to the treatment at the time of relapse. A platinum-based chemotherapy must be considered for patients with stages > I, advanced disease, or yolk sac histology (all stages); three cycles of 5-day platinum-etoposide-bleomycin (PEB) is the most used regimen for completely resected stage I disease, whereas four cycles are recommended for more advanced disease (Pectasides et al. 2008). Patients who show resistance to a platinum-based chemotherapy may receive VAC (vincristine/actinomycin D/cyclophosphamide) or paclitaxel plus gemcitabine or gemcitabine plus oxaliplatin as salvage therapy. On the other hand, in SCST patients with early stage disease the rule of adjuvant chemotherapy is controversial. In advanced stages, debulking surgery is the cornerstone treatment, even in relapsed disease, and a platinum-based chemotherapy, such as PEB regimen, is used.In the future, the role of new target agents, that are already studied in testicular cancer, such as antiangiogenic agents or tyrosine kinase inhibitors or immune-checkpoint inhibitors, could be investigated also in these rare tumors (Manchana et al. 2010).

2.6 Conclusions and Future Perspectives

For decades, the OC treatment consisted in debulking surgery followed by platinum-based chemotherapy. However, the most notable exception to the absence of new treatment options has been the introduction of maintenance therapy with bevacizumab, that showed an improved PFS and OS in the subset of high-risk patients (González-Martín et al. 2019a, b). In the last decade, the PARP inhibitors agents have changed this scenario. Several clinical trials have shown benefits of these drugs in recurrent OC, and they have been approved as a maintenance therapy in patients who have responded to platinum-based chemotherapy, regardless of *BRCA* status. The paradigm of *BRCA* mutation has been exceeded by the definition of "*BRCAness phenotype*" in patients with HR-deficient tumors. The HR-deficiency status characterizes not only the HGSOC, but also the other subtypes, and this biomarker could be useful in this setting in the future, to refine the patients' selection. Although the most recent clinical trials used the same HRD test (i.e., MyChoice test), even if considering different parameters to define HRD patients, it will be crucial to incorporate available and reproducible test in clinical practice in order to give to an high number of patients the chance to be treated with PARP inhibitors. More recently, the VELIA (Coleman et al. 2019), PRIMA (González-Martín et al. 2019a, b), and PAOLA-1 (Ray-Coquard et al. 2019) trials have given for the first time the chance to use PARP inhibitors in first-line setting. The efficacy of those agents was shown in the whole population, with the magnitude of benefit that varies widely among subgroups, highlighting the need to identify specific biological subtypes into clinical practice. On the other hand, the use of PD-L1/PD-1 inhibitors has demonstrated preliminary but very modest activity in EOC, suggesting an opportunity for combination therapies and in biomarker-selected patients. The rationale of using immunotherapy with PARP inhibitors is the association between the high neoantigens load and the high tumor mutational burden with the increasing of TILs and the high expression of PD1/PD-L1 in HRD tumors (Strickland et al. 2016). Ongoing clinical trials (such as ATHENA [NCT03522246], DUO-O [NCT03737643], BGOG/ENGOT-ov43 [NCT03740165], and FIRST [NCT03602859] trial) are assessing the maintenance therapy based on PARP inhibitors in combination with immune-checkpoint inhibitors.Another chance of therapy is the combination of immunotherapy with antiangiogenic agents, given the immunoregulatory effects of VEGF on endothelial and microenvironment cells (Gavalas et al. 2012). Further fields of investigation include defining how "moving" PARP inhibitors in first-line treatment setting can impact on use in recurrent disease and if the patients can benefit from a re-challenge with the same or different drugs. In this setting, the ongoing OReO trial (NCT03106987) has the aim to define the efficacy of olaparib maintenance re-treatment in patients with recurrence EOC, who have had disease progression following maintenance therapy with PARP inhibitors (see Box 2.1 for further reading).

Box 2.1 Recommended reading

Lheureux S, et al. *Epithelial ovarian cancer: Evolution of management in the era of precision medicine.* CA Cancer J Clin. 2019 Jul;69(4):280–304.	https://doi.org/10.3322/caac.21559
Naumann RW, et al. *Phase III trials in ovarian cancer: The evolving landscape of front line therapy.* GynecolOncol. 2019 May;153(2):436–444.	https://doi.org/10.1016/j.ygyno.2019.02.008
Franzese E, et al. *PARP inhibitors in ovariancancer.* CancerTreat Rev. 2019 Feb;73:1–9.	https://doi.org/10.1016/j.ctrv.2018.12.002
Cortez AJ, et al. *Advances in ovarian cancer therapy.* CancerChemotherPharmacol. 2018 Jan;81(1):17–38.	https://doi.org/10.1007/s00280-017-3501-8
Haunschild CE, Tewari KS. *The current landscape of molecular profiling in the treatment of epithelial ovarian cancer.* GynecolOncol. 2020 Oct 11:S0090-8258(20)33953-6.	https://doi.org/10.1016/j.ygyno.2020.09.043
Le Saux O, et al. *Challenges for immunotherapy for the treatment of platinum resistant ovarian cancer.* SeminCancerBiol. 2020 Sep 12:S1044-579X(20)30193-0.	https://doi.org/10.1016/j.semcancer.2020.08.017
Curtin NJ, Szabo C. *Poly(ADP-ribose) polymerase inhibition: past, present and future.* NatRevDrugDiscov. 2020 Oct;19(10):711–736.	https://doi.org/10.1038/s41573-020-0076-6
Rottenberg S, et al. *The rediscovery of platinum-based cancer therapy.* NatRevCancer. 2020 Oct 30.	https://doi.org/10.1038/s41568-020-00308-y
Slomovitz B, et al. *Low-grade serous ovarian cancer: State of the science.* GynecolOncol. 2020 Mar;156(3):715-725.	https://doi.org/10.1016/j.ygyno.2019.12.033
McMullen M, et al. *New approaches for targeting platinum-resistant ovarian cancer.* Semin Cancer Biol. 2020 Aug 29:S1044-579X(20)30186-3.	https://doi.org/10.1016/j.semcancer.2020.08.013

Conflicts of Interest EFG has personal fees from Novartis. AP has personal fees from Servier, Eli-Lilly, and MSD. All the fees are not connected with the present work. The other authors have no conflict of interest to declare.

Authors' Contribution APe and DT coordinated the development of the chapter and shared a preliminary outline, refined with the inputs of EFG and APa. APe, DT, EFG, and APa contributed to writing and revising the proofs; they also provided reciprocal feedback. The final draft was reviewed and approved by all the authors. The contents of the chapter reflect the authors' perspectives and not of their institutions of affiliation.

References

Aghajanian C, Blank SV, Goff BA et al (2012) OCEANS: a randomized, double-blind, placebo-controlled phase III trial of chemotherapy with or without bevacizumab in patients with platinum-sensitive recurrent epithelial ovarian, primary peritoneal, or fallopian tube cancer. J Clin Oncol 30:2039–2045

Alberts DS, Liu PY, Hannigan EV et al (1996) Intraperitoneal cisplatin plus intravenous cyclophosphamide versus intravenous cisplatin plus intravenous cyclophosphamide for stage III ovarian cancer. N Engl J Med 335:1950–1955

Armstrong DK, Bundy B, Wenzel L et al (2006) Intraperitoneal cisplatin and paclitaxel in ovarian cancer. N Engl J Med 354:34–43

Arts-de Jong M, de Bock GH, van Asperen CJ et al (2016) Germline BRCA1/2 mutation testing is indicated in every patient with epithelial ovarian cancer: a systematic review. Eur J Cancer 61:137–145

Aust S, Seebacher-Shariat V (2020) Screening for ovarian cancer: is there still hope? Memo 13:189–192. https://doi.org/10.1007/s12254-019-00563-2

Babaier A, Ghatage P (2020) Mucinous cancer of the ovary: overview and current status. Diagnostics (Basel) 10(1):52. https://doi.org/10.3390/diagnostics10010052

Baumann P, West SC (1998) Role of the human RAD51 protein in homologous recombination and double-stranded-break repair. Trends Biochem Sci 23:247–251

Bell J, Brady MF, Young RC et al (2006) Randomized phase III trial of three versus six cycles of adjuvant carboplatin and paclitaxel in early stage epithelial ovarian carcinoma: a Gynecologic Oncology Group study. Gynecol Oncol 102(3):432–439

Benigno BB, Burrell MO, Daugherty P, Hernandez P (2010) A phase II nonrandomized study of nab-paclitaxel plus carboplatin in patients with recurrent platinum-sensitive ovarian or primary peritoneal cancer. J Clin Oncol 28:5011

Bentivegna E, Gouy S, Maulard A et al (2016) Fertility-sparing surgery in epithelial ovarian cancer: a systematic review of oncological issues. Ann Oncol 27(11):1994–2004

Berek JS, Hacker NF, Lagasse LD et al (1983) Survival of patients following secondary cytoreductive surgery in ovarian cancer. Obstet Gynecol 61(2):189–193

Bodelon C, Killian JK, Sampson JN et al (2019) Molecular classification of epithelial ovarian cancer based on methylation profiling: evidence for survival heterogeneity. Clin Cancer Res 25 (19):5937–5946. https://doi.org/10.1158/1078-0432.CCR-18-3720

Bookman MA, Brady MF, McGuire WP et al (2009) Evaluation of new platinum-based treatment regimens in advanced-stage ovarian cancer: a Phase III Trial of the Gynecologic Cancer Intergroup. J Clin Oncol 27(9):1419–1425. https://doi.org/10.1200/JCO.2008.19.1684

Brahmer JR, Tykodi SS, Chow LQ et al (2012) Safety and activity of anti-PD-L1 antibody in patients with advanced cancer. N Engl J Med 366(26):2455–2465

Brand AH, DiSilvestro PA, Sehouli J, Berek JS (2017) Cytoreductive surgery for ovarian cancer: quality assessment. Ann Oncol 28(Suppl_8):viii25–viii29. https://doi.org/10.1093/annonc/mdx448

Bray F, Ferlay J, Soerjomataram I et al (2018) Global cancer statistics 2018: GLOBOCAN estimates of incidence and mortality worldwide for 36 cancers in 185 countries. CA Cancer J Clin 68(6):394–424

Burger RA, Brady MF, Bookman MA et al (2011) Incorporation of bevacizumab in the primary treatment of ovarian cancer. N Engl J Med 365:2473–2483

Cannistra SA (2004) Cancer of the ovary. N Engl J Med 351:2519–2529

Cass I, Baldwin RL, Varkey T et al (2003) Improved survival in women with BRCA-associated ovarian carcinoma. Cancer 97:2187–2195

Chan JK, Tian C, Fleming GF et al (2010) The potential benefit of 6 vs. 3 cycles of chemotherapy in subsets of women with early-stage high-risk epithelial ovarian cancer: an exploratory analysis of a Gynecologic Oncology Group study. Gynecol Oncol 116(3):301–306

Chapman JR, Taylor MR, Boulton SJ (2012) Playing the end game: DNA double-strand break repair pathway choice. Mol Cell 47(4):497–510

Cheasley D, Wakefield MJ, Ryland GL, Allan PE, Alsop K, Amarasinghe KC et al (2019) The molecular origin and taxonomy of mucinous ovarian carcinoma. Nat Commun 10(1):3935. https://doi.org/10.1038/s41467-019-11862-x

Chen S, Parmigiani G (2007) Meta-analysis of BRCA1 and BRCA2 penetrance. J Clin Oncol 25 (11):1329–1333

Chung YW, Kim S, Hong JH et al (2019) Overexpression of HER2/HER3 and clinical feature of ovarian cancer. J Gynecol Oncol 30(5):e75. https://doi.org/10.3802/jgo.2019.30.e75

Clamp AR, James EC, McNeish IA et al (2019) Weekly dose-dense chemotherapy in first-line epithelial ovarian, fallopian tube, or primary peritoneal carcinoma treatment (ICON8): primary progression free survival analysis results from a GCIG phase 3 randomised controlled trial. Lancet 394(10214):2084–2095. https://doi.org/10.1016/S0140-6736(19)32259-7

Coleman RL, Brady MF, Herzog TJ et al (2017) Bevacizumab and paclitaxel-carboplatin chemotherapy and secondary cytoreduction in recurrent, platinum-sensitive ovarian cancer (NRG Oncology/Gynecologic Oncology Group study GOG-0213): A multicentre, open-label, randomised, phase 3 trial. Lancet Oncol 18:779–791. https://doi.org/10.1016/S1470-2045(17) 30279-6

Coleman R, Enserro D, Spirtos NM et al (2018) A phase III randomized con-trolled trial of secondary surgical cytoreduction (SSC) followed by platinum-based combination chemotherapy (PBC), with or without bevacizumab (B) in platinum-sensitive, recurrent ovarian cancer (PSOC): a NRG oncology/gynecologic oncology group (GOG) study. J Clin Oncol 36 (15_Suppl):5501

Coleman RL, Fleming GF, Brady MF et al (2019) Veliparib with first-line chemotherapy and as maintenance therapy in ovarian cancer. N Engl J Med 381:2403–2415. https://doi.org/10.1056/NEJMoa1909707

Collinson F, Qian W, Fossati R et al (2014) Optimal treatment of early-stage ovarian cancer. Ann Oncol 25(6):1165–1171. https://doi.org/10.1093/annonc/mdu116

Colombo N, Pecorelli S (2003) What have we learned from ICON1 and ACTION. Int J Gynecol Cancer 13:140–143

Colombo N, Guthrie D, Chiari S et al (2003) International Collaborative Ovarian Neoplasm (ICON) collaborators. J Natl Cancer Inst 95(2):125–132

Colombo N, Conte PF, Pignata S et al (2016) Bevacizumab in ovarian cancer: focus on clinical data and future perspectives. Crit Rev Oncol Hematol 97:335–348. https://doi.org/10.1016/j.critrevonc.2015.08.017

Colombo N, Sessa C, du Bois A et al (2019) ESMO-ESGO consensus conference recommendations on ovarian cancer: pathology and molecular biology, early and advanced stages, borderline tumours and recurrent disease. Ann Oncol 30(5):672–705

Coleridge SL, Bryant A, Lyons TJ et al (2019) Chemotherapy versus surgery for initial treatment in advanced ovarian epithelial cancer. Cochrane Database Syst Rev 10:CD005343

Curtin NJ (2005) PARP inhibitors for cancer therapy. Expert Rev Mol Med 7:1–20

Dai CH, Li J, Chen P et al (2015) RNA interferences targeting the Fanconi anemia/BRCA pathway upstream genes reverse cisplatin resistance in drug-resistant lung cancer cells. J Biomed Sci 22:77

Dalton HJ, Fleming ND, Sun CC et al (2017) Activity of bevacizumab-containing regimens in recurrent low-grade serous ovarian or peritoneal cancer: a single institution experience. Gynecol Oncol 145(1):37–40. https://doi.org/10.1016/j.ygyno.2017.01.027

Darzynkiewicz Z, Traganos F, Wlodkowic D (2009) Impaired DNA damage response–an Achilles' heel sensitizing cancer to chemotherapy and radiotherapy. Eur J Pharmacol 625(1–3):143–150

Della Pepa C, Tonini G, Santini D et al (2015) Low Grade Serous Ovarian Carcinoma: from the molecular characterization to the best therapeutic strategy. Cancer Treat Rev 41(2):136–143. https://doi.org/10.1016/j.ctrv.2014.12.003

Disis ML, Taylor MH, Kelly K et al (2019) Efficacy and safety of avelumab for patients with recurrent or refractory ovarian cancer: phase 1b results from the JAVELIN solid tumor trial. JAMA Oncol 5(3):393–401. https://doi.org/10.1001/jamaoncol.2018.6258

Drew Y (2015) The development of PARP inhibitors in ovarian cancer: from bench to bedside. Br J Cancer 113:S3–S9

du Bois A, Quinn M, Thigpen T et al (2005) 2004 consensus statements on the management of ovarian cancer: final document of the 3rd international Gynecologic Cancer intergroup ovarian Cancer consensus conference (GCIG OCCC 2004). Ann Oncol 16(Suppl 8):viii7–viii12

du Bois A, Reuss A, Pujade-Lauraine E et al (2009) Role of surgical outcome as prognostic factor in advanced epithelial ovarian cancer: a combined exploratory analysis of 3 prospectively randomized phase multicenter trials: by the Arbeitsgemeinschaft Gynaekologische Onkologie Studiengruppe Ovarialkarzinom (AGO-OVAR) and the Grouped' Investigateurs Nationaux pour les Etudes des Cancers de l'Ovaire (GINECO). Cancer 115(6):1234–1244.173

DuBois A, Sehouli J, Vergote I et al (2020) Randomized phase III study to evaluate the impact of secondary cytoreductive surgery in recurrent ovarian cancer: final analysis of AGO DESKTOP III/ENGOT-ov20. J Clin Oncol 38(15_Suppl):6000

Eustermann S, Wu W-F, Langelier M-F et al (2015) Structural basis of detection and signaling of DNA single-strand breaks by human PARP-1. Mol Cell 60:742–754. https://doi.org/10.1016/j.molcel.2015.10.032

Fader AN, Java J, Krivak TC et al (2014) The prognostic significance of pre- and post-treatment CA-125 in grade 1 serous ovarian carcinoma: a Gynecologic Oncology Group study. Gynecol Oncol 132(3):560–565

Fancello L, Gandini S, Pelicci PG, Mazzarella L (2019) Tumor mutational burden quantification from targeted gene panels: major advancements and challenges. J Immunother Cancer 7(1):183

Farley J, Brady WE, Vathipadiekal V et al (2013) Selumetinib in women with recurrent low-grade serous carcinoma of the ovary or peritoneum: an open-label, single-arm, phase 2 study. Lancet Oncol 14(2):134–140. https://doi.org/10.1016/S1470-2045(12)70572-7

Farmer H, McCabe N, Lord CJ et al (2005) Targeting the DNA repair defect in BRCA mutant cells as a therapeutic strategy. Nature 434:917–921. https://doi.org/10.1038/nature03445

Ferrandina G, Ludovisi M, Lorusso D et al (2008) Phase III trial of gemcitabine compared with pegylated liposomal doxorubicin in progressive or recurrent ovarian cancer. J Clin Oncol 26 (6):890–896

Ferrara N, Hillan KJ, Gerber HP, Novotny W (2004) Discovery and development of bevacizumab, an anti-VEGF antibody for treating cancer. Nat Rev Drug Discov 3(5):391–400. https://doi.org/10.1038/nrd1381

Fleming JS, Beaugié CR, Haviv I (2006) Incessant ovulation, inflammation and epithelial ovarian carcinogenesis: revisiting old hypotheses. Mol Cell Endocrinol 247(1–2):4–21. https://doi.org/10.1016/j.mce.2005.09.014

Fong P, Boss D, Yap T et al (2009) Inhibition of poly(ADP-ribose) polymerase in tumors from BRCA mutation carriers. N Engl J Med 361:123–134

Friedlander M, Russell K, Millis SZ et al (2015) Molecular profiling of mucinous epithelial ovarian carcinomas (mEOC): opportunities for clinical trials. J Clin Oncol 33:5540

Gabrilovich DI, Nagaraj S (2009) Myeloid-derived suppressor cells as regulators of the immune system. Nat Rev Immunol 9(3):162–174

Gasparri ML, Bardhi E, Ruscito I et al (2017) PI3K/AKT/mTOR pathway in ovarian cancer treatment: are we on the right track? GeburtshilfeFrauenheilkd 77(10):1095–1103. https://doi.org/10.1055/s-0043-118907

Gatta G, van der Zwan JM, Casali PG et al (2011) Rare cancers are not so rare: the rare cancer burden in Europe. Eur J Cancer 47(17):2493–2511. https://doi.org/10.1016/j.ejca.2011.08.008

Gavalas N, Tsiatas M, Tsitsilonis O et al (2012) VEGF directly suppresses activation of T cells from ascites secondary to ovarian cancer via VEGF receptor type 2. Br J Cancer 107:1869–1875. https://doi.org/10.1038/bjc.2012.468

Gershenson DM (2016) Low-grade serous carcinoma of the ovary or peritoneum. Ann Oncol 27 (Suppl_1):i45–i49

Gershenson DM, Bodurka DC, Coleman RL et al (2017) Hormonal maintenance therapy for women with low-grade serous cancer of the ovary or peritoneum. J Clin Oncol 35 (10):1103–1111

Gershenson DM, Miller A, Brady W et al (2019) A randomized phase II/III study to assess the efficacy of trametinib in patients with recurrent or progressive low-grade serous ovarian or peritoneal cancer. Ann Oncol 30(Suppl_5):v851–v934. https://doi.org/10.1093/annonc/mdz394

González-Martín A, Oza AM et al (2019a) Exploratory outcome analyses according to stage and/or residual disease in the ICON7 trial of carboplatin and paclitaxel with or without bevacizumab for newly diagnosed ovarian cancer. Gynecol Oncol 152:53–60

González-Martín A, Pothuri B, Vergote I et al (2019b) Niraparib in patients with newly diagnosed advanced ovarian cancer. N Engl J Med 381:2391–2402. https://doi.org/10.1056/NEJMoa1910962

Goodell V, Salazar LG, Urban N et al (2006) Antibody immunity to the p53 oncogenic protein is a prognostic indicator in ovarian cancer. J Clin Oncol 24(5):762–768

Gras E, Catasus L, Argüelles R et al (2001) Microsatellite instability, MLH-1 promoter hypermethylation, and frameshift mutations at coding mononucleotide repeat microsatellites in ovarian tumors. Cancer 92:2829–2836

Grisham R, Monk JB, Banerjee S et al (2019) 1 MILO/ENGOT-OV11: Phase-3 study of binimetinib versus physician's choice chemotherapy (PCC) in recurrent or persistent low-grade serous carcinomas of the ovary, fallopian tube, or primary peritoneum. Int J Gynecol Cancer 29:A1

Grossman DC, Curry SJ, Owens DK et al (2018) Screening for ovarian cancer: US preventive services task force recommendation statement. JAMA 319:588–594

Guan B, Mao TL, Panuganti PK et al (2011) Mutation and loss of expression of ARID1A in uterine low-grade endometrioid carcinoma. Am J Surg Pathol 35:625–632. https://doi.org/10.1097/PAS.0b013e318212782a. PMID: 21412130

Harter P, du Bois A, Hahmann M et al (2006) Surgery in recurrent ovarian cancer: the Arbeitsgemeinschaft Gynaekologische Onkologie (AGO) DESKTOP OVAR trial. Ann Surg Oncol 13(12):1702–1710

Harter P, Sehouli J, Lorusso D et al (2019) A randomized trial of lymphadenectomy in patients with advanced ovarian neoplasms. N Engl J Med 380(9):822–832

Heckl M, Schmoeckel E, Hertlein L et al (2018) The ARID1A, p53 and ß-catenin statuses are strong prognosticators in clear cell and endometrioid carcinoma of the ovary and the endometrium. PLoS One 13(2):e0192881. https://doi.org/10.1371/journal.pone.0192881

Hirst JE, Gard GB, Mcillroy K et al (2009) High rates of occult fallopian tube cancer diagnosed at prophylactic bilateral salpingo-oophorectomy. Int J Gynecol Cancer 19(5):826–829

Hunn J, Rodriguez GC (2012) Ovarian cancer: etiology, risk factors, and epidemiology. Clin Obstet Gynecol 55(1):3–23

Hunter SM, Anglesio MS, Ryland GL et al (2015) Molecular profiling of low grade serous ovarian tumours identifies novel candidate driver genes. Oncotarget 6(35):37663

Ishida S, McCormick F, Smith-McCune K, Hanahan D (2010) Enhancing tumor-specific uptake of the anticancer drug cisplatin with a copper chelator. Cancer Cell 17(6):574–583
Itamochi H, Oishi T, Oumi N et al (2017) Whole-genome sequencing revealed novel prognostic biomarkers and promising targets for therapy of ovarian clear cell carcinoma. Br J Cancer 117 (5):717–724. https://doi.org/10.1038/bjc.2017.228
Javle M, Curtin NJ (2011) The role of PARP in DNA repair and its therapeutic exploitation. Br J Cancer 105(8):1114–1122
Jones S, Wang TL, Shihe M et al (2010) Frequent mutations of chromatin remodeling gene ARID1A in ovarian clear cell carcinoma. Science 330:228–231
Kaelin WG Jr (2005) The concept of synthetic lethality in the context of anticancer therapy. Nat Rev Cancer 5:689. https://doi.org/10.1038/nrc1691
Kajiyama H, Suzuki S, Utsumi F et al (2019) Comparison of long-term oncologic outcomes between metastatic ovarian carcinoma originating from gastrointestinal organs and advanced mucinous ovarian carcinoma. Int J Clin Oncol 24:950–956
Karin LCM (2001) Mammalian MAP kinase signalling cascades. Nature 410:37–40
Kaye S, Lubinski J, Matulonis U et al (2012) Phase II, open-label, randomized, multicenter study comparing the efficacy and safety of olaparib, a poly(ADP-ribose) polymerase inhibitor, and pegylated liposomal doxorubicin in patients with BRCA1 or BRCA2 mutations and recurrent ovarian cancer. J Clin Oncol 30:372–379
Khanna KK, Jackson SP (2001) DNA double-strand breaks: signaling, repair and the cancer connection. Nat Genet 27(3):247. https://doi.org/10.1038/85798
Konstantinopoulos PA, Ceccaldi R, Shapiro GI, D'Andrea AD (2015) Homologous recombination deficiency: exploiting the fundamental vulnerability of ovarian cancer. Cancer Discov 5:1137–1154. https://doi.org/10.1158/2159-8290.CD-15-0714
Kurman RJ, Shih IM (2016) The dualistic model of ovarian carcinogenesis: revisited, revised, and expanded. Am J Pathol 186(4):733–747
Kurman RJ, Carcangiu ML, Herrington CS, Young RH (2014) WHO classification of tumours of female reproductive organs, 4th edn. Springer, New York
Lawrie TA, Winter-Roach BA, Heus P, Kitchener HC (2015) Adjuvant (post-surgery) chemotherapy for early stage epithelial ovarian cancer. Cochrane Database Syst Rev 12:CD004706
Ledermann J, Harter P, Gourley C et al (2012) Olaparib maintenance therapy in platinum-sensitive relapsed ovarian cancer. N Engl J Med 366:1382–1392
Ledermann JA, Raja FA, Fotopoulou C et al (2013) Newly diagnosed and relapsed epithelial ovarian carcinoma: esmo clinical practice guidelines. Ann Oncol 24(Suppl 6):vi24–vi32
Ledermann JA, Drew Y, Kristeleit RS (2016) Homologous recombination deficiency and ovarian cancer. Eur J Cancer 60:49–58
Lindemann K, Kristensen G, Mirza MR et al (2016) Poor concordance between CA-125 and RECIST at the time of disease progression in patients with platinum-resistant ovarian cancer: analysis of the AURELIA trial. Ann Oncol 27(8):1505–1510
Lindor NM, Guidugli L, Wang X et al (2012) A review of a multifactorial probability-based model for classification of BRCA1 and BRCA2 variants of uncertain significance (VUS). Hum Mutat 33:8–21. https://doi.org/10.1002/humu.21627
Longo DL (2019) Personalized medicine for primary treatment of serous ovarian cancer. N Engl J Med 381(25):2471–2474. https://doi.org/10.1056/NEJMe1914488
Manchana T, Ittiwut C, Mutirangura A, Kavanagh JJ (2010) Targeted therapies for rare gynaecological cancers. Lancet Oncol 11:685–693
Mangili G, Sigismondi C, Gadducci A et al (2011) Outcome and risk factors for recurrence in malignant ovarian germ cell tumors: a MITO-9 retrospective study. Int J Gynecol Cancer 21:1414–1142
Markman M, Bundy BN, Alberts DS et al (2001) Phase III trial of standard-dose intravenous cisplatin plus paclitaxel versus moderately high-dose carboplatin followed by intravenous paclitaxel and intraperitoneal cisplatin in small-volume stage III ovarian carcinoma: an

intergroup study of the Gynecologic Oncology Group, Southwestern Oncology Group, and Eastern Cooperative Oncology Group. J Clin Oncol 19:1001–1007
Mateo J, Moreno V, Gupta A et al (2016) An adaptive study to determine the optimal dose of the tablet formulation of the PARP inhibitor Olaparib. Target Oncol 11:401–415
Matsuo K, Machida H, Grubbs BH et al (2018) Trends of low grade serous ovarian carcinoma in the United States. J Gyncol Oncol 29(1):e15
Matulonis UA, Shapira-Frommer R, Santin AD et al (2019) Antitumor activity and safety of pembrolizumab in patients with advanced recurrent ovarian cancer: results from the phase II KEYNOTE-100 study. Ann Oncol 30(7):1080–1087
Mazzarella L, Morganti S, Marra A et al (2020) Master protocols in immuno-oncology: do novel drugs deserve novel designs? J Immunother Cancer 8(1):e000475. https://doi.org/10.1136/jitc-2019-000475
Mehta A, Haber JE (2014) Sources of DNA double-strand breaks and models of recombinational DNA repair. Cold Spring Harb Perspect Biol 6:a016428. https://doi.org/10.1101/cshperspect.a016428
Mirza M, Monk B, Herrstedt J et al (2016) Niraparib maintenance therapy in platinum-sensitive, recurrent ovarian cancer. N Engl J Med 375:2154–2164
Miyamoto S, Kakutani S, Sato Y et al (2018) Drug review: pazopanib. Jpn J Clin Oncol 48 (6):503–513. https://doi.org/10.1093/jjco/hyy053
Momenimovahed Z, Tiznobaik A, Taheri S, Salehiniya H (2019) Ovarian cancer in the world: epidemiology and risk factors. Int J Women's Health 11:287–299. https://doi.org/10.2147/IJWH.S197604
Monk BJ, Herzog TJ, Kaye SB et al (2012) Trabectedin plus pegylated liposomal doxorubicin (PLD) versus PLD in recurrent ovarian cancer: overall survival analysis. Eur J Cancer 48 (15):2361–2368
Monk BJ, Grisham RN, Banerjee S et al (2020) MILO/ENGOT-ov11: binimetinib versus physician's choice chemotherapy in recurrent or persistent low-grade serous carcinomas of the ovary, fallopian tube, or primary peritoneum. J Clin Oncol 2020:JCO2001164. https://doi.org/10.1200/JCO.20.01164
Moore K, Colombo N, Scambia G et al (2018) Maintenance olaparib in patients with newly diagnosed advanced ovarian cancer. N Engl J Med 379(26):2495–2505. https://doi.org/10.1056/NEJMoa1810858
Moschetta M, George A, Kaye SB, Banerjee S (2016) BRCA somatic mutations and epigenetic BRCA modifications in serous ovarian cancer. Ann Oncol 27:1449–1455. https://doi.org/10.1093/annonc/mdw142
Murthy P, Muggia F (2019) PARP inhibitors: clinical development, emerging differences, and the current therapeutic issues. Cancer Drug Resist 2:665–679. https://doi.org/10.20517/cdr.2019.002
NCCN guidelines v1 2020. Ovarian cancer. nccn.org. Accessed 8 Aug 2020
Ntanasis-Stathopoulos I, Fotopoulos G, Tzanninis IG, Kotteas EA (2016) The emerging role of tyrosine kinase inhibitors in ovarian cancer treatment: a systematic review. Cancer Investig 34:313–339. https://doi.org/10.1080/07357907.2016.1206117
O'Neill CJ, Deavers MT, Malpica A et al (2005) An immunohistochemical comparison between low-grade and high-grade ovarian serous carcinomas: significantly higher expression of p53, MIB1, BCL2, HER-2/neu, and C-KIT in high-grade neoplasms. Am J Surg Pathol 29 (8):1034–1041
Okuno S, Sato H, Kuriyama-Matsumura K et al (2003) Role of cystine transport in intracellular glutathione level and cisplatin resistance in human ovarian cancer cell lines. Br J Cancer 88 (6):951–956
Park HJ, Kim DW, Yim GW et al (2013) Staging laparoscopy for the management of early-stage ovarian cancer: a meta-analysis. Am J Obstet Gynecol 209(1):58.e1–e8

Patel JN, Braicu I, Timms KM et al (2018) Characterisation of homologous recombination deficiency in paired primary and recurrent high-grade serous ovarian cancer. Br J Cancer 119:1060–1066

Pectasides D, Pectasides E, Kassanos D (2008) Germ cell tumors of the ovary. Cancer Treat Rev 34:427–441

Pennington KP, Walsh T, Harrell MI et al (2014) Germline and somatic mutations in homologous recombination genes predict platinum response and survival in ovarian, fallopian tube, and peritoneal carcinomas. Clin Cancer Res 20:764–775

Perren TJ, Swart AM, Pfisterer J et al (2011) A phase 3 trial of bevacizumab in ovarian cancer. N Engl J Med 365:2484–2496

Pfisterer J, Weber B, Reuss A et al (2006) Randomized phase III trial of topotecan following carboplatin and paclitaxel in first-line treatment of advanced ovarian cancer: a gynecologic cancer intergroup trial of the AGO-OVAR and GINECO. J Natl Cancer Inst 98(15):1036–1045

Piccart MJ, Bertelsen K, James K et al (2000) Randomized intergroup trial of cisplatin–paclitaxel versus cisplatin–cyclophosphamide in women with advanced epithelial *ovarian cancer: three-year results*. JNCI 92(*9*):699–708. https://doi.org/10.1093/jnci/92.9.699

Pignata S, Scambia G, Ferrandina G et al (2011) Carboplatin plus paclitaxel versus carboplatin plus pegylated liposomal doxorubicin as first-line treatment for patients with ovarian cancer: the MITO-2 randomized phase III trial. J Clin Oncol 29(27):3628–3635

Pignata S, Scambia G, Katsaros D et al (2014) Carboplatin plus paclitaxel once a week versus every 3 weeks in patients with advanced ovarian cancer (MITO-7): a randomised, multicentre, open-label, phase 3 trial. Lancet Oncol 15(4):396–405

Pignata S, Lorusso D, Scambia G et al (2015) Pazopanib plus weekly paclitaxel versus weekly paclitaxel alone for platinum-resistant or platinum-refractory advanced ovarian cancer (MITO 11): a randomised, open-label, phase 2 trial. Lancet Oncol 16(5):561–568

Pignata S, Scambia G, Bologna A et al (2017) Randomized controlled trial testing the efficacy of platinum-free interval prolongation in advanced ovarian cancer: the MITO-8, MaNGO, BGOG-Ov1, AGO-Ovar2.16, ENGOT-Ov1, GCIG Study. J Clin Oncol 35(29):3347–3353

Pignata S, Lorusso D, Joly F et al (2018) Chemotherapy plus or minus bevacizumab for platinum-sensitive ovarian cancer patients recurring after a bevacizumab containing first line treatment: the randomized Phase 3 trial: MITO16B-MaNGO OV2B-ENGOT OV17. J Clin Oncol 36:5506. https://doi.org/10.1200/JCO.2018.36.15_suppl.5506)

Poveda AM, Selle F, Hilpert F et al (2015) Bevacizumab combined with weekly paclitaxel, pegylated liposomal doxorubicin, or topotecan in platinum-resistant recurrent ovarian cancer: analysis by chemotherapy cohort of the randomized Phase III AURELIA trial. J Clin Oncol 33 (32):3836–3838

Prakash R, Zhang Y, Feng W, Jasin M (2015) Homologous recombination and human health: the roles of BRCA1, BRCA2, and associated proteins. Cold Spring Harb Perspect Biol 7:016600. https://doi.org/10.1101/cshperspect.a016600

Prat J, FIGO Committee on Gynecologic Oncology (2014) Staging classification for cancer of the ovary, fallopian tube, and peritoneum. Int J Gynaecol Obstet 124(1):1–5. https://doi.org/10.1016/j.ijgo.2013.10.001

Prat J, D'Angelo E, Espinosa I (2018) Ovarian carcinomas: at least five different diseases with distinct histological features and molecular genetics. Hum Pathol:11–27

Pujade-Lauraine E, Wagner U, Aavall-Lundqvist E et al (2010) Pegylated liposomal Doxorubicin and Carboplatin compared with Paclitaxel and Carboplatin for patients with platinum-sensitive ovarian cancer in late relapse. J Clin Oncol 28(20):3323–3329

Pujade-Lauraine E, Hilpert F, Weber B et al (2014) Bevacizumab combined with chemotherapy for platinum-resistant recurrent ovarian cancer: the AURELIA open-label randomized phase III trial. J Clin Oncol 32:1302–1308. https://doi.org/10.1200/JCO.2013.51.4489

Pujade-Lauraine E, Ledermann JA, Selle F et al (2017) Olaparib tablets as maintenance therapy in patients with platinum-sensitive, relapsed ovarian cancer and a BRCA1/2 mutation (SOLO2/

ENGOT-Ov21): a double-blind, randomised, placebo-controlled, phase 3 trial. Lancet Oncol 18:1274–1284. https://doi.org/10.1016/S1470-2045(17)30469-2

Pujade-Lauraine E, Fujiwara K, Ledermann JA et al (2019) Avelumab alone or in combination with pegylated liposomal doxorubicin versus pegylated liposomal doxorubicin alone in platinum-resistant or refractory epithelial ovarian cancer: primary and biomarker analysis of the phase III JAVELIN Ovarian 200 trial. Gynecol Oncol 154:21–22

Querleu D, Planchamp F, Chiva L et al (2017) European Society of Gynaecological Oncology (ESGO) guidelines for ovarian cancer surgery. Int J Gynecol Cancer 27(7):1534–1542

Ray-Coquard I, Pautier P, Pignata S et al (2019) Olaparib plus bevacizumab as first-line maintenance in ovarian cancer. N Engl J Med 381:2416–2428

Ricci AD, Rizzo A, Novelli M et al (2020) Specific toxicity of maintenance olaparib versus placebo in advanced malignancies: a systematic review and meta-analysis. Anticancer Res 40:597–608. https://doi.org/10.21873/anticanres.13989

Roy R, Chun J, Powell SN (2012) BRCA1 and BRCA2: different roles in a common pathway of genome protection. Nat Rev Cancer 12:68–78. https://doi.org/10.1038/nrc3181

Rustin GJ, van der Burg ME, Griffin CL et al (2010) Early versus delayed treatment of relapsed ovarian cancer (MRC OV05/EORTC 55955): a randomised trial. Lancet 376(9747):1155–1163

Ryan NAJ, Evans DG, Green K, Crosbie EJ (2017) Pathological features and clinical behavior of Lynch syndrome-associated ovarian cancer. GynecolOncol 144(3):491–495. https://doi.org/10.1016/j.ygyno.2017.01.005

Schreiber V, Dantzer F, Ame JC, de Murcia G (2006) Poly(ADP-ribose): novel functions for an old molecule. Nat Rev Mol Cell Biol 7:517–528

Shen J, Ju Z, Zhao W et al (2018) ARID1A deficiency promotes mutability and potentiates therapeutic antitumor immunity unleashed by immune checkpoint blockade. Nat Med 24 (5):556–562. https://doi.org/10.1038/s41591-018-0012-z

Shimada M, Kigawa J, Ohishi Y et al (2009) Clinicopathological characteristics of mucinous adenocarcinoma of the ovary. Gynecol Oncol 113(3):331–334

Shoji T, Komiyama S, Kigawa J et al (2018) An open-label, randomized, phase II trial evaluating the efficacy and safety of standard of care with or without bevacizumab in platinum-resistant epithelial ovarian, fallopian tube, or primary peritoneal cancer patients previously treated with bevacizumab for front-line or platinum-sensitive ovarian cancer: rationale, design, and methods of the Japanese Gynecologic Oncology Group Study JGOG3023. BMC Cancer 18:771

Sidaway P (2020) MSI-H: a truly agnostic biomarker? Nat Rev Clin Oncol 17:68

Singer G, Shih IM, Truskinovsky A et al (2003a) Mutational analysis of K-ras segregates ovarian serous carcinomas into two types: invasive MPSC (low-grade tumor) and conventional serous carcinoma (high grade tumor). Int J Gynecol Pathol 22(1):37–41

Singer G, Oldt R III, Cohen Y et al (2003b) Mutations in BRAF and KRAS characterize the development of low-grade ovarian serous carcinoma. J Natl Cancer Inst 95(6):484–486

Slomovitz B, Gourley C, Carey MS et al (2020) Low-grade serous ovarian cancer: state of the science. Gynecol Oncol 156(3):715–725. https://doi.org/10.1016/j.ygyno.2019.12.033

Storey DJ, Rush R, Stewart M et al (2008) Endometrioid epithelial ovarian cancer: 20 years of prospectively collected data from a single center. Cancer 112(10):2211–2220. https://doi.org/10.1002/cncr.23438

Strickland KC, Howitt BE, Shukla SA et al (2016) Association and prognostic significance of BRCA1/2-mutation status with neoantigen load, number of tumor-infiltrating lymphocytes and expression of PD-1/PD-L1 in high grade serous ovarian cancer. Oncotarget 7(12):13587–13598

Stuart GC, Kitchener H, Bacon M et al (2011) 2010 Gynecologic Cancer InterGroup (GCIG) consensus statement on clinical trials in ovarian cancer: report from the Fourth Ovarian Cancer Consensus Conference. Int J Gynecol Cancer 21(4):750–755

Tang M, O'Connell RL, Amant F et al (2019) PARAGON: a phase II study of anastrozole in patients with estrogen receptor-positive recurrent/metastatic low-grade ovarian cancers and serous borderline tumors. Gynecol Oncol 154:531–538

TCGA (2011) Integrated genomic analyses of ovarian carcinoma. Nature 474:609–615

Telli ML, Timms KM, Reid J et al (2016) Homologous recombination deficiency (HRD) score predicts response to platinum-containing neoadjuvant chemotherapy in patients with triple-negative breast cancer. Clin Cancer Res 22:3764–3773

Toss A, Tomasello C, Razzaboni E et al (2015) Hereditary ovarian cancer: not only BRCA 1 and 2 genes. Biomed Res Int 2015:341723. https://doi.org/10.1155/2015/341723

Trimbos JB (2000) Staging of early ovarian cancer and the impact of lymph node sampling. Int J Gynecol Cancer 10(S1):8–11

Trimbos JB, Parmar M, Vergote I et al (2003) International Collaborative Ovarian Neoplasm trial 1 and Adjuvant ChemoTherapy in Ovarian Neoplasm trial: two parallel randomized phase III trials of adjuvant chemotherapy in patients with early-stage ovarian carcinoma. J Natl Cancer Inst 95(2):105–112

Trimbos JB, Timmers P, Pecorelli S et al (2010) Surgical staging and treatment of early ovarian cancer: long-term analysis from a randomized trial. J Natl Cancer Inst 102(13):982–987. https://doi.org/10.1093/jnci/djq149

United States of America Food and Drug Administration (FDA) (2018) Bevacizumab data sheet. Accessed at: https://www.accessdata.fda.gov/drugsatfda_docs/label/2018/125085s323lbl.pdf. Accessed 4 sept 2020

United States of America Food and Drug Administration (FDA) (2020a) FDA approves niraparib for first-line maintenance of advanced ovarian cancer. https://www.fda.gov/drugs/drug-approvals-and-databases/fda-approves-niraparib-first-line-maintenance-advanced-ovarian-cancer. Accessed 4 Sept 2020

United States of America Food and Drug Administration (FDA) (2020b) FDA approves olaparib plus bevacizumab as maintenance treatment for ovarian, fallopian tube, or primary peritoneal cancers. https://www.fda.gov/drugs/drug-approvals-and-databases/fda-approves-olaparib-plus-bevacizumab-maintenance-treatment-ovarian-fallopian-tube-or-primary. Accessed 30 July 2020

Varga A, Piha-Paul S, Ott PA et al (2019) Pembrolizumab in patients with programmed death ligand 1-positive advanced ovarian cancer: analysis of KEYNOTE-028. Gynecol Oncol 152 (2):243–250

Vasey PA, Jayson GC, Gordon A et al (2004) Phase III randomized trial of docetaxel-carboplatin versus paclitaxel-carboplatin as first-line chemotherapy for ovarian carcinoma. J Natl Cancer Inst 96(22):1682–1691

Vergote I, De Brabanter J, Fyles A et al (2001) Prognostic importance of degree of differentiation and cyst rupture in stage I invasive epithelial ovarian carcinoma. Lancet 357(9251):176–182

Vergote I, Coens C, Nankivell M, EORTC; MRC CHORUS study investigators et al (2018) Neoadjuvant chemotherapy versus debulking surgery in advanced tubo-ovarian cancers: pooled analysis of individual patient data from the EORTC 55971 and CHORUS trials. Lancet Oncol 19(12):1680–1687

Vergote I, du Bois A, Floquet A et al (2019) Overall survival results of AGO-OVAR16: a phase 3 study of maintenance pazopanib versus placebo in women who have not progressed after first-line chemotherapy for advanced ovarian cancer. Gynecol Oncol 155(2):186–191. https://doi.org/10.1016/j.ygyno.2019.08.024

Vineyard MA, Daniels MS, Urbauer DL et al (2011) Is low-grade serous ovarian cancer part of the tumor spectrum of Hereditary Breast and Ovarian Cancer? Gynecol Oncol 120(2):229–232

Wagner U, Marth C, Largillier R et al (2012) Final overall survival results of phase III GCIG CALYPSO trial of pegylated liposomal doxorubicin and carboplatin vs paclitaxel and carboplatin in platinum-sensitive ovarian cancer patients. Br J Cancer 107(4):588–591

Walker JL, Brady MF, Wenzel L et al (2019) Randomized trial of intravenous versus intraperitoneal chemotherapy plus bevacizumab in advanced ovarian carcinoma: an NRG oncology/gynecologic oncology group study. J Clin Oncol 37(16):1380–1390

Walsh CS (2015) Two decades beyond BRCA1/2: homologous recombination, hereditary cancer risk and a target for ovarian cancer therapy. Gynecol Oncol 137(2):343–350. https://doi.org/10.1016/j.ygyno.2015.02.017

Wong KK, Lu KH, Malpica A et al (2007) Significantly greater expression of ER, PR, and ECAD in advanced-stage low-grade ovarian serous carcinoma as revealed by immunohistochemical analysis. Int J Gynecol Pathol 26(4):404–409

Yates MS, Meyer LA, Deavers MT et al (2011) Microscopic and early-stage ovarian cancers in brca1/2 mutation carriers: Building a model for early BRCA-associated tumorigenesis. Cancer Prev Res 4(3):463–470

Zhang L, Conejo-Garcia JR, Katsaros D et al (2003) Intratumoral T cells, recurrence, and survival in epithelial ovarian cancer. N Engl J Med 348(3):203–213

Zhang Y, Luo G, Li M (2019) Global patterns and trends in ovarian cancer incidence: age, period and birth cohort analysis. BMC Cancer 19:984. https://doi.org/10.1186/s12885-019-6139-6

Zhao Y, Adjei AA (2014) The clinical development of MEK inhibitors. Nat Rev Clin Oncol 11 (7):385–400. https://doi.org/10.1038/nrclinonc.2014.83

3 The Hallmarks of Ovarian Cancer: Actionable Genetics, Targetable Pathways, and Predictive Biomarkers

Khalid El Bairi, Ouissam Al Jarroudi, and Said Afqir

Abstract

The development of the conceptual cancer hallmarks has deeply changed our understanding of cancer initiation, progression, and metastasis. Moreover, this pivotal effort is a milestone that provided the scientific rationale for developing new cancer biomarkers and anticancer drugs. In ovarian cancer (OC), the ten cancer hallmarks described by *Hanahan and Weinberg* were investigated in translational studies for prognostic and predictive biomarker discovery. In addition, several interventional clinical trials used these principles to explore the clinical efficacy of several chemotherapeutic and targeted agents such as antiangiogenics and PARP inhibitors. Promisingly, survival outcomes in women with OC were improved with the arrival of novel single agents and combinatorial approaches. In this chapter, the clinical impact of genetics, biomarkers, and therapy in OC is reviewed based on the hallmarks of cancer. We particularly present a special emphasis on druggable targets investigated in phase II/III clinical trials for OC.

Keywords

Ovarian cancer · Hallmarks · Genetics · Therapy · Biomarkers · Outcomes

K. El Bairi (✉) · O. Al Jarroudi · S. Afqir
Department of Medical Oncology, Mohammed VI University Hospital, Oujda, Morocco

Faculty of Medicine and Pharmacy, Mohammed Ist University, Oujda, Morocco
e-mail: k.elbairi@ump.ac.ma

K. El Bairi (ed.), *Ovarian Cancer Biomarkers*,
https://doi.org/10.1007/978-981-16-1873-4_3

3.1 Introduction

With the advent of next-generation sequencing platforms, emerging ovarian cancer (OC) genomic data illustrated important druggable pathways that enabled the successful development of various novel anticancer molecules such as PARP inhibitors (PARPi) and antiangiogenics. Until this time, the dualistic origins and pathogenesis of OC are still debated because of the changing evidence reported in the literature every year (Klotz and Wimberger 2017; Soong et al. 2018). OC is widely regarded as a genetic disease in which the accumulation of mutations is a key driver of its pathogenesis. Targetable genetic alterations reported in OC (Petrillo et al. 2016) might be classified according to the next-generation hallmarks of cancer as previously defined by Hanahan and Weinberg's influential manuscripts (Hanahan and Weinberg 2000, 2011; De Palma and Hanahan 2012; Hanahan and Coussens 2012; Lambert et al. 2017). These hallmarks are defined as "*acquired functional capabilities that allow cancer cells to survive, proliferate, and disseminate; these functions are acquired in different tumor types via distinct mechanisms and at various times during the course of multistep tumorigenesis*" (Hanahan and Weinberg 2011). In this perspective, the present chapter will be discussed according to this promising model. Moreover, a special and central spotlight will be given to the translation of these alterations in cancer drug discovery and biomarkers development based on recent observational and interventional human trials.

3.2 Actionable Hallmarks of Ovarian Cancer

3.2.1 Synthetic Lethality Beyond Genomic Instability

DNA damages and subsequent alterations in cell repair mechanisms are the principal causes that favor tumorigenesis. These are notable results of tumor mutational instability enabling proliferative properties to cancer cells. Genomic instability is the most studied cancer hallmark until today. Repair pathways of DNA damages are complex and encompass several genes of the family of homologous recombination repair (HRR), non-homologous end-joining, and single-strand annealing (De Picciotto et al. 2016). In OC, BReast CAncer (*BRCA*), RAD51 recombinase (*RAD51*), and partner and localizer of BRCA2 (*PALB2*) orchestrate HRR and are found mutated particularly in patients with high-grade serous histology (Lord and Ashworth 2012). Mutations in these tumor suppressor genes drive genomic instability which is a well-known characteristic that predicts outcomes in several cancers including OC. Remarkably, mutations in these genes—namely pathogenic actionable *BRCA1* and *BRCA2* variants—render women with OC particularly sensitive to chemotherapy (see Chaps. 4 and 7) and also PARPi (Le Page et al. 2020), a recently emerged concept known as synthetic lethality. Of note, synthetic lethality induced by PARPi followed by senolytic agents has proven to be synergistic preclinically and therefore, combinatorial approaches using this approach seem to be promising (Topatana et al. 2020). Furthermore, a durable response to immune-checkpoint blockade can be achieved based on genomics. OC patients with HRR deficiency have a notable infiltration of immune infiltrates which correlate with greater improvement in overall survival (OS) (Keenan et al. 2019; Morse et al. 2019).

The development of PARPi based on this hallmark is a milestone in OC therapy. Various PARPi were approved worldwide for treating OC as a treatment and/or maintenance therapy based on landmark studies (Mirza et al. 2020). PARPi were initially investigated in three randomized phase III trials (NOVA, SOLO-2, and ARIEL-3) as maintenance treatment for patients with recurrent OC after platinum-based chemotherapy (Mirza et al. 2018). NOVA was a double-blind phase III trial that randomized OC patients with platinum-sensitive and recurrent disease to receive niraparib as monotherapy or placebo in a 2:1 fashion with progression-free survival (PFS) as a primary endpoint (Mirza et al. 2016). In this trial, 553 women were enrolled including 203 participants with germline mutated *BRCA* and other 350 participants with non-mutated *BRCA*. Median PFS in niraparib arm was significantly longer as compared to the placebo group ($p < 0.001$) with a manageable bone-marrow toxicity profile by dose reduction. In the germline mutated *BRCA* cohort, women treated with niraparib had 21 months of PFS as compared to 5.5 months in those treated with placebo (HR: 0.27; 95% CI: 0.17–0.41). Furthermore, patients with HRR deficiency (HRD) beyond *BRCA* also benefited from niraparib treatment within an increase of median duration of PFS by 9 months (HR: 0.38; 95% CI: 0.24–0.59) (Mirza et al. 2016). Following these promising findings for niraparib which is the only PARPi approved as maintenance therapy regardless of *BRCA* status, olaparib, another PARPi given as tablets was investigated in the SOLO-2/ENGOT-Ov21 phase III trial (Pujade-Lauraine et al. 2017). This study was a randomized, placebo-controlled and enrolled 295 platinum-sensitive and recurrent OC with *BRCA1* or *BRCA2* mutations to receive olaparib or placebo (2:1 ratio). Median PFS was significantly longer in the arm treated with olaparib than the placebo arm (19.1 vs 5.5 months, HR: 0.30, CI: 0.22–0.41, $p < 0.0001$) (Pujade-Lauraine et al. 2017). Long-term benefit from this oral therapy as a maintenance therapy for relapsed OC was markedly noticed as demonstrated by the latest updated OS data presented at ASCO20 virtual meeting (Poveda et al. 2020). Final OS in this trial showed that maintenance olaparib provided an improved median OS of 12.9 months as compared to placebo after a median follow-up of 65 months (Poveda et al. 2020). Rucaparib was studied in the randomized and placebo-controlled ARIEL-3 phase III trial ($n = 564$, 2:1 ratio) as a maintenance therapy for patients with recurrent platinum-sensitive who had received two regimens of platinum-based chemotherapy (Coleman et al. 2017a, b). Patients with mutated *BRCA* OC had superior median PFS (22.9 vs 5.4 months; HR: 0.23, 95% CI: 0.16–0.34, $p < 0.0001$). In addition, patients with HRD carcinoma also benefited from recuparib (13.6 vs 5.4 months; HR: 0.32, 0.24–0.42, $p < 0.0001$). With a hazard ratio of 0.36, clinically meaningful benefits of recuparib was also noticed in the intention-to-treat population ($p < 0.0001$) (Coleman et al. 2017a, b).

In the recurrent setting, ARIEL-2 was an open-label multicenter phase II trial that investigated rucaparib in 206 women with recurrent and platinum-sensitive high-grade serous OC (Swisher et al. 2017). The median PFS of patients in the *BRCA* mutant cohort after treatment with rucaparib was 12.8 months. In the other cohorts, median PFS was 5.7 months and 5.2 months in patients with high and low loss of heterozygosity, respectively (Swisher et al. 2017). QUADRA is another phase II trial ($n = 463$) that was planned to investigate the clinical efficacy of niraparib as a single agent in the fourth or later line of treating recurrent OC (Moore et al. 2019a). Enrolled heavily pretreated patients were mainly resistant or refractory to platinum-based chemotherapy ($n = 151$ and $n = 161$, respectively). Median follow-up for OS exceeds 1 year with a manageable hematological toxicity profile, as expected (Moore et al. 2019a). More recently, SOLO-3 randomized FDA-mandated confirmatory phase III was designed to look at response rates for PARP inhibitor olaparib versus one of the non-platinum drugs used in this setting including pegylated liposomal doxorubicin, paclitaxel, gemcitabine, or topotecan (Penson et al. 2020). This study randomly assigned 266 recurrent OC patients with platinum-sensitive disease and *BRCA* mutant tumors to receive olaparib or single non-platinum chemotherapy and the objective response rate (ORR) was its primary endpoint. ORR in this population was significantly higher (72.2%) compared to chemotherapy (51.4%). In heavily pretreated women who had received at least two prior lines of chemotherapy, ORR was also superior in the olaparib arm (84.6% vs 61.5%). Median PFS also favored olaparib, which resulted in significantly improved outcomes (HR: 0.62; $p = 0.013$; 13.4 vs 9.2 months) (Penson et al. 2020). However, as mentioned above, this phase III compared a PARPi versus non-platinum drugs in a platinum-sensitive setting without a control using platinum-based chemotherapy. Therefore, this strategy should be reserved for OC patients who are not candidates for platinum-based chemotherapy.

Four randomized phase III clinical trials using PARPi have been conducted for newly diagnosed OC in the first-line setting (SOLO-1, PAOLA-1, PRIMA, and VELIA) (for review, see: Franzese et al. 2020; Mirza et al. 2020; Lee and Matulonis 2020). These trials were all in the front-line setting and had PFS as the primary endpoint but with differences in terms of the composition of their control arms, the timing of the use of PARP inhibition, and platinum-resistance status (Mirza et al. 2020). SOLO-1 was a double-blind phase III trial that randomly allocated patients with newly diagnosed OC and *BRCA* mutant tumors to receive olaparib as a maintenance treatment or placebo in a 2:1 fashion after clinical response platinum-based chemotherapy (Moore et al. 2018c). After a median follow-up of 41 months of the 391 enrolled participants, a reduction of risk of disease progression or death by 70% was noticed in the olaparib arm as compared to placebo (HR: 0.30; 95% CI: 0.23–0.41; $p < 0.001$) (Moore et al. 2018c). Of note, this study excluded all patients without *BRCA* mutant tumors and also not permitted a prior exposure to bevacizumab. Niraparib was studied as monotherapy for maintenance after response to first-line chemotherapy in the randomized and placebo-controlled PRIMA phase III trial ($n = 733$) (González-Martín et al. 2019). Half of the enrolled participants had homologous recombination deficient tumors in which PFS was statistically and clinically meaningful as compared to the placebo arm (21.9 vs 10.4 months; HR: 0.43; 95% CI: 0.31–0.59; $p < 0.001$). Moreover, PFS in the intention-to-treat population was also improved (13.8 vs 8.2 months; HR: 0.62; 95% CI: 0.50–0.76;

$p < 0.001$) (González-Martín et al. 2019). The efficacy of veliparib in the first-line induction treatment was assessed in the VELIA study (Coleman et al. 2019). 1140 patients with previously untreated OC received carboplatin and paclitaxel in combination with veliparib followed by veliparib for maintenance or without veliparib as maintenance in the experimental arm and the standard of care plus placebo and placebo maintenance in the control arm (1:1:1 ratio). Median PFS in *BRCA*-mutated women was significantly superior to the control group and achieved 34.7 vs 22 months (HR: 0.44; 95% CI: 0.28–0.68; $p < 0.001$). Notably, the population of patients with homologous recombination deficiency also benefited from veliparib (HR: 0.68; 95% CI: 0.56–0.83; $p < 0.001$). The findings of this study suggest that first-line induction therapy using carboplatin, paclitaxel, and veliparib followed by veliparib maintenance is superior in terms of PFS as compared to the classical doublet protocol alone (Coleman et al. 2019). PAOLA-1 examined the clinical benefits of adding olaparib to bevacizumab in the first-line maintenance after response to chemotherapy plus bevacizumab in OC patients *BRCA* mutation status (Ray-Coquard et al. 2019). 806 eligible patients received either olaparib or placebo in a randomized fashion (2:1). Median PFS was increased with the use of olaparib in combination with bevacizumab as compared to bevacizumab and placebo (HR: 0.59; 95% CI: 0.49–0.72; $p < 0.001$). The hazard ratio for progression or death in women with positive tumors for homologous recombination deficiency (including *BRCA*) treated with olaparib was 0.33 suggesting a substantial benefit from this combination (Ray-Coquard et al. 2019). Currently, this doublet is considered as the standard of care for first-line maintenance regardless of *BRCA* and HRR deficiency.

Building on this, these landmark studies were successful in providing evidence supporting the use of PARPi in various OC treatment settings. This is further supported by recent multiple meta-analyses of randomized and controlled trials discussed in this section (Tomao et al. 2019; Ruscito et al. 2020; Lin et al. 2021; Hao et al. 2021). Future head-to-head comparisons of PARPi and combinatorial approaches with other anticancer drugs including antiangiogenics and immune-checkpoint blockers will be promising to improve OC care (Veneris et al. 2020) and are a research priority. Moreover, synthetic lethality appears to play a principal role in selecting patients to benefit from the development of PARPi. Knowledge on HRR including *BRCA* mutations seems to be important in conferring sensitivity to these agents. The accuracy of currently available genetic testing procedures needs to be improved in the future. More details on this hallmark can be found in the other chapters of this book.

3.2.2 Tumor Promoting Inflammation

It is well established that inflammation substantially contributes to the supply of protumoral state as well as in the progression of malignancies (Diakos et al. 2014; Taniguchi and Karin 2018). During cancer progression and metastasis, a large number of tumor cells undergo necrotic cell death which drives the recruitment of immune inflammatory cells that can actively promote cancer invasiveness by acting on angiogenesis and cell proliferation mechanisms (Hanahan and Weinberg 2011). In the ovaries, several events that majorly delay inflammation such as parity (Fortner et al. 2018), oral contraceptives use (Collaborative Group on Epidemiological Studies of Ovarian Cancer 2008; Cibula et al. 2011; Havrilesky et al. 2013), and non-steroidal anti-inflammatory drugs are associated with a reduced risk of OC (Trabert et al. 2018) and improved outcomes in OC patients (Verdoodt et al. 2018). On the other hand, events causing inflammation such as endometriosis have been suggested to increase OC risk (Pearce et al. 2012; Wendel et al. 2018). The link between cancer and inflammation has been investigated in both epidemiological and experimental studies and it was subsequently confirmed through anti-inflammatory therapies that were relatively effective in chemopreventive approaches as suggested by numerous recent meta-analyses (Qiao et al. 2018; Zhang et al. 2016a; Wang et al. 2015; Huang et al. 2014a). Inflammation can damage DNA by releasing reactive oxygen species (ROS) which may cause considerable structural and functional changes such as somatic mutations during the multistep carcinogenesis (Kawanishi et al. 2017). Oxidative stress has been linked to cancer initiation and progression by inducing genome instability through DNA damage or by its mutagenic effects (Aguilera and García-Muse 2013). High concentrations of ROS at the site of damage cause DNA DSBs, mutations in tumor suppressor genes and proto-oncogenes which promote carcinogenesis (Kruk and Aboul-Enein 2017; Kawanishi et al. 2017). Interestingly, various molecular changes associated with repeated hemorrhage-associated oxidative stress during carcinogenesis of high-grade serous OC may explain some pieces of the puzzle (Kobayashi et al. 2017). Retrograde menstruations were proposed as a possible driver of high-grade serous OC by accumulation of genetic alterations in some key genes such as *CCNE1* (Kroeger and Drapkin 2016), *EZH2* (Li and Zhang 2013), *ALDH1A1* (Chui et al. 2014), and *PAX2* (Song et al. 2013) that have key roles in tissue differentiation and carcinogenesis (reviewed by Kobayashi et al. 2017). In addition, fimbrial cells of the fallopian tube may also be a target of ROS (Kobayashi et al. 2017) and are currently considered as a possible origin of high-grade serous OC (Karnezis et al. 2017). Mature ovarian follicles and their fluids (a rich source of ROS) during ovulation were also recently emerged as another probable inflammatory factor that may affect ovarian malignant transformation by causing DNA double-strand breaks and upregulation of inflammatory pathways (Bahar-Shany et al. 2014; Huang et al. 2015). Moreover, cyclooxygenase 2 (COX-2) was found to be highly expressed in OC and correlated with tumor grade (Zhang et al. 2019a). Moreover, COX-2 seems to enhance the capability of cancer cells for proliferation and invasiveness and also confers cisplatin-resistance (Zhang et al. 2019a; Deng et al. 2020). In animal studies, COX-2 inhibition by celecoxib was found to reduce the invasion and growth of OC cells (Li et al. 2012; Wang et al. 2018). This concept was introduced into interventional clinical trials for OC with two published randomized phase II studies using the COX-2 inhibitor celecoxib in combination with carboplatin. Heavily pretreated OC patients were enrolled in a single-arm phase II study to evaluate the clinical activity of oral celecoxib combined with carboplatin (NCT01124435) (Legge et al. 2011). ORR was 28.9% including three complete and ten partial responses with median PFS and OS of 5 and

13 months, respectively, and a well-tolerated toxicity profile (Legge et al. 2011). DoCaCel study was another randomized phase II clinical trial that investigated celecoxib as a combination with docetaxel and carboplatin compared to up-front chemotherapy alone in the first-line setting for stage IC to IV OC (Reyners et al. 2012). After a median follow-up of 32.2 months, median PFS and OS were similar in both arms (14.3 and 34 months respectively). However, no conclusions can be drawn as most patients discontinued celecoxib earlier because of skin reactions (Reyners et al. 2012). Recently, celecoxib was given with metronomic chemotherapy using oral cyclophosphamide for patients with recurrent epithelial OC (Gupta et al. 2019). No difference in terms of medial OS was noticed between the combination group compared to cyclophosphamide alone ($p = 0.95$) (Gupta et al. 2019). Celecoxib is currently investigated in combination with chemotherapy in other ongoing clinical trials for OC (NCT02432378, NCT00538031). Moreover, acetylsalicylic acid (aspirin), another COX-2 inhibitor is being explored for preventing venous thromboembolism among women with OC receiving neoadjuvant chemotherapy (NCT04352439). Aspirin is also used in a randomized phase II study of atezolizumab, bevacizumab, and aspirin for recurrent platinum-resistant OC in the ongoing EORTC-1508 ($n = 122$) (NCT02659384).

3.2.3 Sustaining Proliferative Signaling

3.2.3.1 PI3K/AKT/mTOR Pathway

Phosphoinositol 3-kinase (PI3K)/protein kinase B (AKT)/mammalian target of rapamycin (mTOR) signaling pathway is implicated in various required cell functions such as cell growth, vesicle trafficking, metabolism control, survival, mobility, and angiogenesis and is triggered by cell surface tyrosine kinase receptors (RTKs) (Bilanges et al. 2019; Li et al. 2014; Ghigo et al. 2012). This central signaling axis involves PI3K, the major downstream transducer RTKs, and allows activation of AKT by phosphorylation, which in turn activates downstream effector serine/threonine-protein kinase mTOR. PI3K is composed of eight isoforms divided into class I, class II, and class III PI3Ks that generate lipid messengers involved in signal transduction of intracellular trafficking (Vanhaesebroeck et al. 2010). Oncogenic *PIK3CA* is one of the most commonly mutated genes in human cancers and encodes for enzymatic PI3K protein activated by extracellular signals essentially growth factors (Fruman and Rommel 2014). The negative regulation of PI3K signaling is mainly driven by phosphatase and tensin homolog (*PTEN*) and inositol polyphosphate 4-phosphatase type II (*INPP4B*) tumor suppressor genes (LoRusso 2016). Notably, Loss of *PTEN* or *INPP4B* leads to prolonged activation of AKT which directly activates mTOR complex (mTORC) by phosphorylation. Therefore, this leads to activation of eukaryote translation initiation factor 4E binding protein-1 (4EBP-1) and ribosomal S6 kinase-1 (S6K-1) with protein synthesis as a result which is required for cell-cycle progression and growth (Laplante and Sabatini 2012; Mabuchi et al. 2015).

Upregulation of PI3K/AKT/mTOR pathway can occur as a result of overactivation, modifications in the downstream targets of PI3K and mutations in their regulatory and/or catalytic domains (Mabuchi et al. 2015). Notably, PI3K/AKT/mTOR axis plays a central function in the proliferation and progression of OC (Petrillo et al. 2016; Aziz et al. 2018a). According to the TCGA study, genetic aberrations in PI3K pathway suggested that 45% of OC cases harbor this alteration (Cancer Genome Atlas Research Network 2011). These aberrations include incident mutations and amplifications in key oncogenes *PIK3CA* (12%, 46% in clear cell OC), *PIK3R1* (3.8%), *AKT1* (2%), *AKT2* (13.3%), and *mTOR* (1.9%) (reviewed by Mabuchi et al. 2015). Mutations in *PIK3CA* are frequent (51%) especially in ovarian clear cell carcinomas (a distinct and relatively rare histopathologic subtype of epithelial OC) as found by a recent study using whole-exome sequencing technology (Murakami et al. 2017). Not previously reported *PIK3R1* mutations (8%) in the same tumor histology were also found which suggest that integrated genomic profiling using NGS may be useful in understanding the molecular genetics of this aggressive subtype of OC (Murakami et al. 2017). Similarly, in another NGS report enrolling more clear cell OC patients ($n = 48$), *PIK3CA* mutations were found in 50% of cases (Shibuya et al. 2018). Importantly, *PIK3CA* missense mutations were found significantly associated with improved OS in OC patients with clear cell histology (Rahman et al. 2012). In addition, clear cell ovarian tumors with mutated *PIK3CA* are likely to have hyalinized/mucoid stroma which is a potential risk of paraneoplastic thromboembolism (Kato et al. 2018). Amplification of *PIK3CA* is also seen in recurrent OC suggesting maintained alteration of this pathway during progression and metastasis (Li et al. 2019a). Taken together this high mutation frequency of *PIK3CA* gene in clear cell OC, this signature is of great significance as a biomarker for diagnosis and prognosis and should be investigated in further studies. Alterations in tumor suppressor genes *PTEN* (protein loss or downregulation) and *INPP4B* have also been reported in OC and account for 77% (Martins et al. 2014) and 79% (protein loss) (Salmena et al. 2015), respectively. Importantly, *PTEN* loss was found as an early event in OC and it induces fallopian tube tumor initiation and invasion via a mechanism involving upregulation of *WNT4*, a key gene in cell migration (Russo et al. 2018). Moreover, INPP4B and PTEN loss were found significantly associated with worse outcomes in OC (Gewinner et al. 2009; Skírnisdóttir and Seidal 2011; Salmena et al. 2015; Patch et al. 2015), however, data from other reports were not in line with these findings (McCormick et al. 2016; Bakkar et al. 2015).

Notably, Cai et al. assessed the clinical significance of this pathway in OC based on a meta-analytic approach that included 20 eligible studies (PTEN: 11, PI3K: 5, AKT: 11) and 2499 patients with epithelial OC (Cai et al. 2014). High PI3K and protein AKT expressions were found associated with reduced OS (PI3K—HR: 1.44, 95% CI: 1.08–1.91; AKT—HR: 1.60, 95% CI: 1.26–2.04) (Cai et al. 2014). In terms of PFS, OC patients with high PI3K and protein AKT expressions were related to poor outcomes (PI3K—HR: 3.35, 95% CI: 1.14–9.82; AKT—HR: 1.65, 95% CI: 1.07–2.55) (Cai et al. 2014). Accordingly, the currently available evidence is insufficient to recommend these biomarkers as predictors of prognosis and additional updated meta-analyses and translational prospective studies are warranted.

Drugging the components of the PI3K/AKT/mTOR signaling cascade has been extensively investigated in various human clinical trials according to the U.S. National Library of Medicine database (http://www.clinicaltrials.gov). mTOR inhibition using temsirolimus alone or combined with other anticancer drugs tested in early dose-finding phase I trials showed manageable toxicity profile as well as some signals of clinical activities in gynecological cancers including OC (Temkin et al. 2010; Boers-Sonderen et al. 2014; Piha-Paul et al. 2014; Kyriakopoulos et al. 2016). Previously, Behbakht et al. conducted a phase II trial to study the efficacy of weekly intravenous temsirolimus in 60 patients with persistent and recurrent epithelial OC and other peritoneal carcinomas that have received at least 1–3 chemotherapy regimens (Behbakht et al. 2011). The modest activity was seen in this setting including 24.1% of patients that had a PFS $\geq$ 6 months and 9.3% with partial response (Behbakht et al. 2011). Moreover, Emons et al. enrolled women ($n = 22$) with platinum-refractory/resistant OC to receive weekly intravenous temsirolimus in a phase II trial (AGO-GYN8; NCT01460979) but unfortunately, it didn't meet its predefined efficacy endpoint (Emons et al. 2016). Recently, everolimus, an oral mTOR inhibitor, was combined in another phase II trial with the aromatase inhibitor letrozole in relapsed estrogen receptor-positive high-grade OC in both platinum-resistant and sensitive settings (Colon-Otero et al. 2017). Promisingly, this study enrolling 20 OC patients found a 47% 12-week PFS rate with this combination (median PFS: 3.9 months; 95% CI: 2.8–11.0 and median OS: 13 months) (Colon-Otero et al. 2017). More recently, Tew et al. randomized 150 OC patients in a phase II trial (GOG186-G; NCT00886691) with a recurrent or persistent disease to receive bevacizumab combined with oral everolimus versus bevacizumab alone (Tew et al. 2018). In this study, PFS was the primary endpoint and was not significantly improved in the everolimus arm compared to bevacizumab alone (5.9 vs 4.5 months, HR: 0.95; 95% CI: 0.66–1.37, $p = 0.39$) (Tew et al. 2018). Furthermore, similar findings were noted for median OS (16.6 vs 17.3 months, respectively, HR: 1.16; 95% CI: 0.72–1.87, $p = 0.55$) (Tew et al. 2018). Unfortunately, this combination associating mTOR inhibitor everolimus and bevacizumab demonstrated higher rates of serious adverse events ($\geq$ grade 3) including gastrointestinal perforation and it was not effective in this indication (Tew et al. 2018). Therefore, it is not recommended for further clinical exploration in patients with recurrent OC. Biological rationale and additional clinical data about mTOR inhibition in gynecologic cancers can be found in a recent review (Kassem and Abdel-Rahman 2016).

Preliminary evidence of targeting this pathway by inhibiting AKT has also shown some anticipation in developing new therapeutics for high-grade OC (Fu et al. 2012). Perifosine, a small-molecule AKT inhibitor developed by AEterna Zentaris, was previously tested in platinum and taxane resistant or refractory high-grade OC in combination with docetaxel and showed some signals of activity as well as a good tolerability profile in this phase I trial (Fu et al. 2012). Perifosine monotherapy was also tested in a phase II trial based on a basket design using *PIK3CA* mutational status for recurrent OC patients' stratification (Hasegawa et al. 2017). The modest activity was seen in OC patients with mutated *PIK3CA* including disease control rates (40%) compared with wild-type status (12.5%) (Hasegawa et al. 2017). Therapeutic advances regarding AKT axis blockade using small molecules and biologics are reviewed elsewhere (in general, by Mattmann et al. 2011 and in gynecologic malignancies, by Bregar and Growdon 2016). Antitumor activity of PI3K inhibition using the Genentech's pictilisib (GDC-0941) designed to be used orally was initially found to have some clinical signs of efficacy in patients with platinum-refractory OC exhibiting PTEN loss and *PIK3CA* amplification (Sarker et al. 2014). When combined with MEK1/2 inhibitor trametinib, PI3K inhibition by buparlisib (BKM120, Array BioPharma and Novartis) given daily has shown promising response in OC patients with mutated *KRAS* (Bedard et al. 2015). However, these positive results were invalidated by the serious toxicity profile found in this phase Ib (NCT01155453) trial including grade 3/4 adverse events (Bedard et al. 2015). Furthermore, combined inhibition of PI3K and PARP in vitro (Wang et al. 2016a) provided the first evidence of synergistic activity that was tested in a phase I trial (Matulonis et al. 2016). Remarkably, the association of PI3K inhibitor buparlisib with PARP inhibitor olaparib demonstrated clinical benefits in breast and OC subjects with both germline mutated and wild-type *BRCA* (Matulonis et al. 2016). Recently, the use of olaparib with the PI3K inhibitor alpelisib confirmed the synergistic effects of this combination (Konstantinopoulos et al. 2019). In this dose-escalation and dose-expansion phase Ib trial (NCT01623349), the authors observed preliminary clinical evidence of the efficacy of this association with 36% of patients having a partial response and 50% with stable disease, which merits further investigation in epithelial OC (Konstantinopoulos et al. 2019). To date, clinical data on this topic are not mature enough to conduct large randomized phase III trials. As a final point, until to date, most sequencing reports have provided discordant mutation frequencies in genes related to this pathway which makes developing targeted drugs difficult as they play an important role in drug resistance. Therapeutic interventions in this OC pathway showed some promise that should be evaluated in future clinical trials with potential predictive biomarkers for better patients' selection.

3.2.3.2 RAS Pathway

The RAS/RAF/MEK/ERK cascade is a receptor tyrosine kinase-dependent signaling axis that links intracellular gene expression pathways to extracellular stimuli (De Luca et al. 2012). It enhances key cellular activities including proliferation, survival, migration, cell-cycle regulation, and other cell functions by phosphorylation/dephosphorylation mechanisms. The dysfunction of this pathway by genetic alterations has been linked to several human malignancies including type I epithelial OC (Spreafico et al. 2017; Della Pepa et al. 2015) and contributes to the hallmarks of cancer by sustaining proliferative signaling. The canonical RAS/RAF/MEK/ERK cascade is initiated by signals such as binding ligands (growth factors, cytokines, etc.) to the corresponding receptor at the cell membrane level. The RAS family of proteins includes three important members, KRAS, NRAS, and HRAS which are located downstream of receptors. The downstream mediators RAF isoforms are protein kinases activated by the binding of small G proteins of the RAS family to their N-terminal region. Basically, activated RAS recruits and activates RAF which in turn phosphorylates MEK1/2 leading to ERK activation. Activated ERK1/2 has a wide variety of cytosolic and nuclear targets that induce inappropriate cell proliferation and metabolism, survival, and mobility (Papa et al. 2018; Liu et al. 2018). Deregulation of this pathway mainly by constitutive activation of RAS and RAF proteins has been well studied in most solid cancers (reviewed elsewhere: Khan et al. 2018).

Recent studies suggest that *KRAS* mutations are found in clear cell OC with a prevalence ranging from 13% to 16.7% (Shibuya et al. 2018; Zannoni et al. 2014, 2016). *KRAS* and *BRAF* mutations are rare in high-grade serous OC but are proposed to be an important driver of its cancer biology (Cancer Genome Atlas Research Network 2011). In low-grade serous OC, *BRAF* mutations are less common and represent 5% (Turashvili et al. 2018), which is contradictory with the previous data suggesting 33% prevalence (Singer et al. 2003). Based on targeted exome and whole-genome sequencing, Moujaber et al. find that 13.8% of low-grade serous OC patients had somatic mutations in the *BRAF* gene (Moujaber et al. 2018). However, this difference in mutation frequency may be due to the difference in the enrollment of patients with this relatively rare OC subtype as well as the variability of clinical stages of included samples. Moreover, low-grade serous OC is known for remarkable mutated *KRAS* (35%) (Singer et al. 2003). In summary, *KRAS* and *BRAF* mutations are more likely to be associated with low-grade serous and clear cell OC (Prat et al. 2018; DeFazio et al. 2016; Kaldawy et al. 2016; Russel and McCluggage 2004). Very few reports have investigated the prognostic value of these genetic alterations in OC. Earlier, Wong et al. found based on a cohort of 91 OC samples that low-grade serous tumors with mutant-*BRAF* and *KRAS* are likely to have improved clinical outcomes (Wong et al. 2010). In addition, patients with this chemoresistant disease harboring mutated *BRAF* had better OS as compared to patients with wild-type *KRAS* and *BRAF* status (Grisham et al. 2012). Recently, it was reported that low-grade serous OC patients with mutated *BRAF* or *KRAS* have significantly improved OS compared with wild-type patients (106.7 vs 66.8 months, respectively; $p = 0.018$) (Gershenson et al. 2015). Unexpectedly, these findings are conflicting with the recent results in the Chinese patients in which neither *KRAS* nor *BRAF* mutations were found to be prognostic biomarkers (Xu et al. 2017). In addition, mutated *KRAS* was found to predict chemosensitivity to anticancer drug decitabine (an FDA approved DNA methyltransferase inhibitor) (Stewart et al. 2015) but the real clinical impact of these two mutated signatures (*KRAS* and *BRAF*) is still inconclusive because of the small number of enrolled cases and therefore, should be replicated in larger cohorts.

The blockade of the components of this pathway by the recently developed inhibitors, trametinib (mekinist®, Novartis), dabrafenib (tafinlar®, GlaxoSmithKline), and vemurafenib (zelboraf®, Plexxikon and Hoffmann-La Roche) has demonstrated significant clinical benefits in various cancers such as advanced melanoma (Luther et al. 2019; Dhillon 2016) and lung cancer (Kelly 2018) especially when combined with other anticancer agents. In OC, preclinical findings indicating the efficacy of MEK inhibitors in cancer cell lines (Simpkins et al. 2018; Pétigny-Lechartier et al. 2017; Fernández et al. 2016, 2019; Gruosso et al. 2015; Cossa et al. 2014; Sheppard et al. 2013; Katagiri et al. 2010) have provided biological rationale of using MEK blockade in human clinical trials. In this perspective, selumetinib (AZD6244; Array BioPharma and AstraZeneca), a potent orally available small molecule that inhibits MEK1/2 enzymes, was recently granted orphan drug designation by the FDA for treating uveal melanoma, thyroid cancer, and neurofibromatosis (AdisInsight (Springer) website, https://adisinsight.springer.com/drugs/800019504, accessed 25/01/2019). It was investigated in OC in a single-arm phase II trial (NCT00551070) enrolling women with recurrent low-grade serous ovarian or peritoneal tumors (Farley et al. 2013). This pretreated population experienced a PFS of 11 months and 63% of patients had PFS > 6 months which merit further development of this drug in this chemoresistant OC (Farley et al. 2013). Interestingly, a dramatic response to selumetinib was seen in a patient with mutated *KRAS* recurrent low-grade serous OC who showed a durable response for more than 7 years (Takekuma et al. 2016). Selumetinib is being investigated by M.D. Anderson Cancer Center and AstraZeneca in a phase I trial (NCT03162627) combined with PARP inhibitor olaparib for patients with advanced endometrial, ovarian, and other solid malignancies with altered RAS pathway and is still recruiting (estimated study completion date: 2026). In addition, selumetinib combined with fulvestrant (Faslodex®), an estrogen receptor antagonist developed by AstraZeneca, showed potential for this association in reversing resistance in positive estrogen receptor OC (Hew et al. 2015) which illustrates a promising use in upcoming early human studies. MEK blockade by binimetinib (MEK162; Array BioPharma), another inhibitor of this pathway, has shown an interesting prolongation of response duration (31 months) in a woman with advanced/recurrent low-grade serous OC that was enrolled in the MILO phase III trial (NCT01849874) and having mutated *KRAS* (Han et al. 2018). Additionally, evidence of binimetinib activity in OC has been achieved in a phase Ib trial (NCT01649336) combining this drug with paclitaxel particularly in patients with known altered MEK pathway (Grisham et al. 2018). MILO phase III randomized and parallel-assignment clinical trial is currently being conducted to assess the efficacy of binimetinib as monotherapy versus best physician choice (paclitaxel, topotecan, or PLD) in women ($n = 360$, estimated) with recurrent or persistent low-grade serous OC in North America, Europe, and Australia (NCT01849874). MILO study completion date is estimated in September 2019. Trametinib is another potential oral inhibitor of MEK enzymes that have exhibited impressive response rates with dabrafenib combo in treating solid cancers especially unresectable or metastatic melanoma with *BRAF* $^{V600E/K}$ mutations (Long et al. 2017a, b; Abdel-Rahman et al. 2016). In OC, doublet PI3K/MEK inhibition using buparlisib in combination with trametinib has been studied in phase Ib trial (NCT01155453) and demonstrated promising clinical signals of activity (76% of disease control rate) in patients with mutated *KRAS* (Bedard et al. 2015). To date, only two case reports have reported dramatic response to trametinib combined with dabrafenib or metformin in selected patients with low grade and clear cell histology harboring *KRAS* and *BRAF* mutations and therefore, highlighting the need for clinical trials with predefined basket designs (Mendivil et al. 2018; Castro et al.

2015). This underscores the need for predictive biomarkers for this pathway blockade to identify OC patients who are most likely to derive durable clinical benefit. A phase III randomized trial (NCT02101788) is being conducted by the NCI (National Cancer Institute) that will enroll an estimated number of 260 recurrent or progressive low-grade OC patients with cross-over assignment. In this trial, PFS is the primary endpoint with intention-to-treat analysis and patients will be randomized to receive trametinib or clinician's choice (topotecan, paclitaxel, letrozole, tamoxifen, or PLD). Importantly, this trial will also assess various genetic testing by NGS for various genes related to this pathway such as KRAS in addition to circulating cell-free tumor DNA and their correlation with tumor response. Patient recruitment with this rare histological subtype is the major challenging barrier. Taken together, targeting this pathway in this subtype of OC is at the beginning and promising treatments are to come in the near future (for a detailed review in this topic, see: McLachlan et al. 2016a, b).

3.2.3.3 Cyclin E1

Cyclin 1 protein is encoded by the *CCNE1* gene and constitutes a core signaling that accelerates G1/S transition by binding cyclin-dependent kinases (CDK) (Kanska et al. 2016). Principally, CDK2 is the main partner of CCNE1 and plays a key role in various cell functions such as cell-cycle progression, DNA replication, transcription, and repair (Wood and Endicott 2018; Kanska et al. 2016). Interactions of CCNE1 and their associated CDK can provoke modifications in their ATP-binding pockets which enables access of target substrates. Briefly, CDK enzymes are activated by Cdc25 which in turn phosphorylates Cdc25 by positive feedback to generate active CDK/cyclins required for cell-cycle control (Kanska et al. 2016). Negative regulation of this signaling is ensured by cell-cycle inhibitors p21 and p27, key mediators of *TP53*-mediated damage response as well as TGF-β/SMAD pathway (reviewed in detail elsewhere: Kanska et al. 2016).

Increased oncogenic CCNE1/CDK2 kinase activity is involved in the mitogenic transformation of various cancers such as hepatocellular carcinoma (Bayard et al. 2018; Sonntag et al. 2018), lung cancer (Huang et al. 2012), breast cancer (Lundgren et al. 2015), endometrial and uterine cancers (Kuhn et al. 2014), and OC (Kuhn et al. 2016). *CCNE1* genetic deregulation by amplification is an early event in the genesis of fallopian tube-derived high-grade serous OCs (Karst et al. 2014; Kuhn et al. 2016). Genetically altered *CCNE1* is found in about 20% of OCs (Nakayama et al. 2010). Notably, OC patients with *CCNE1* amplifications tend to have poor survival (Nakayama et al. 2010; Cancer Genome Atlas Research Network 2011; Ayhan et al. 2017; Zhao et al. 2018) and are chemoresistant to standard chemotherapy (Patch et al. 2015; Etemadmoghadam et al. 2009). Recently, various reports have confirmed this association which supports the use of altered *CCNE1* as a prognosticator and predictive biomarker of treatment failure in OC management. In this perspective, an early study by Etemadmoghadam et al. found that *CCNE1* copy number gain is significantly associated with poor PFS and OS in a cohort of 43 advanced serous ovarian tumors (Etemadmoghadam et al. 2010). Similarly and based on primary tumors data, another study by the previous team showed that high-grade OC patients with amplified *CCNE1* showed short OS and their tumors were associated with polyploidy (Etemadmoghadam et al. 2013a), a substantial driver of chemotherapy resistance (Kuznetsova et al. 2015; Mittal et al. 2017). Moreover, this study has also demonstrated that cell polyploidy drives resistance to inhibition of CCNE1 partner CDK2 and therefore may be used to identify a subset of OC patients that are likely to benefit from anti-CDK agents under development (Etemadmoghadam et al. 2013a). Of note, polyploidy arises from genome doubling, early during cancer evolution and is highly common across various cancers with poor prognosis (Bielski et al. 2018). Likewise, another recent study suggests that tumors from high-grade serous OC patients ($n = 41$) with short survival are characterized by focal copy number gain of *CCNE1* in addition to wild-type *BRCA* status (Yang et al. 2018). In a relatively large cohort that enrolled 262 high-grade serous OC, amplified-*CCNE1* tumors were found associated with genome instability as well as poor clinical outcomes as compared with the non-amplified group (Aziz et al. 2018b). Unlike previously discussed reports and contrary to the expectations, Pils et al. demonstrated in a cohort of 172 serous epithelial OC tissues that amplified-*CCNE1* has no impact on clinical outcomes (Pils et al. 2014). Surprisingly, based on Cox model, high *CCNE1* gene expression was found to be significantly an independent predictive biomarker of prolonged OS in stage III/IV OC patients (Pils et al. 2014). One possible explanation is that ovarian tumors harboring *CCNE1* alterations may have other important genetic signatures that influence survival and therapy response and have to be considered as well because of the substantial heterogeneity within and between OC patients. More recently, co-amplification of *CCNE1* and *BRD4* (bromodomain and extraterminal 4) was found in OC patients with worse OS (Petersen et al. 2020). In addition, this report also confirmed the role of high protein expression of cyclin E in conferring platinum-resistance ($p = 0.016$) (Petersen et al. 2020). These discordant results came from small study cohorts which limit definitive answers to the prognostic and predictive value of this oncogene in OC. Hopefully, more conclusive data are awaited especially from randomized and controlled trials that are investigating *CCNE1* in OC as a biomarker for patients' stratification. Based on promising anticancer activity of bortezomib (a proteasome inhibitor) in *CCNE1*-amplified high-grade serous OC (Etemadmoghadam et al. 2013b), this amplification is being used as a predictor of response rate in a currently recruiting phase II trial (NCT03509246) that will evaluate the efficacy of bortezomib combined with PLD for platinum-resistant OC patients with wild-type *BRCA* status. In addition, two other phase I/II trials (NCT02797977; NCT02797964) conducted by Sierra Oncology, Inc. are recruiting patients with advanced cancers including OC and will investigate SRA737 agent (a checkpoint kinase 1 inhibitor) based on various genetic signatures including altered *CCNE1* and *BRCA* to predict sensitivity to this new anticancer drug.

Remarkable advances regarding pharmacological inhibition of the kinase components of this pathway were recently achieved especially in breast cancer with the promising results from phase III trials (NCT01958021, NCT01942135) testing inhibitors of cyclin-dependent kinases (CDK) 4/6 including palbociclib (Ibrance®, Pfizer) (Verma et al. 2016) and ribociclib (Kisqali®, Novartis)

(Hortobagyi et al. 2016). In OC, preclinical investigation of dinaciclib (MK-7965, Merck & Co), a CDK2 inhibitor, showed synergistic anticancer activity when combined with AKT inhibitors in CCNE1-amplified tumors (Au-Yeung et al. 2016). In addition, a combination of ribociclib and cisplatin followed by ribociclib maintenance demonstrated potential antitumor response in both in vitro and in vivo high-grade serous OC model (Iyengar et al. 2018). Currently, there is one phase I clinical trial (NCT02897375) recruiting patients with advanced cancers including OC and will assess the safety of palbociclib combined with cisplatin or carboplatin. Ribociclib is also being evaluated in OC in combination with immunotherapy (PDR001) and hormone therapy (fulvestrant) in a phase I trial (NCT03294694) as well as in another phase I trial (NCT03056833) in combination with paclitaxel/carboplatin and is still currently recruiting patients. Until this time, only one phase II trial (NCT03673124, $n = 51$) by the Gynecologic Oncology Group (GOG—http://www.gog.org) in collaboration with Pfizer is planned to evaluate the efficacy of palbociclib combined with letrozole in women with recurrent low-grade serous OC and it is estimated to provide first results in July 2021. Promisingly, these recent signs of progress in understanding this proliferative signaling have illuminated potential targets and biomarkers to guide drug selection and are currently used in developing novel targeted agents for OC.

3.2.3.4 EGFR Pathway

Historically, epidermal growth factor receptor (EGFR) and its related proteins including human epidermal receptor (HER2) have been extensively studied for more than three decades and their critical role in epithelial cell development and cancer has been elucidated since 1978 (for review see: Mitsudomi and Yatabe 2010; Arteaga and Engelman 2014). Moreover, family members of EGFR proteins are important targets of multiple anticancer drugs such as monoclonal antibodies and small-molecule tyrosine kinase inhibitors that were successfully developed for treating various epithelial cancers including gynecological cancers (Reyes et al. 2014). The interaction between the four EGFR family transmembrane protein receptors through homodimerization and heterodimerization, as a result of ligand binding and/or receptor mutations, directly affects downstream key cell signaling pathways by activating many genes responsible for tumor cell proliferation, survival, and invasion (Sigismund et al. 2017). Studies reporting overexpression of EGFR in epithelial OC suggest a range of 4–100% of cases (Teplinsky and Muggia 2015). Importantly, EGFR and HER protein (or gene) members, especially HER2, are suggested to have an impact on the prognosis of OC as demonstrated by recent studies (Despierre et al. 2015; Demir et al. 2014; Shang et al. 2017a) and an up-to-date meta-analysis (Luo et al. 2018). However, blockade of EGFR in randomized controlled trials (RCTs) comparing targeted anti-EGFR drugs with or without standard chemotherapy in epithelial OC patients as first-line or as maintenance has demonstrated a marginal gain in survival outcomes (Morrison et al. 2018).

3.2.3.5 Folate Receptor Pathway

Folate is a vitamin with fundamental roles in DNA synthesis and methylation, and also recombination repair (Rizzo et al. 2018). Cellular intake of folates is achieved throughout its contact with the reduced folate carrier transporter or by endocytosis facilitated by folate receptor alpha (FR-α) glycoprotein (Zhao et al. 2011). FR-α is encoded by the FOLR1 gene located on chromosome 11 (11q13.4). FR-α is a high affinity glycosylphosphatidylinositol membrane-anchored protein that binds and transports physiological levels of folate into cells (Rizzo et al. 2018). FR-α is suggested to affect chemoresistance via regulating the expression of apoptosis-related signaling proteins, Bcl-2 and Bax (Chen et al. 2012). A higher FR-α expression was found to be an important biomarker for prognosis and response to therapy in several aggressive solid cancers such as pancreatic ductal adenocarcinoma (Cai et al. 2017), triple-negative breast cancer (Ginter et al. 2017), and recurrent, platinum-resistant and refractory OC (Martin et al. 2017; Rubinsak et al. 2018). Furthermore, OC patients who express an increased level of FR-α have poor response to chemotherapy ($p = 0.021$) as well as poor disease-free interval (HR: 2.45; 95% CI: 1.16–5.18, $p = 0.02$) and OS (HR: 3.6; 95% CI: 0.93–13.29, $p = 0.03$) (Chen et al. 2012). Promisingly, recent studies provided rational therapeutic targeting of FR-α in OC as showed by several human clinical trials using monoclonal antibodies (Armstrong et al. 2013), vaccines (Kalli et al. 2018), and novel class antibody-drug conjugates (ADC) (Stewart and Cristea 2019). Recently, Armstrong et al. enrolled 54 OC patients with platinum-sensitive disease in phase II open-label trial comparing the anti-FR-α farletuzumab (MORAb-003) weekly as monotherapy versus in combination with standard carboplatin and taxanes (paclitaxel 175 mg/m^2 or docetaxel 75 mg/m^2) every 3 weeks (six cycles) followed by farletuzumab as maintenance (Armstrong et al. 2013). Notably, adding farletuzumab to carboplatin and taxanes improved the response rate and duration of response in this setting (Armstrong et al. 2013). Following these promising results, a phase III randomized and controlled trial (NCT00849667) was conducted to evaluate treatment with farletuzumab versus placebo in 1100 recurrent and sensitive OC but it didn't show any statistically significant difference between the arms (Vergote et al. 2016). Interestingly, attempts to develop immunity against FR-α in OC based on peptide vaccines were also investigated and showed motivating results (Kalli et al. 2018). In this perspective, a phase I trial (NCT01606241) that tested the safety of FR-α peptide vaccine and enrolled OC patients with no evidence of disease after completed standard therapy found that this strategy is well-tolerated and that FR-α T-cell immunogenic response was developed over the vaccination course which was observed and persisted for at least 12 months (Kalli et al. 2018). In addition, Yeku et al. assessed this strategy in a phase II trial (NCT02764333) using TPIV200 vaccine (Tapimmune Inc.), a polypeptide multi-epitope against FR-α, in combination with anti-PD-L1 durvalumab (Imfinzi®, AstraZeneca) for patients with platinum-resistant or refractory OC (Yeku et al. 2018). This promising combination with an immune-checkpoint inhibitor was found safe and opened a new era for OC vaccines. FR-α-based therapeutic targeting in OC has benefited from the innovative ADC as well (Moore et al. 2018a). Briefly, ADC are newly developed anticancer drugs and are based on engineered complexes composed of a monoclonal antibody directed against cancer cell antigens such as (FR-α and CD30), a biologically active cytotoxic drug and a linker (Moore et al. 2018a; Beck et al. 2017). This method enables a targeted delivery and cancer-killing ability with reduced toxicity by allowing discrimination between healthy and cancer tissues (Beck et al. 2017). There are currently various randomized and controlled trials investigating ADCs in human cancers such as brentuximab vedotin (Adcetris®, Seattle Genetics) and ado-trastuzumab emtansine (Kadcyla®, Genentech) as well as mirvetuximab soravtansine (IMGN853, ImmunoGen) for OC particularly for platinum-resistant patients. Mirvetuximab soravtansine is an ADC that binds to FR-α to deliver a powerful anti-microtubule (maytansinoid) drug into cancer cells (Moore et al. 2018a). Phase I dose-finding and safety trials demonstrated manageable toxicity (grade 1 or 2 fatigue, blurred vision, and diarrhea) and encouraging preliminary clinical activity in OC (Moore et al. 2017, 2018b). Recently, results of FORWARD II (expansion cohort, NCT02606305) phase Ib trial combining mirvetuximab soravtansine with immune-checkpoint inhibitor pembrolizumab (Keytruda®, Merck) were presented at ESMO 2018 meeting and showed potential signals of clinical activity in recurrent platinum-resistant setting (Matulonis et al. 2018). Promisingly, FORWARD I phase III multicenter trial conducted by ImmunoGen, Inc. in collaboration with Gynecologic Oncology Group is enrolling 333 women with platinum-resistant advanced OC in a randomized fashion (NCT02631876). This trial compared the efficacy of mirvetuximab soravtansine versus the investigator's choice of chemotherapy (paclitaxel, pegylated liposomal doxorubicin (PLD), or topotecan) in FR-α-positive patients and with PFS as a primary endpoint (study design reviewed by Moore et al. 2018a). Recently, the findings of this pivotal trial showed significant improvements in the arm treated with mirvetuximab soravtansine in terms of ORR (24% vs 10% in the controlled arm; $p = 0.014$) but without improved PFS in the intention to treat population (HR: 0.981; $p = 0.897$) (Moore et al. 2019b). The data on OS (as of August 2019) showed a benefice for this antibody-drug conjugate in patients selected based on high expression of FR-α (16.4 vs 12.0 months; HR: 0.678, $p = 0.048$) (Moore et al. 2019b). Two additional phase III trials (MIRASOL/NCT04209855, SORAYA/NCT04296890) with a large sample size for this setting are currently ongoing. Moreover, approaches using combinations such as mirvetuximab soravtansine and bevacizumab yielded promising findings for this difficult-to-treat population (O'Malley et al. 2020; Fowler 2020). Furthermore, academic clinical trials are also currently ongoing to study the early efficacy of mirvetuximab soravtansine in combination with PARP inhibitors and chemotherapy (NCT02996825/cohort C; NCT03552471).

In another effort for this setting, vintafolide (a folate-vinca (desacetylvinblastine hydrazide) conjugate; Endocyte®) that targets tumors with positive FR-α was tested in phase III trials (Ledermann et al. 2015; Assaraf et al. 2014). In this perspective, PRECEDENT is a phase II trial (NCT00722592) that has been conducted to randomize 149 women (intention to treat population) with platinum-resistant OC to receive intravenous vintafolide + PLD versus PLD alone (Naumann et al. 2013). Some marginal improvement in terms of PFS in the vintafolide arm was seen in this difficult to treat setting (5.0 vs 2.7 months, HR: 0.63; 95% CI: 0.41–0.96, $p = 0.031$) (Naumann et al. 2013). However, the interim analysis of the following PROCEED phase III trial (NCT01170650) didn't provide significantly improved outcomes with this treatment and therefore, the study was stopped to enroll more patients (Oza et al. 2015b). This strategy particularly using mirvetuximab soravtansine may represent a promising hope for targeting this pathway in platinum-resistant OC (for further reading, see: Bergamini et al. 2016; Scaranti et al. 2020; El Bairi et al. 2021). This hallmark of OC and particularly this drug target seem to have a promising future as a therapeutic strategy for this aggressive gynecological cancer.

3.2.4 Evading Growth Suppressors

3.2.4.1 TP53 Network

Mutated *TP53* events are still by far the most prevalent in cancer since the discovery of this tumor suppressor gene in 1979 (Soussi 2010). Every year, thousands of papers are published and provided notable novel findings regarding p35 functions, genetic variants as well as possible therapeutic interventions. There are more than 70,000 articles recorded on PubMed/Medline until today along with 140 clinical trials on the US ClinicalTrials.gov database (accessed 25 February 2019). Moreover, there is a rich source of data related to this gene and important databases were created for this purpose such as the IARC TP53 Database (http://p53.iarc.fr/) and The UMD TP53 Database (https://p53.fr/tp53-database) providing updated information for the scientific community working on this hot subject (for review, see: Leroy et al. 2014; Bouaoun et al. 2016). The *TP53* gene encodes for p53 protein with suppressive cell functions and is the most studied anti-oncogene to date (Aubrey et al. 2016). P53 protein has binding transcription factor activity and can bind to various promoter elements of key human genes to regulate their expression. Particularly, *TP53* fundamentally controls cell proliferation and maintains the integrity of the human genome and is linked to all cancer hallmarks previously described by Hanahan and Weinberg in 2011 (Hanahan and Weinberg 2011; Aubrey et al. 2016). Briefly, in normal conditions, low p53 levels are maintained by negative regulation of MDM2 (murine double minute 2), an E3 ubiquitin ligase, that represses p53 transcriptional function and also enables its degradation by the proteasome (Vijayakumaran et al. 2015). Furthermore, p53 acts on several target genes that mediate cell-cycle arrest, DNA repair, apoptosis, and autophagy in the presence of activating stimuli such as oncogene expression and DNA damage.

While somatic *TP53* gene alterations are frequent in several cancers (Hainaut and Pfeifer 2016), germline mutations predispose to a wide spectrum of early-onset cancers such as Li-Fraumeni and Li-Fraumeni-like syndromes (Guha and Malkin 2017; Andrade et al. 2017). According to the TCGA project, OCs are characterized predominantly (96%) by mutated *TP53* in almost all sequenced tumors (Cancer Genome Atlas Research Network 2011). *TP53* gene alterations reported in cancer are represented mainly by point mutations and are dominated by missense mutations (exons 5–8) particularly in breast and OCs (Silwal-Pandit et al. 2017). Tumor cells with mutated *TP53* can control the gene expression associated with tumorigenesis, including proliferation, migration, and invasiveness (Kang et al. 2013; Lee et al. 2015; Ren et al. 2016; Ahn et al. 2017; Xu et al. 2019). Mutated *TP53* upregulates the expression of several pro- and anti-apoptotic genes, such as *MYC, FAS, BCL2L, NFkB2*, and *ABCB1* (Brosh and Rotter 2009). Recent evidence from sequencing reports of low stage tumors suggests that deleterious *TP53* mutations alongside tetraploidy and homologous recombination repair defects are the earliest events in the pathogenesis of high-grade serous OC (Flesken-Nikitin et al. 2013; Chien et al. 2015; Huang et al. 2015; Labidi-Galy et al. 2017; Soong et al. 2019).

Based on previous studies that assessed the clinical relevance of linking *TP53* mutations with the prognosis of OC (Kang et al. 2013; Rechsteiner et al. 2013; Nadkarni et al. 2013; Wong et al. 2013; Wojnarowicz et al. 2012; McAlpine et al. 2012; Köbel et al. 2010; Bernardini et al. 2010), various recent studies have provided evidence regarding their impact on survival outcomes and response to treatments. In this regard, the $TP53^{K351N}$ variant was found to be associated with platinum-resistance to neoadjuvant chemotherapy in advanced OC (Zhang et al. 2014). Notably, this mutation independently predicted disease-free survival in this setting (Zhang et al. 2014). Mechanistically, it seems that mutated *TP53* induces genome instability and chromosome 7 accumulation in addition to *MDR1* gene amplification favors chemoresistance (Zhang et al. 2017). Recently, these findings were confirmed in a large prospective cohort (Ghezelayagh et al. 2020). In fact, *TP53* mutations, which account for 87.9% in high-grade OC, were found associated with platinum sensitivity even after adjusting for *BRCA*-mutated status (OR: 0.41, 95% CI: 0.17–0.99; $p = 0.048$) but not with survival outcomes (Ghezelayagh et al. 2020). However, several authors have recently demonstrated that *TP53* also impacts the survival of OC patients. Based on the Cancer Genome Atlas (TCGA) data, Seagle et al. demonstrated that *TP53* hot spot mutations in epithelial high-grade serous OC confer differential OS outcomes (Seagle et al. 2015). Patients with R248 codon had the worse OS, followed by those with any other codons, R175 codon, and R273 codon which had the highest OS ($p = 0.04$). Moreover, the authors also showed their in vitro experimentation that *TP53* mutations confer resistance to the antimicrotubules paclitaxel, epothilone B, and ixabepilone (Seagle et al. 2015). In another TCGA-based study, the co-occurrence of mutated *TP53* and *BRCA* in serous OC was found to be associated with improved survival as compared to *TP53* or *BRCA* alone (Li et al. 2019b). However, the latest cohort report by Mandilaras et al. demonstrated that these mutations have no impact on a first platinum-free interval or OS (Mandilaras et al. 2019). To date, the prognostic impact of loss or gain of functions of *TP53* in OC is still conflicting. Therapeutically, targeting the TP53 pathway was also investigated in early clinical trials for OC. A phase II trial (NCT01164995) that investigated AZD1775 (a WEE1 kinase inhibitor developed by Merck®) given orally in combination with carboplatin in patients with *TP53*-mutated resistant or refractory OC to first-line chemotherapy showed encouraging signs of efficacy (Leijen et al. 2016). The toxicity profile was manageable and was mainly represented by fatigue, nausea, thrombocytopenia, diarrhea, and vomiting. In the 21 evaluated patients for efficacy, the overall response was 43% including one patient that had a prolonged complete response. In addition, median PFS and OS were 5.3 and 12.6 months, respectively, in this difficult-to-treat population (Leijen et al. 2016). More recently, Oza et al. conducted a double-blind phase II trial (NCT01357161) to investigate the efficacy of oral adavosertib (AZD1775) or placebo in association with carboplatin and paclitaxel in OC patients with platinum-sensitive disease and enriched with mutated *TP53* (Oza et al. 2020). The addition of adavosertib to chemotherapy was found to improve PFS (HR: 0.63; 95% CI: 0.38–1.06); $p = 0.08$, meeting the predefined significance threshold <0.2 (Oza et al. 2020). More recently, the clinical activity of adavosertib in combination with gemcitabine in platinum-resistant or refractory OC was investigated in a randomized and placebo-controlled phase II trial (NCT02151292) (Lheureux et al. 2021). Median PFS in women treated with adavosertib and gemcitabine was significantly superior compared to gemcitabine monotherapy (HR: 0.55; 95% CI: 0.35–0.90, $p = 0.015$). Regarding OS, the experimental arm median OS was 11.4 months compared to 7.2 months in the control group treated with gemcitabine (HR: 0.56; 95% CI: 0.35–0.91, $p = 0.017$). However, despite this hope for this setting with poor outcomes, this study results introduced clinically significant adverse events (Lheureux et al. 2021). These works highlight the important role of *TP53* in OC and may be a promising targetable pathway for drug discovery in this cancer.

3.2.4.2 Retinoblastoma Protein Signaling

Historically, the retinoblastoma gene (*RB1*) was initially discovered in the 80th and was the first isolated human tumor suppressor gene (Lee et al. 1987). *RB1* gene is located at chromosome 13 (13q14.2) and is a key player in the control processes of cell-cycle progression in cooperation with other tumor suppressors such as *BRCA* and *TP53* (Di Fiore et al. 2013). Notable functions including cell-cycle arrest, cell death, genomic stability, differentiation, and a plethora of other cellular roles are regulated by this triplet of anti-oncogenes (Dick and Rubin 2013; Manning and Dyson 2012). Negative regulators of RB1 function by phosphorylation encompass cyclin D, CDK4, and CDK6 and allow G1/S transition by activation of the E2F family of transcription factors (transcribe a range of genes required for S phase) which therefore enable mitogenic release (reviewed in detail by Sherr and McCormick 2002; Dick and Rubin 2013).

RB1 loss is not only implicated in the development of retinoblastoma but is also related to the initiation and progression of several pediatric and adult cancers such as OC (Li et al. 1991; Takenaka et al. 2015; Stover et al. 2016; Jia and Zhao 2019). In addition to germline and somatic alterations of *RB1* observed in many cancers, a previous analysis of three case-control studies suggested that single nucleotide polymorphisms in three common variants of this gene may be also associated with an increased risk to develop invasive OC (Braem et al. 2011; Song et al. 2006). Data from the TCGA study found that *RB1* expression is deregulated in 67% of high-grade serous OC cases (The Cancer Genome Atlas Research Network 2011). A recent report using NGS found a prevalence of 29% of copy number variation of *RB1* gene in recurrent OC (Du et al. 2018) but there is still a lack of sequencing studies focusing on the prevalence of its genetic alterations in primary tumors. To date, most

OC genome sequencing projects focused only on the prognostic value of *RB1* for chemoresistance and survival outcomes (Garsed et al. 2018; Du et al. 2018; Patch et al. 2015; Takenaka et al. 2015; Milea et al. 2014). Gene breakage or homozygous deletion in *RB1* in OC was found recently to be associated with exceptional response to platinum-based treatment mainly in patients with improved PFS (Garsed et al. 2018). Gene breakage is a type of genetic alteration due to high levels of replication stress and causes a defect in DNA repair mechanisms which may explain possible sensitivity to various treatments. This previous study further assessed RB1 protein loss based on immunohistochemistry in a cohort of 313 OC patients including 91 exceptional responders and found a significant association with long PFS (35%, $p < 0.001$) as compared with unselected OC cases (Garsed et al. 2018). Moreover, Kaplan-Meier survival analysis suggested that exceptional responders to treatment with RB1 protein loss had better survival when their tumors harbor HRR deficiency ($p = 0.03$) (Garsed et al. 2018) which is consistent with a previous large cohort of high-grade serous OC (Milea et al. 2014).

3.2.5 Activating Invasion and Metastasis

Metastasis is a fatal hallmark of cancer. Patients with advanced cancer die often because of metastatic disease. This inevitable and organotropic process, particularly in OC, involves a complex interaction between intrinsic tumor characteristics and surrounding stroma (Welch and Hurst 2019). In OC, neoplastic progression into the peritoneal cavity was widely considered to be different as compared with other solid cancers. In fact, OC cells metastasize through a route using passive spread known as trans-coelomic dissemination (Barbolina 2018; Tan et al. 2006) in which multicellular spheroids adhere to mesothelial cells in the peritoneal cavity to build secondary metastatic sites. However, recent findings also suggest that hematogenous dissemination into the omentum can be also seen via circulating tumor cells (Yeung et al. 2015; Pradeep et al. 2014). Peritoneal metastases in OC are responsible for poor patients' prognosis. Various molecular signaling pathways involved in epithelial-to-mesenchymal transition (EMT), angiogenesis, and motility were defined and investigated to understand metastasis and offer therapeutic interventions and biomarkers to predict outcomes.

3.2.5.1 Cadherins

Cadherins family of cell-surface glycoproteins are involved in the calcium-dependent cell–cell adhesion that sustains the integrity of epithelial cells and tissue architecture and are found in most mammalian tissues (Gloushankova et al. 2017; Shamir and Ewald 2015). Cadherins constitute with other proteins (such as integrins and cytoskeleton proteins) molecular complexes known as adherens junctions that mediate intercellular adhesive interactions involved in various cell functions including adhesion (Klezovitch and Vasioukhin 2015), polarity (Ebnet et al. 2018), mechanotransduction (Leckband and de Rooij 2014), trafficking and migration (Collins and Nelson 2015; Brüser and Bogdan 2017), as well as communication with extracellular matrix (ECM) (Ferreira et al. 2015). Deregulation of cadherin signaling by mutations, loss, methylation, damage or by other signaling pathways such as FGF2 plays a central role in cancer progression by promoting EMT which is a key characteristic of epithelial tumor cell invasion into the surrounding microenvironment and spread to distant organs (Sawada et al. 2008; Gheldof and Berx 2013; Lau et al. 2013; Wang et al. 2016b; Kourtidis et al. 2017; Wong et al. 2018). In addition, cadherin also forms a complex with β-catenin and supports its canonical oncogenic cell growth activity (Shahbazi and Perez-Moreno 2015). Cadherin molecules can be divided into type I [E-encoded by *CDH1* gene and N-encoded by *CDH2* gene] and are found in tissues with a high degree of intercellular cohesion such as human epithelia and type II expressed in cells with motility features (Pal et al. 2018). There are also other cadherins with potential impact on cancer progression such as VE and FAT cadherins and are reviewed elsewhere (Ashaie and Chowdhury 2016; Zhang et al. 2016b). In ovarian tissues, it was previously suggested that fallopian tube epithelia express more likely E-cadherin while ovarian surface epithelium (derived from mesoderm) expresses N-cadherin (Qiu et al. 2017; Adler et al. 2015; Koensgen et al. 2010; Hudson et al. 2008; Ahmed et al. 2007). However, cadherin expression is considered heterogeneous (Klymenko et al. 2017a) and it is admitted that well-differentiated OC express E-cadherin, while advanced and metastatic tumors display N-cadherin upregulation, a concept known as cadherin switching that favors metastasis (Patel et al. 2003; Hazan et al. 2004; Cheung et al. 2010) and is observed during EMT involved in intraperitoneal seeding of OC cells (Klymenko et al. 2017b; van Baal et al. 2018). In OC, other altered cadherins were also investigated such as P-cadherin which was previously found to facilitate the dissemination of tumor cell aggregates into the peritoneum (Usui et al. 2014) (for review, see: Vieira and Paredes 2015; Roggiani et al. 2016). The loss of cell–cell adhesion by cadherin alterations is therefore implicated in malignant transformation and invasive behaviors of OC as suggested by several latest studies (Chmelarova et al. 2018; Chen et al. 2017; Teng et al. 2015; Du et al. 2014; Huang et al. 2014b; Wang et al. 2014; Wakahashi et al. 2013). Importantly, downregulation of cadherins is regarded as an essential event in OC progression and aggressiveness and predicts poor outcomes (Yu et al. 2017; Peng et al. 2012). Based on immunohistochemistry and tissue microarray, Takai et al. analyzed tumor samples from 174 primary tumors and 34 metastases from OC patients for EMT markers (E-cadherin and its inhibitor Snail) and their associations with outcomes (Takai et al. 2014). Patients with EMT-positive markers (reduced E-cadherin and nuclear Snail expression) were likely to have peritoneal dissemination than those with negative status ($p < 0.05$) (Takai et al. 2014). Remarkably, in multivariate analysis, EMT-positive status was significantly associated with PFS ($p < 0.05$) and OS ($p < 0.01$) (Takai et al. 2014). Moreover, another report assessed the prognostic value of E-cadherin expression in advanced-stage high-grade serious OC patients ($n = 98$) treated with platinum-based chemotherapy and found that positive E-cadherin by immunostaining predicts better outcomes (Miše et al. 2015). Positive E-cadherin tumors were found significantly associated with improved response to first-line platinum-based treatment ($p < 0.001$) as well as better PFS and OS ($p < 0.001$ for both) (Miše et al. 2015). In addition, positive E-cadherin expression predicts drug sensitivity to platinum ($p <$ 0.001) and improved OS ($p = 0.01$) in multivariate analysis (Miše et al. 2015). Notably, a recent analysis from the Japanese Gynecologic Oncology Group (JGOG) (3016A1 study) of 201 high-grade serous OC cases showed that patients with mesenchymal transition phenotype have the worst prognosis (PFS: 1.4 years and OS: 3.6 years) (Murakami et al. 2019). A similar conclusion was drawn by a recent meta-analysis that included 1720 OC patients and found that reduced E-cadherin expression correlates with poor OS (pooled HR: 1.74, 95% CI: 1.40–2.17) and PFS (HR: 1.45, 95% CI: 1.12–1.86) (Yu et al. 2017). However, important heterogeneity ($I^2_{statistic} = 57.0\%, p = 0.003$) among studies enrolled for OS analysis was noted and may be explained by the difference in E-cadherin detection methods that were used by studies and their related cut-off point variations (Yu et al. 2017).

In an attempt to target this signaling axis, various therapeutic interventions were investigated (Wong et al. 2018; Mrozik et al. 2018) but their use in clinical research is still at the beginning. In OC, Bialucha et al. examined the anticancer activity of an antibody-drug conjugate HKT288 targeting tumor-associated antigen cadherin 6 (Bialucha et al. 2017). First-in-human HKT288 is an immunoconjugate consisting of a human monoclonal antibody against cadherin 6 conjugated to a maytansine-based cytotoxic agent developed by Novartis and was tested in a phase I trial for OC and renal carcinoma (NCT02947152) (currently terminated). Importantly, HKT288 showed durable anticancer activity in xenografts derived from ovarian and renal cancer patients (Bialucha et al. 2017). Of note, cadherin 6 is responsible for cancer metastatic behavior (Gugnoni et al. 2017) and correlates with poor prognosis (Ma et al. 2018b). Hence, drugging this EMT pathway merits further evaluation in OC.

3.2.5.2 ZEB1 and ZEB2 Axis

ZEB (zinc finger E-box-binding homeobox) 1 and 2 are transcription factors with pleiotropic roles especially in regulating the EMT process via mechanisms involving cell plasticity (Zhang et al. 2019b; Caramel et al. 2018; Krebs et al. 2017). ZEB DNA-binding proteins family promotes metastasis by repressing epithelial markers such as E-cadherins and activating mesenchymal cell programs (Simeone et al. 2018; Fardi et al. 2019; Zhang et al. 2019b). In addition, invasiveness of OC is enhanced when ZEB proteins are upregulated by various factors such as placental growth factor (PLGF) (Song et al. 2016), MAGI1-IT1 long non-coding RNA (Gao et al. 2019), TGF-β (Rafehi et al. 2016), and miR-429 (Chen et al. 2011). Various reports have indicated that high expression of these ZEB1/2 markers provides important prognostic information in OC (Yoshihara et al. 2009; Prislei et al. 2015; Wu et al. 2016; Yan et al. 2017; Sakata et al. 2017; Zhang et al. 2018). Previously and based on gene expression profiling of 43 OC tissues, Yoshihara et al. showed that high ZEB2 expression is an independent factor of poor PFS (HR: 1.37; 95% CI: 1.07–1.78, $p = 0.014$) and OS (HR: 1.53; 95% CI: 1.05–2.22, $p = 0.027$) on Cox multivariate analysis (Yoshihara et al. 2009). Later, another report that enrolled a cohort of 143 OC patients found that high ZEB2 mRNA expression is significantly correlated with poor survival outcomes as compared to patients with low ZEB2 mRNA expression (PFS: 16 vs 23 months, $p = 0.035$, OS: 42 vs 70 months, $p = 0.002$) (Prislei et al. 2015). Recently, a retrospective study from Yan et al. aimed to examine ZEB2 expression as a prognostic biomarker in OC based on tissue samples from 64 epithelial tumors, 36 benign tumors, and 28 normal specimens (Yan et al. 2017). Positive expression of ZEB2 was significantly increased in OC as compared to benign tumors and associated with differentiated histology and FIGO stage as well ($p = 0.002$ for both) (Yan et al. 2017). Furthermore, patients with positive expression of ZEB2 had worse OS ($p = 0.002$) (Yan et al. 2017). However, this prognostic significance disappeared in Cox multivariate analysis (HR: 1.496; 95% CI: 0.567–3.948, $p = 0.416$) (Yan et al. 2017).

In addition to its prognostic value, ZEB1 was found recently to mediate chemoresistance to platinum in OC cells by downregulating solute carrier family 3 member 2 (SLC3A2) (Cui et al. 2018). SLC3A2 is a cell-surface transporter and transmembrane glycoprotein involved in intracellular calcium levels control and is mainly expressed in rapidly proliferating cells (Fotiadis et al. 2013). Also, SLC3A2 was found to induce migration and invasion (Wang et al. 2017a). ZEB1 downregulates SLC3A2, and thus may likely induce dormancy and senescence of tumor cells which are known hallmarks of resistance to anticancer therapy (Yeh and Ramaswamy 2015; Endo and Inoue 2019). However, this concept is not discussed deeply yet in the current literature. Therapeutically, Sakata et al. demonstrated based on an in vitro and in vivo study that ZEB1 inhibition restored sensitivity to paclitaxel in resistant OC cells (Sakata et al. 2017). Similarly, suppression of ZEB1 in other cancers displayed potent anticancer properties in resistant cells (Peng et al. 2019; Ren et al. 2013). This signaling axis has an important link with EMT and OC patients' outcomes and there is growing evidence supporting the role of ZEB1/ZEB2 axis in other malignant cellular processes such as stemness, senescence, and cell death (Caramel et al. 2018). Therefore, additional studies are needed to better understand this signaling pathway in cell biology in general and particularly in cancer.

3.2.5.3 EpCAM

Epithelial cell adhesion molecule (EpCAM, also known as CD326) is a cell–cell adhesion glycoprotein involved in various cellular pathways including cell integrity, proliferation, signaling, and migration (Yahyazadeh Mashhadi et al. 2019; Schnell et al. 2013). EpCAM was reported to be highly expressed in various tumors of epithelial origin (Spizzo et al. 2011; for review, see: Herreros-Pomares et al. 2018). Of note, in vitro assessment found that this marker promotes invasion during the EMT process especially in cancer cells with non-mesenchymal phenotype (Martowicz et al. 2012). Phenotypic immunostaining of EpCAM in human tumors suggests stable or high expression in tumor-associated stem cells, effusions, and metastases (Patriarca et al. 2012). Moreover, germline *EPCAM* deletion in colorectal tissues causes *MSH2* epigenetic silencing which predisposes to Lynch syndrome (Pathak et al. 2019; Tutlewska et al. 2013). The presence of this molecule on circulating tumor cells is becoming a potential candidate for real-time profiling of human cancers (de Wit et al. 2019; Loeian et al. 2019) including OC (Van

Berckelaer et al. 2016) based on liquid biopsy approaches (Grover et al. 2014). Highly expressed EpCAM in OC stages is well documented. Previously, a retrospective study detected EpCAM in all OC subtypes and FIGO stages (Köbel et al. 2008). Furthermore, this can also be seen in recurrent ovarian tumors and metastases (Bellone et al. 2009). Clinical impact and prognostic value of EpCAM overexpression in OC were investigated in three recent studies and suggest favorable outcomes (Battista et al. 2014; Woopen et al. 2014; Tayama et al. 2017). Battista et al. evaluated the expression of EpCAM in a cohort of 117 OC and found a significant independent prognostic value for this biomarker in terms of disease-specific survival (HR: 0.408, 95% CI: 0.197–0.846; $p = 0.016$) on multivariate analysis (Battista et al. 2014). Similarly, another German report that enrolled tissue samples from 74 OC patients mostly with advanced FIGO stages found that overexpressed EpCAM is significantly associated with improved PFS ($p = 0.040$) and better response to chemotherapy ($p = 0.048$) (Woopen et al. 2014). In addition, EpCAM was found to predict OS ($p = 0.022$) (Woopen et al. 2014). Findings from a recent large Japanese study by Tayama et al. ($n = 168$) confirmed these data (Tayama et al. 2017). Kaplan-Meier curves of OS stratified by EpCAM expression found significant difference between high and low groups (HR: 2.17; 95% CI: 1.22–3.88; $p = 0.008$) (Tayama et al. 2017). However, these cohorts of OC patients that assessed EpCAM as a prognostic biomarker were retrospective in their design and exploratory in their nature and therefore, their findings must be interpreted with caution.

Therapeutically, EpCAM is a potential target for anticancer therapy that was investigated using trifunctional bispecific antibodies such as catumaxomab (Removab®) (Krishnamurthy and Jimeno 2018; Frampton 2012) and small-molecule inhibitors (Tretter et al. 2018) particularly for malignant ascites in peritoneal carcinomatosis (Knödler et al. 2018). Catumaxomab was developed by Neovii Biotech® (a German pharmaceutical company) and evaluated in phase II/III prospective trial (NCT00836654) that randomized 258 patients ($n = 129$ for OC) to receive catumaxomab combined with paracentesis against control of patients treated with paracentesis alone for recurrent malignant ascites (Heiss et al. 2010). Modest clinically meaningful improvement was reached in terms of puncture-free survival which was longer in the group treated with catumaxomab as compared to the control arm (median 46 vs 11 days; $p < 0.0001$) as well as in terms of median time to next paracentesis (77 vs 13 days; $p < 0.0001$) (Heiss et al. 2010). Moreover, catumaxomab was found to improve ascites symptoms and quality of life of OC patients with a chemotherapy-refractory setting in a single-arm open-label multicenter US phase II trial ($n = 32$; NCT00326885) (Berek et al. 2014). In platinum-resistant disease, this drug has slight anticancer activity as suggested by a phase IIa of the AGO trialists (NCT00189345) (Baumann et al. 2011). Catumaxomab given as an intraperitoneal infusion was approved by the US FDA and the EMA in Europe in early 2009 but withdrawn later for marketing since 2014 for insolvency concerns (https://neovii.com/neovii-completes-marketing-authorisation-withdrawal-of-removab-in-the-european-union/?cn-reloaded=1. Accessed 19/06/2019).

3.2.6 Enabling Replicative Immortality

In physiological conditions, mutant cells are suppressed by a blockade of their proliferation and eliminated by immunity. On some occasions, these cells can be immortal by additional (epi)genetic events that progress their phenotype into highly malignant cells that in turn can induce senescence and escape from tumor suppression (Moiseeva et al. 2020). The viable state of cancer cell senescence (also called cytostasis or dormancy) classically presents as a growth arrest but with the retained proliferative ability for survival, a well-known cancer condition called cellular plasticity (Damen et al. 2020). Accordingly, dormant/proliferative cancer cells have unlimited replicative potential. Telomere dysfunction and oncogenic and exogenic-induced stresses are the principal causes that stimulate cell senescence (Yaswen et al. 2015). Notably, the presence of senescent cells in cancer clones is associated with recurrent disease, metastatic dissemination, and poor outcomes (Damen et al. 2020). This hallmark is less investigated in OC for therapeutic approaches. However, its involvement in tumorigenesis and prognosis seems to be important. After front-line chemotherapy, OC cells can escape and survive to repopulate the initial tumors (Telleria 2013). This repopulation phenomenon encompasses transient cells with a senescent phenotype that drive relapse (Telleria 2013). Recently, Lam et al. demonstrated that signaling mechanisms of chemoresistance in OC and dormancy are linked (Lam et al. 2020). Chemoresistant OC cells had an enhanced survival by senescence (Lam et al. 2020). Telomere shortening in OC, which is regulated by telomerase—a prominent enzymatic activity of cancer cells, is involved in genomic instability that introduces additional mutations. During this event, end-to-end fusions in chromosomes were observed and can induce genome instability and bypass host cellular protection. Telomere shortening was remarkably noticed in serous tubal intraepithelial carcinomas, a precursor of high-grade serous OC (Kuhn et al. 2010). Moreover, this alteration was also observed in tubo-ovarian dysplastic lesions (Chen et al. 2013). This suggests that telomere shortening occurs earlier during ovarian tumorigenesis and is a selective mechanism of cancer cell immortality. The use of telomerase by tumor cells to maintain their telomere length and integrity has been an attractive druggable target. In addition, the pharmacological elimination of dormant cells has also been investigated using the so-called senolytic/senostatic drugs (Wyld et al. 2020). In this perspective, preclinical combinatorial approaches using these drugs and the standard OC chemotherapy were investigated (Meng et al. 2012; Stamelos et al. 2013; Wyld et al. 2020). Targeted inhibition of telomerase activity in OC using BIBR1532 and carboplatin was found to block the formation of spheroid-forming cells in vitro (Meng et al. 2012). Moreover, the preclinical use of navitoclax, an orally bioavailable Bcl-2 inhibitor directed against senescent cells, demonstrated an improved efficacy against OC cells when combined with paclitaxel-carboplatin therapy (Stamelos et al. 2013). Of note, the combination of paclitaxel and navitoclax was also previously shown to have a synergistic effect against OC cells (Wong et al. 2012). In OC patients, the high expression of Bcl-x(L) which induces senescence mediated chemoresistance and the use of these drugs reduced resistant cells (Wong et al. 2012). Clinically, this approach was investigated in a phase II trial (MONAVI-1/NCT02591095) using the single-agent navitoclax in 47 women with platinum-resistant/refractory recurrent OC. The preliminary findings of this trial in 44 patients assessable for efficacy showed a long response in 11 subjects treated with chemotherapy after navitoclax in addition to 12 patients that had high response (Brachet et al. 2017). This suggests that this agent may reverse platinum-resistance in this difficult-to-treat population (McMullen et al. 2020). However, the findings of the blockade of this hallmark in OC which are mainly based on few preclinical studies are not convincing yet. Telomere shortening not only drives tumor cell senescence but is also involved in genome instability (Bär and Thum 2017). The model of "*too little of it can kill you but too much of it can kill you too*" enlightens well the difficulty of targeting this hallmark in cancer and the timing of its inhibition seems to be crucial (Bär and Thum 2017). As the mechanisms of replicative immortality interfere with those of "evading growth suppressors," the previous chapter discussing TP53 and RB pathways adds more details on this subject. For further reading, see: Książek (2020), Sikora et al. (2020), Saleh et al. (2020), and Moiseeva et al. (2020).

3.2.7 Inducing Angiogenesis

Without doubt, this hallmark accounts for the most relevant achievements and the most potential exploited compounds in cancer. Pathologic angiogenesis has a principal role in the growth and metastasis of solid tumors. This process is biologically supported by a network of pathways and growth factors dominated by vascular endothelial growth factor (VEGF) (Apte et al. 2019). Tumor hypoxia is a central regulator of VEGF expression through HIF and other hypoxia-related factors and genes such as platelet-derived growth factor (PDGF) and oncogenic mutations that synchronize VEGF-related signaling pathways (Apte et al. 2019). The VEGF/VEGF-R1/R2 canonical signaling induces vascular permeability, cell proliferation, migration, and survival via the activation of several kinases. An important number of studies demonstrated that VEGF expression has a prognostic value in OC. Previously, pooled data from a meta-analysis of 19 studies showed that VEGF overexpression is associated with reduced OS in OC (Hui and Meng 2015). Moreover, another meta-analysis of 16 studies also demonstrated that serum and tissue expression of VEGF is an independent predictor of poor PFS in OC (Yu et al. 2013).

Blockade of angiogenesis in OC resulted in promising findings. Bevacizumab is a neutralizing anti-VEGF monoclonal antibody approved for treating OC. Bevacizumab was investigated in several phase III trials for OC including ICON-7 (Perren et al. 2011; Oza et al. 2015a), GOG-0213 (Coleman et al. 2017a, b), GOG-0218 (Burger et al. 2011; Tewari et al. 2019), OCEANS (Aghajanian et al. 2012), and AURELIA (Pujade-Lauraine et al. 2014) for patients with newly diagnosed or recurrent disease. The FDA and EMA approvals of this anticancer drug were based on the promising findings of these landmark trials particularly GOG-0218. This phase III trial was designed to show the superiority of adding bevacizumab to standard chemotherapy in the front-line setting. The investigators tested this hypothesis using three-arm placebo-controlled study that compared standard chemotherapy alone, chemotherapy plus bevacizumab, and chemotherapy plus bevacizumab followed by bevacizumab as maintenance in a population of 1873 women (Burger et al. 2011). The results of this study showed an increase in PFS by 4 months (but not in OS) in the arm adding bevacizumab to the standard carboplatin and paclitaxel treatment of advanced OC (Burger et al. 2011). Similarly, ICON-7 was a phase III trial that explored the benefits of bevacizumab in combination with the standard of care (Perren et al. 2011). This trial randomly assigned 1528 patients with OC to receive bevacizumab in association with carboplatin and paclitaxel or chemotherapy alone. PFS was also improved in this trial favoring the addition of bevacizumab to the standard of care (HR: 0.81; 95% CI: 0.70–0.94; $p = 0.004$) (Peeren et al. 2011).

In recurrent disease, OCEANS was a phase III ($n = 484$) placebo-controlled study that explored the addition of bevacizumab to carboplatin and gemcitabine as compared to this doublet alone in the platinum-sensitive setting (Aghajanian et al. 2012). Median PFS was superior in the bevacizumab arm (12.4 vs 8.4 months; HR: 0.484; 95% CI: 0.388–0.605; $p < 0.0001$) (Aghajanian et al. 2012). In the GOG-0213 phase III trial ($n = 674$) that was powered for OS, a clinically meaningful difference of OS by 5 months was noticed in the bevacizumab group as compared to chemotherapy alone (Coleman et al. 2017a, b). In addition, the investigators confirmed the benefits of bevacizumab plus gemcitabine and carboplatin concerning the PFS (Coleman et al. 2017a, b). In the platinum-resistant setting, the efficacy of bevacizumab in combination with non-platinum chemotherapy was explored in the AURELIA phase III trial ($n = 361$) (Pujade-Lauraine et al. 2014). This study showed an improvement in median PFS and ORR in the bevacizumab-containing arm (6.7 months vs 3.4 months and 27.3% and 11.8%, respectively) (Pujade-Lauraine et al. 2014). Based on these data, bevacizumab was also approved for the treatment of both platinum-sensitive and resistant recurrent OC, but not for refractory setting.

Cediranib is another antiangiogenic drug that was investigated in OC (Orbegoso et al. 2017). This molecule is an oral antiangiogenic vascular endothelial growth factor receptor 1–3 (VEGFR1–3) inhibitor. The efficacy of cediranib was explored in women with relapsed platinum-sensitive OC in the ICON-6 phase III trial ($n = 486$) (Lederman et al. 2016). PFS was improved in the group of patients treated with cediranib given with chemotherapy and continued as a maintenance treatment but with added adverse events including voice changes, diarrhea, neutropenia, and hypothyroidism which were the most common causes of treatment discontinuation (Lederman et al. 2016). In a randomized phase II study, cediranib was given in association with olaparib in comparison with olaparib alone in a population of 90 patients with platinum-sensitive OC (Liu et al. 2019a). Median PFS was doubled in the intention-to-treat population of the combination group (16.5 vs 8.2 months, HR: 0.5, $p = 0.007$) and also in the subgroup with wild-type/unknown germline *BRCA* status (23.7 vs 5.7 months, $p = 0.002$) (Liu et al. 2019a). These encouraging results provided the rationale to investigate the combination of cediranib and olaparib in the ongoing ICON-9 phase III trial which will randomize 618 women with relapsed platinum-sensitive OC following a response to platinum-based chemotherapy to receive this association or olaparib alone as maintenance treatment (Elyashiv et al. 2021). PFS and OS are co-primary endpoints of this clinical trial and it is estimated to be completed in 2024 (Elyashiv et al. 2021).

Pazopanib, an oral multikinase inhibitor of VEGFR and also platelet-derived growth factor receptor (PDGFR), was investigated in OC in the AGO-OVAR16 phase III trial (du Bois et al. 2014). This study randomized 940 women with advanced OC who did not progress after first-line platinum-taxane chemotherapy to receive pazopanib or placebo as maintenance treatment (1:1). The hazard ratio for progression or death was 0.77 (95% CI: 0.64–0.91; $p = 0.0021$) with a median PFS of 17.9 months in pazopanib arm versus 12.3 months in patients treated with placebo. An interim analysis in 35.6% of patients did not show a significant difference in terms of survival (du Bois et al. 2014). Similarly, no improvements in median OS were noticed (Vergote et al. 2019a). Nintedanib is another tyrosine kinase inhibitor of VEGFR that has been studied for the standard first-line in advanced OC (du Bois et al. 2016). In this perspective, AGO-OVAR 12 phase III explored the efficacy of the combination of standard paclitaxel and carboplatin with nintedanib versus the doublet and placebo for newly diagnosed advanced OC. In this study, 1366 women were randomly assigned to receive one of the two combinations in a 2:1 fashion. The nintedanib group has statistically significantly increased median PFS as compared to the control (17.2 vs 16.6 months, HR: 0.84; 95% CI: 0.72–0.98, $p = 0.024$) but without a clinically meaningful improved PFS (0.6 months benefit). In addition, this combinatorial regimen was associated with more gastrointestinal adverse events (du Bois et al. 2016). This big clinical trial for chemo-naïve OC patients is a good example of overpowered negative clinical trials in which statistical difference has no value over clinical significance. Other angiogenic targets such as angiopoietins 1 and 2 and Tie2 receptor were also explored for therapeutic strategies. Trebananib is an inhibitor of this pathway that was studied in phase III trials for OC. TRINOVA-1, TRINOVA-2, and TRINOVA-3 were randomized phase III clinical trials that studied the combination of trebananib with standard chemotherapy or single agents, paclitaxel and PLD for first-line and recurrent settings but without providing clinically meaningful improvements in median PFS (Monk et al. 2014; Marth et al. 2017; Vergote et al. 2019b). The exploration of antiangiogenics in OC is also being studied in other ongoing phase III trials. Other details on combinatorial synergistic approaches particularly immune-checkpoint blockade can be found in Sect. 2.9 (*Avoiding Immune Destruction*).

3.2.8 Resisting Cell Death

Classically, the regulation of cell death encompasses two major circuits, the extrinsic pathway that receives extracellular signals through death receptors and the intrinsic program that engages p53 after DNA damage. Basically, the activation of cell death leads to progressive activation of caspases that causes proteolysis. However, cancer cells resist natural programmed cell death to avoid their elimination by host defense mechanisms. The deregulated machinery of apoptosis in cancer involves several strategies to avoid inducing sensors particularly "*TP53* loss", which suppresses critical damages for cells by activating intracellular signaling of death (Hanahan and Weinberg 2011). Accumulating evidence also demonstrated that cancer cells escape from cell death by increasing the expression of major negative regulators such as Bcl-2 and its relative Bcl-xL or downregulating multiple pro-apoptotic signals (Bax, Bim, and Puma). Also, additional mechanisms allow cancer cells to resist using diverse secondary pathways gained during tumor evolution (for scoping reviews on this topic, see elsewhere: Singh et al. 2019; Carneiro and El-Deiry 2020). Other forms of regulated cell death beyond apoptosis have recently emerged and merit recommended reading elsewhere (Wang et al. 2020; Galluzzi et al. 2017, 2018). In OC, mutated *TP53* is a well-known signature of early events of ovarian carcinogenesis (Kuhn et al. 2012). *TP53* mutations are believed to drive platinum-resistance and were also found to predict disease-free survival (Zhang et al. 2014; Seagle et al. 2015). The value of other cell death-related proteins in OC outcomes seems to be limited. On the one hand, the high expression of the pro-apoptotic Bax was found to prolong survival and predicted platinum sensitivity in OC (Yigit et al. 2012). Regarding Bcl-2, data from the large Danish MALOVA cohort showed that this marker may not be of clinical importance for the prognosis of OC patients (Høgdall et al. 2010). On the other hand, the pro-survival proteins (Bcl-xL and Mcl-1) were found to drive chemotherapy resistance in high-grade serous OC (Stover et al. 2019). Therapeutically, the use of agents that physically interfere with anti-apoptotic proteins via BH3 motifs seems to be a promising approach for cell death induction (so-called BH3 mimetics) (Ashkenazi et al. 2017). The efficacy of these agents was investigated in several preclinical studies. Previously, Simonin et al. showed that Bcl-xL and Mcl-1 cooperate to protect OC cells against oncogenic stress and cell death induced by chemotherapy (Simonin et al. 2009). These findings were later confirmed suggesting that their concomitant inhibition may be effective in OC (Brotin et al. 2010; Lincet et al. 2013). The exploitation of calcium signaling via calmodulin inhibition in combination with the BH3 mimetic ABT-737 was found to induce apoptosis by sensitizing OC cells (Bonnefond et al. 2015). A human pilot study by the team of *Stéphanie Lheureux* was conducted to explore predictive biomarkers of ABT-737 in patients with high-grade serous OC (NCT01440504) (Lheureux et al. 2015). Relevant markers of response were established to select patients for clinical trial design, and this includes Bim, Mcl-1, and phospho-Erk1/2 (Lheureux et al. 2015).

This has provided a rationale for investigating other antagonists to disrupt this pathway. The association of the Bcl-2 selective inhibitor WEHI-539 and the BH3 mimetic ABT-737 showed synergistic effects in potentiating the anticancer activity of carboplatin in vitro using various OC cells by inducing caspase 3/7 and PARP cleavage (Abed et al. 2016). Similarly, the combination of a PARP inhibitor (BMN-673) and BH3 mimetic ABT-263 also showed synergistic cytotoxic effects against OC cells by increasing the expression of Bim, a pro-apoptotic protein

(Yokoyama et al. 2017). Recently, Iavarone et al. explored the therapeutic blockade of MEK/ERK signaling based on cobimetinib (GDC-0973) combined to ABT-263 using patient-derived xenograft models of high-grade serous OC (Iavarone et al. 2019). The results of this report showed greater inhibition of tumor growth as compared to the single agent. Moreover, baseline levels of pro-apoptotic protein BIM and/or pERK were predictors of drug response suggesting their potential value as biomarkers (Iavarone et al. 2019). More recently, a strategy using drug repurposing of naftopidil to increase the expression of BH3-only proteins including Bim, Puma, and Noxa resulted in sensitizing patient-derived organoid models from OC patients to ABT-737 and the MEK inhibitor trametinib (Florent et al. 2020a). Of note, naftopidil is an α_1-adrenergic receptor antagonist used in benign prostatic hyperplasia management (reviewed by Florent et al. 2020b). The area of preclinical research on BH3 mimetics as single agents or in combination with other targeted therapeutics in OC seems to be highly active. To the best of our knowledge, there is only one BH3 mimetic that has been investigated in a clinical trial for OC (NCT02591095). MONAVI-1 was a French open-label phase II trial that studied navitoclax (ABT-263) given daily in a population of OC patients with platinum-resistant disease. Early signs of efficacy of this monotherapy were revealed in 11 patients that were treated with chemotherapy; therefore, confirming that this BH3 mimetic is a potent sensitizer (Brachet et al. 2017). More details on this hallmark in OC can be found in Sects. 2.4 and 2.6 (*Evading Growth Suppressors* and *Enabling Replicative Immortality*).

3.2.9 Avoiding Immune Destruction

Escape from host mechanisms of defense involving immune surveillance is an emerging hallmark of cancer (Hanahan and Weinberg 2011). Tumor cells avoid immunological killing by overexpressing immune-checkpoints such as programmed death-ligand 1 (PD-L1) and cytotoxic T-lymphocyte antigen-4 (CTLA-4) (Fig. 3.1), infiltration of immunosuppressive cells such as regulatory T lymphocytes (T^{reg}), and disruption of antigen processing and presentation machinery (Tang et al. 2020). As in other cancers, the tumor microenvironment of OC contains various cellular components of clinical value including tumor-infiltrating cells (TILs), tumor associated macrophages (TAMs), tumor associated neutrophils (TANs), cancer-associated fibroblasts (CAFs), and a variety of other cells (Macpherson et al. 2020). The prognostic value of these immune suppressive infiltrates as biomarkers was extensively studied in OC (Macpherson et al. 2020). A recent meta-analysis of 19 studies ($n = 6004$) pooled data of TILs in high-grade serous OC and demonstrated a significant association with OS and PFS (Hao et al. 2020). Indeed, intratumor and stromal TILs were favorably correlated to survival outcomes in this setting. Hence, these updated results confirmed the previous findings of Hwang's meta-analysis and other earlier TILs studies (Hwang et al. 2012; Webb et al. 2016; James et al. 2017; Wang et al. 2017b; Buderath et al. 2019). Recent additional reports on this topic also showed the benefits of high TILs in women with high-grade

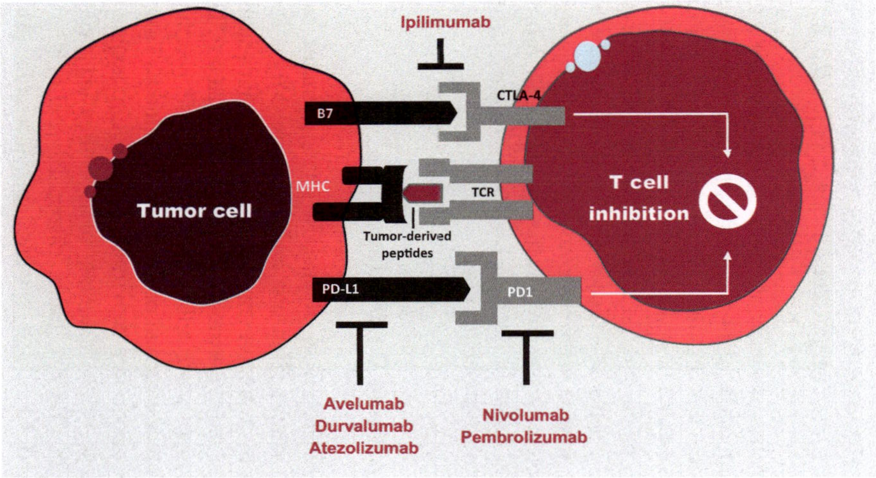

Fig. 3.1 Overview of immune-checkpoint blockade used in ovarian cancer clinical trials. Abbreviations: *CTLA-4* cytotoxic T-lymphocyte-associated protein 4, *MHC* major histocompatibility complex, *PD1* programmed death 1, *PD-L1* programmed death-ligand 1, *TCR* T cell receptor

serous OC. Martin de la Fuente et al. reported that patients with higher CD3, PD-L1, and PD-1 had significantly longer OS (Martin de la Fuente et al. 2020). Moreover, high expression of TILs was also found to have a positive impact on survival in OC (Martin de la Fuente et al. 2020). TILs in OC are most prevalent in tumors with high-grade histology (Chen et al. 2020). Improved PFS and immune response in OC patients with positive PD-L1 was also seen in advanced FIGO stages (Chen et al. 2020). OCs have frequently deficient homologous recombination systems with or without *BRCA* mutations. This allows tumors a notable expression of neo-antigens which in turn are marked indicators of an immune response in solid cancers (Fumet et al. 2020; Cormedi et al. 2020) and OC (Strickland et al. 2016; Le Saux et al. 2020). Therefore, these data are of important significance for investigating immunotherapy in this setting. The recent introduction of immune-oncology in clinical practice has revolutionized our current management of cancer. The advent of immune-checkpoint inhibitors (ICIs) and their predictive biomarkers for patients' selection has deeply changed outcomes in some cancers previously known to be aggressive (El Bairi et al. 2020; Keenan et al. 2019; Ribas and Wolchok 2018). Stunning successes with some cancers such as melanomas (Pasquali et al. 2018), metastatic colorectal cancer with microsatellite instability (André et al. 2020), and lung cancer (Almutairi et al. 2019), little benefits have been reported in OC (Le Saux et al. 2020). The therapeutic arsenal using immune-checkpoint blockade is a recent development in the design of novel clinical trials for OC using combinatorial approaches (Le Saux et al. 2020). OC is classically regarded as a "cold tumor" characterized by decreased levels of TILs (Le Saux et al. 2020). Therefore, response to ICIs in OC has been commonly reported to be low. Initial phase I/II studies that were conducted to investigate ICIs in OC have shown modest improvement in outcomes.

Experience with pembrolizumab (an anti-programmed death-1 (PD-1) monoclonal antibody) in phase I clinical trials as monotherapy for solid cancers (KEYNOTE-028/NCT02054806) demonstrated a durable antitumor response with a manageable safety and toxicity profile in patients with advanced PD-L1-positive OC (Varga et al. 2019). Following these early signs of efficacy, a two-cohort phase II study was conducted in patients with recurrent and advanced OC (KEYNOTE-100/NCT02674061). Cohort A included 285 patients that received 1–3 lines of therapy and cohort B ($n = 91$) received 4–6 lines of treatments (Matulonis et al. 2019). Pembrolizumab as a single agent at a dose of 200 mg was given every 3 weeks for both cohorts. ORR and disease control rate in cohort A were 7.4% and 37.2%, respectively, and 9.9% and 37.4% in cohort B. Notably, a higher response was observed in patients with a combined positive score (CPS) ≥ 1 (10% vs. 4.1% for CPS < 1). In addition, PFS in both cohorts was 2.1 months. The toxicity profile in this study was consistent with the previous experience with this agent (Matulonis et al. 2019). As expected, modest response was demonstrated for this novel monotherapy in this setting. However, a historical case report showed a complete response in an OC patient treated with pembrolizumab alone and harboring *PD-L1* gene structural variations (Bellone et al. 2018). The authors observed a notable complete response in a patient with recurrent advanced chemoresistant high-grade serous OC that progressed on all standard therapies. Whole exome sequencing of the surgical specimens showed a low tumor mutational load/megabase with a remarkable structural variation of *PD-L1* gene causing unusual PD-L1 surface expression. This was markedly associated with high infiltration of CD4 and CD8 TILs, macrophages, and B lymphocytes suggesting immune escape (Bellone et al. 2018). To test the hypothesis that PARP inhibitors may increase the expression of PD-L1 (Jiao et al. 2017; Sato et al. 2017); and therefore the response to pembrolizumab, the TOPACIO/KEYNOTE-162 phase I/II trial (NCT02657889) investigated this approach in patients with platinum-resistant disease (Konstantinopoulos et al. 2019). This study was a single-arm and open-label and used pembrolizumab in combination with oral niraparib (200 mg daily for both) every 3 weeks. ORR and disease control rates were 18% and 65%, respectively. Moreover, three complete responses and eight partial responses were noticed regardless of prior bevacizumab exposure or *BRCA* status (Konstantinopoulos et al. 2019). Recently, the biomarker analysis of this study identified *PD-L1 and PD-L2* amplification as determinants of exceptional response in some patients of this trial (Färkkilä et al. 2020). In another phase II non-comparative trial (NCT02865811; $n = 23$), Lee et al. showed that the combination of pembrolizumab with PLD has a manageable toxicity profile and provided a preliminary evidence of its clinical activity including 26.1% of ORR in the population of patients with platinum-resistant OC (Lee et al. 2020). Moreover, the combination of pembrolizumab with metronomic cyclophosphamide and bevacizumab in another phase II trial (NCT02853318; $n = 40$) also demonstrated clinical benefits in OC patients with recurrent disease including >12 months of durable response in 25% of the treatment population that encompassed mainly platinum-resistant women (Zsiros et al. 2020). However, despite promising, these phase II trials were non-randomized and no comparator was added to their design and therefore, these early signs of efficacy should be interpreted with caution. The ongoing study registered on the US ClinicalTrials database shows more than 70 clinical trials using pembrolizumab used as monotherapy or in combination with other anticancer drugs for OC (www.clinicaltrials.gov, accessed 14/01/2020). The MK-7339-001/KEYLYNK-001/ENGOT-ov43/GOG-3036 is an ongoing phase III trial that may provide definitive and strong evidence for the future use of this agent in OC (NCT03740165). This study randomizes 1086 OC patients with advanced disease to receive the standard carboplatin-paclitaxel with or without pembrolizumab followed by maintenance therapy with the PARP inhibitor olaparib or placebo in the first-line setting. The study uses PFS and OS as primary endpoints and it is expected to be completed in August 2025.

The anti-PD-L1 durvalumab was investigated in OC as a combination with other therapeutics including PARP inhibitors and vaccines. A proof-of-concept phase II trial (NCT02484404; $n = 35$) aimed to assess the efficacy of durvalumab given every 4 weeks in combination with oral olaparib in recurrent and predominantly platinum-resistant OC (Lampert et al. 2020). The ORR was 14% and the disease control rate reached 71%. Moreover, this combination was found to increase the infiltration of TILs and IFNγ/TNFα release, which both are indicators of immunomodulatory response. Moreover, patients with increased IFNγ had superior PFS (HR: 0.37, 95% CI: 0.16–0.87, $p = 0.023$ (Lampert et al. 2020). Durvalumab was also investigated in combination with the folate receptor alpha vaccine TPIV200 in patients with advanced platinum-resistant OC (Zamarin et al. 2020a). The investigators found an increased T cell response to vaccine peptides and prolonged median OS in one patient (21 months) in addition to stable disease in nine patients (Zamarin et al. 2020a). To test the hypothesis that PARP inhibitors create neo-antigens that may upregulate PD-L1 expression, MEDIOLA phase II trial (NCT02734004) was initiated. The initial results of this study that investigated the doublet olaparib and durvalumab and the triplet olaparib, durvalumab, and bevacizumab in non-germline *BRCA*-mutated platinum-sensitive and relapsed OC were recently presented at ESMO 2020 virtual meeting (Drew et al. 2020). Remarkably, ORR and PFS were 77.4% and 14.7 months, respectively, in the cohort treated with the triplet combination as compared to 31.3% of ORR and 5.5 months of PFS with the doublet (Drew et al. 2020). These encouraging results may be supported by the ongoing DUO-O phase III trial investigating the triplet approach ($n = 1254$; NCT03737643) in advanced OC. This is a large randomized multicenter phase III that was designed to evaluate the efficacy of durvalumab combined with the standard platinum-based chemotherapy and bevacizumab followed by durvalumab and bevacizumab as maintenance therapy or durvalumab, bevacizumab, and olaparib. PFS is the primary endpoint of this clinical trial, which is expected to provide preliminary results in November 2025.

Avelumab is another anti-PD-L1 that was investigated in the landmark JAVELIN studies for OC. The phase Ib (NCT01772004) part of this multicohort trial that investigated avelumab in OC was an open-label single-arm study that enrolled 125 participants with recurrent or refractory disease who had received platinum-based chemotherapy (Disis et al. 2019). Avelumab was given at a dose of 10 mg/kg every 14 days until progression assessed by RECIST version 1.1, unacceptable toxicities, or withdrawal from enrollment. After a median follow-up of 26.6 months, confirmed ORR was noticed in 12 patients with 1 and 11 complete and partial responses, respectively. 1-year PFS rate was 10.2% and median OS reached 11.2 months (Disis et al. 2019). The mature data of JAVELIN Ovarian 200 phase III trial (NCT02580058) were discouraging (Pujade-Lauraine et al. 2019). This study randomized 566 OC patients with platinum-resistant or refractory disease to receive avelumab as monotherapy or avelumab + PLD as compared to PLD alone (1:1:1 ratio) (Pujade-Lauraine et al. 2018). No significant differences between the three arms in terms of PFS and OS in the intention-to-treat population were noticed (Pujade-Lauraine et al. 2019). Similarly, the JAVELIN Ovarian 100 (NCT02718417) phase III trial that evaluated avelumab combined with/or following carboplatin-based chemotherapy versus chemotherapy alone in untreated OC patients did not meet its primary endpoint (Ledermann et al. 2020). This trial was stopped due to futility of efficacy at a planned interim analysis.

The ICIs nivolumab (anti-PD-1) and ipilimumab (anti-CTLA-4) were also investigated in OC for both platinum-resistant and sensitive settings. A first phase II clinical trial enrolled 20 patients with platinum-resistant OC to receive intravenous nivolumab every 2 weeks as a monotherapy until disease progression (Hamanishi et al. 2015). The investigators found severe adverse events in two patients and ORR was 15%. Median PFS and OS were 3.5 and 20 months, respectively (Hamanishi et al. 2015). Nivolumab given every 2 weeks was also studied in combination with bevacizumab in a single-arm phase II trial (NCT02873962) (Liu et al. 2019c). This association is believed to have synergistic effects by modulating the tumor microenvironment to turn OC into a "hot tumor" (Tamura et al. 2019). Patients with platinum-sensitive OC seem to benefit much more from this combination as compared to those with platinum-resistance (ORR: 40% vs 16.7%) (Liu et al. 2019c). In another phase II study (NCT02498600), nivolumab was also studied in combination with ipilimumab as compared to nivolumab alone for OC as a dual blockade strategy (Zamarin et al. 2020b). This study included 100 OC patients with recurrent or persistent disease that were randomly allocated to receive monotherapy every 2 weeks or induction double blockade every 3 weeks followed by maintenance monotherapy with nivolumab. The median PFS was doubled in the combination as compared to nivolumab alone (3.9 vs 2 months, respectively, HR: 0.53; 95% CI: 0.34–0.82) (Zamarin et al. 2020b). As in other clinical trials, PD-L1 status didn't predict response to these agents. Therefore, other predictive biomarkers are needed for patients' selection in this setting. A phase III randomized and placebo-controlled four-arm trial (NCT03522246/ATHENA/GOG-3020/ENGOT-ov45) is currently exploring the activity of nivolumab in combination with rucaparib after front-line platinum-based chemotherapy in 1000 newly diagnosed OC patients (Westin et al. 2019). This multicenter study is expected to release its early findings in 2024. Promisingly, this type of combination involving a prior exposure to chemotherapy may be successful. It was recently demonstrated that neoadjuvant chemotherapy boosts local immunity in high-grade serous OC (Jiménez-Sánchez et al. 2020; Mesnage et al. 2017). Moreover, blockade of CTLA-4 within the intact tumor microenvironment in OC was demonstrated to induce tumor-reactive CD8+ tumor-infiltrating lymphocytes (Friese et al. 2020). This may improve the effectiveness of combined strategies after this initial modality.

Atezolizumab is an immune-checkpoint inhibitor of PD-L1 that is currently studied in treating OC (Palaia et al. 2020). A multicenter phase I trial ($n = 12$; NCT01375842) that enrolled women with recurrent epithelial OC evaluated the safety and tolerability profile of atezolizumab used as a single agent (Liu et al. 2019b). Long response duration was observed in two patients only and no new safety signals were identified for atezolizumab (Liu et al. 2019b). Atezolizumab was also investigated in OC in combination with bevacizumab in another phase I trial ($n = 20$; NCT01633970) for platinum-resistant disease (Moroney et al. 2020). ORR was 15% and disease control rate was 55%. Median PFS and OS were 4.9 and 10.2 months, respectively. The prior exposure to treatments and PD-L1 status did not affect response to this combination (Moroney et al. 2020). In preclinical animal models, this combination was found to attenuate resistance to cisplatin by a synergestic suppression of epithelial to mesenchymal transition (Zhang et al. 2019c). To the best of our knowledge, no published findings of phase II trials using this agent in OC are available. All currently ongoing phase II studies on atezolizumab in OC are still in progress at the time of this chapter writing. This makes the ongoing phase III trials on this immune-checkpoint inhibitor in OC questionable in terms of the rationale for conducting large randomized and controlled trials. In this regard, IMagyn050/GOG 3015/ENGOT-OV39 is a large phase III trial (NCT03038100) that will randomize newly diagnosed advanced OC patients to receive either front-line atezolizumab combined with paclitaxel, carboplatin, and bevacizumab or placebo combined with the previous triplet (Moore and Pignata 2019). This trial is expected to enroll 1300 patients and PFS and OS are its co-primary endpoints in the intention-to-treat population and in the subpopulation of patients with positive PD-L1 (Moore and Pignata 2019). The preliminary findings of this study were presented at the ESMO 2020 Virtual Congress and demonstrated that the addition of atezolizumab to the standard of care did not improve PFS in this setting (Moore et al. 2020). The AGO-OVAR 2.29/ENGOT-ov34 is another ongoing phase III (NCT03353831) designed to investigate the clinical activity of atezolizumab combined with non-platinum chemotherapy and bevacizumab (standard of care) versus standard of care plus placebo in platinum-resistant OC (Harter et al. 2020). The estimated sample size of this trial is 664 patients and OS and PFS are its co-primary endpoints and it is currently recruiting patients. In platinum-sensitive OC, the Spanish randomized and controlled phase III ANITA trial (NCT03598270; ENGOT-Ov41/GEICO 69-O) is recruiting patients to receive atezolizumab + platinum-based chemotherapy followed by maintenance by niraparib + atezolizumab (experimental arm) versus a control arm consisting of platinum-based chemotherapy + placebo followed by maintenance by niraparib + placebo (González-Martín et al. 2020). With a sample size of 414 patients and PFS as a primary endpoint, the authors expect to demonstrate a benefit in terms of PFS per RECIST v1.1 criteria with a HR of 0.7 (power: 80%, two-sided p-value $<5\%$) (González-Martín et al. 2020). Atezolizumab is also being studied in the ATALANTE randomized and controlled phase III trial in platinum-sensitive and relapsed OC ($n = 405$, ENGOT-ov29/NCT02891824) (Kurtz et al. 2018). The investigators will compare the efficacy of adding atezolizumab to chemotherapy in combination with bevacizumab as compared to chemotherapy and bevacizumab alone in 2:1 ratio. The primary endpoint is RECIST v1.1-based PFS and the first results are estimated to be released in September 2023. Finally, the use of ICIs as monotherapies in OC didn't show clinically meaningful improvements in OC. However, combinatorial approaches using antiangiogenics or PARP inhibitors with ICIs seem to be promising. These associations are believed to induce an angiogenic tumor access by TILs. Presently, a promising escalating strategy using first-line platinum-based chemotherapy combined with ICIs and antiangiogenics followed by maintenance regimen with ICIs, antiangiogenics, and PARPi is being studied in several phase III trials and is believed to improve survival outcomes in OC.

The clinical evaluation of other immunotherapeutic strategies such as the Toll-like receptor 8 (TLR8) agonist motolimod (NCT01666444) (Monk et al. 2017), the IDO1 inhibitor epacadostat (NCT01685255) (Kristeleit et al. 2017), and the Vigil® DNA engineered immunotherapy (Oh et al. 2016) was not successful in delivering improved outcomes to OC patients.

3.2.10 Deregulating Cellular Energetics

During neoplastic transformation, the deregulated control of the cell cycle involves an adjustment of energetic metabolism to fuel the tumorigenic process (Hanahan and Weinberg 2011). The use of glucose is a characteristic of normal cells, however; the previous works of the German Nobel laureate *Otto Heinrich Warburg* (1883–1970) showed that cancer cells have atypical energy metabolism (Warburg 1930, 1956). Accordingly, even in the presence of oxygen, tumor metabolism is reprogrammed to be dependent of glycolysis and thus the concept of "aerobic glycolysis or Warburg effect" (nicely reviewed elsewhere: Pascal et al. 2020; Scheid et al. 2021; Urbano 2021). This metabolic switch is partially covered by upregulation of glucose membrane transporters such as GLUT-1 which in turn is associated with mutated anti-oncogenes and activated oncogenes such as *Myc* and *RAS* (Hanahan and Weinberg 2011). During hypoxia, tumor cells accentuate their energetic needs based on glycolysis reliance by increasing the levels of hypoxia-inducible factor (HIF)-α (Hanahan and Weinberg 2011). Together, this suggests that this hallmark is essential for angiogenesis and invasion; and consequently the aggressive cancer phenotype (Icard et al. 2018). A previous report showed that GLUT-1 expression is correlated with tumor proliferation and microvessel density, in addition to suboptimal debulking in patients overexpressing this marker and Ki-67 (OR: 3.8, $p = 0.01$) (Semaan et al. 2011). Moreover, GLUT-1 was found associated with tumor cell mitosis (Kim et al. 2012) and its overexpression predicted reduced OS and shorter DFS in epithelial OC (Cantuaria et al. 2001; Cho et al. 2013). In addition, HIF-α in OC, which is released as a homeostatic response to hypoxia, promotes vasculogenic mimicry to induce epithelial to mesenchymal transition (Du et al. 2014). Also, HIF-α expression was found associated with metastasis and reduced 5-year survival and poor OS (Shen et al. 2017; Jin et al. 2014a; Braicu et al. 2014; Shimogai et al. 2008). Notably, several authors have investigated the Warburg effect in OC as a source for energy supply (Zhang et al. 2018; Ma et al. 2018a; Shang et al. 2017b; Jin et al. 2014b). Some of these preclinical studies have also provided potential pharmacological inhibitors of aerobic glycolysis in OC such as ginsenoside (Lu et al. 2020; Zhou et al. 2018), ABT737 (a BH3 mimetic) (Dong et al. 2020), ivermectin (Li et al. 2020), and berberine (Li et al. 2021). One clinical trial has attempted to investigate an inhibitor of these pathways in OC. This was a phase II trial (NCT01652079) that enrolled 63 patients with recurrent platinum-resistant ovarian, fallopian tube, or peritoneal cancer to receive the anti-HIF-1α investigational nanoparticle-drug conjugate CRLX101 (camptothecin as the active molecule) in combination with bevacizumab. The latest available results of this two-stage trial and its preceding preclinical study showed that this combination is synergistic with durable inhibition of HIF-1α (Pham et al. 2015; Krasner et al. 2014, 2015, 2016). Very recently, the combination of EP0057 (formerly CRLX101) with weekly paclitaxel for recurrent or persistent epithelial ovarian, fallopian tube, or primary peritoneal cancer in a phase Ib/II trial (NCT02389985/$n = 30$) demonstrated an ORR of 31.6% in women with prior treatment with bevacizumab and one complete response (Duska et al. 2020). To the best of our knowledge, this study was terminated after the company decision.

3.3 Conclusion

With the emergence of data from large-scale sequencing projects, novel targets were discovered for OC. These actionable molecular alterations enabled enlargement of the current therapeutic arsenal against this aggressive cancer. Moreover, various biomarkers were also explored and seem to be promising for predicting prognosis and therapy response. There is a considerable move to exploit the hallmarks of cancer in improving outcomes and designing novel clinical trials for OC (Fig. 3.2). *Genome Instability, Inducing Angiogenesis, Avoiding Immune Destruction, and Sustaining Proliferative Signaling* were the most influencing hallmarks for the development of landmark phase III trials for OC. This list (Table 3.1) is expected to be extended in the future with newly launched phase III clinical studies which may supply the currently available treatments of OC with additional therapeutic approaches particularly targeted agents. Some signaling pathways that have a notable role in ovarian carcinogenesis were not discussed in this chapter because of the word limit and are illustrated elsewhere in other reviews (for further reading, see Box 3.1).

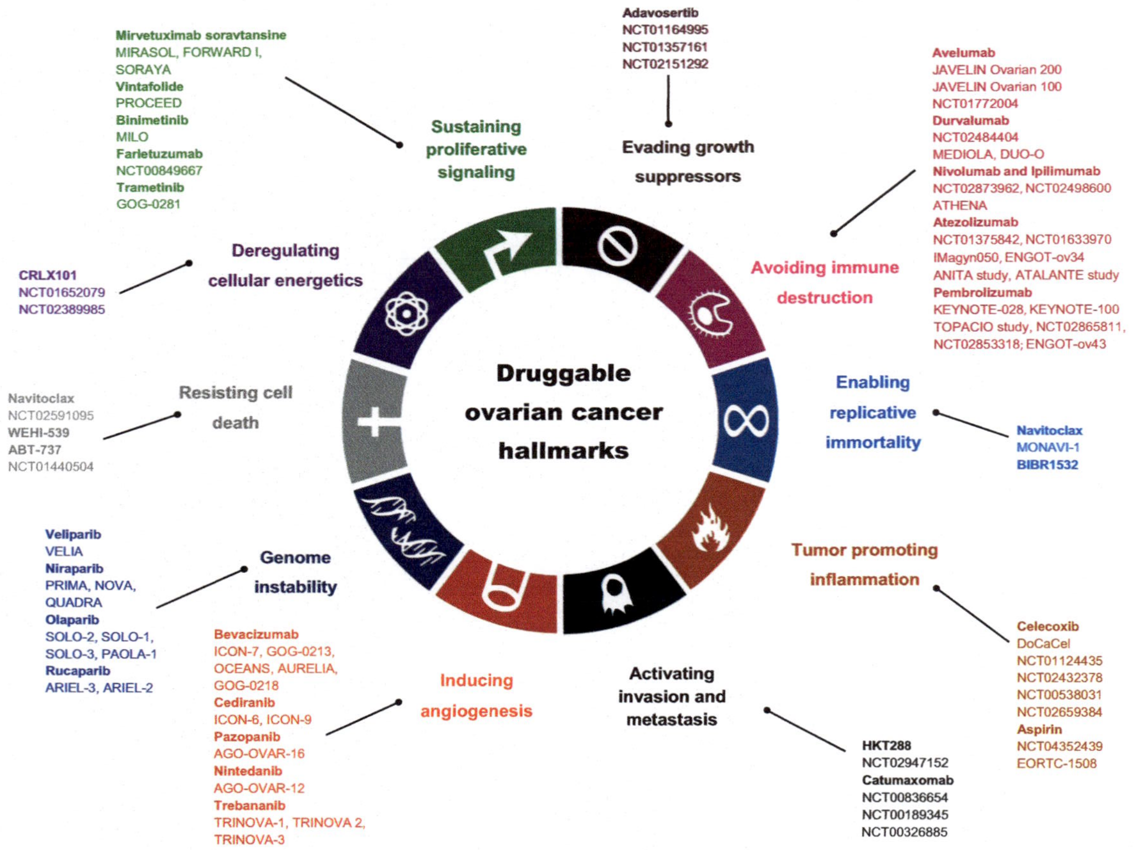

Fig. 3.2 Selected clinical studies using the hallmarks of ovarian cancer for drug development

Table 3.1 Selected phase III trials developed based on the concepts of "Cancer Hallmarks" in ovarian cancer

Cancer hallmarks	Trial name or NCT	Sample size	Anticancer drug	Disease setting	Study status
Genome instability	NOVA	553	Niraparib	Maintenance for recurrent platinum-sensitive	Completed
	SOLO-2	295	Olaparib		
	ARIEL-3	564	Rucaparib		
	SOLO-1	391	Olaparib	Maintenance in newly diagnosed	
	PAOLA-1	806			
	VELIA	1140	Veliparib	First-line and maintenance	
	PRIMA	733	Niraparib	First-line	
	SOLO-3	266	Olaparib	Recurrent platinum-sensitive	
Inducing angiogenesis	ICON-7	1528	Bevacizumab	First-line	Completed
	AURELIA	361		Recurrent platinum-resistant	
	GOG-0218	1873		First-line	
	GOG-0213	674		Recurrent platinum-sensitive	
	OCEANS	484			
	ICON-6	486	Cediranib		
	ICON-9	618			Ongoing
	TRINOVA-1	919	Trebananib	Recurrent	Completed
	TRINOVA-2	223		Recurrent partially platinum-sensitive or resistant	
	TRINOVA-3	1164		First-line	
	AGO-OVAR-12	1366	Nintedanib		
	AGO-OVAR-16	940	Pazopanib	First-line maintenance	

(continued)

Table 3.1 (continued)

Cancer hallmarks	Trial name or NCT	Sample size	Anticancer drug	Disease setting	Study status
Avoiding immune destruction	GOG-3036	1086	Pembrolizumab	First-line	Ongoing
	DUO-O	1254	Durvalumab		
	JAVELIN Ovarian 200	566	Avelumab	Recurrent platinum-resistant	Completed
	JAVELIN Ovarian 100	998		First-line	
	GOG-3020	1000	Nivolumab	First-line	Ongoing
	IMagyn050	1030	Atezolizumab		
	AGO-OVAR 2.29	664		Recurrent platinum-resistant	
	ANITA	414			
	ATALANTE	405		Recurrent platinum-sensitive	
Sustaining proliferative signaling	GOG-0281	260	Trametinib	Recurrent low-grade serous OC	Ongoing
	MIRASOL	430	Mirvetuximab soravtansine	Recurrent platinum-resistant	
	PROCEED	640	Vintafolide		Suspended
	SORAYA	110	Mirvetuximab soravtansine		Ongoing
	FORWARD I	333			Completed
	NCT00849667	1100	Farletuzumab	Recurrent platinum-sensitive	
	MILO	360	Binimetinib	Recurrent or persistent low-grade serous OC	

Box 3.1 Recommended reading of particular interest

Citation	DOI or PMID
Bogani G, et al. *Immunotherapy for platinum-resistant ovarian cancer*. Gynecol Oncol. 2020;158(2):484–488.	https://doi.org/10.1016/j.ygyno.2020.05.681
Madariaga A, et al. *Manage wisely: poly (ADP-ribose) polymerase inhibitor (PARPi) treatment and adverse events*. Int J Gynecol Cancer. 2020;30(7):903–915.	https://doi.org/10.1136/ijgc-2020-001288
Kuroki L, Guntupalli SR. *Treatment of epithelial ovarian cancer*. BMJ. 2020;371:m3773.	https://doi.org/10.1136/bmj.m3773
Moore KN, et al. *PARP inhibition in recurrent ovarian cancer*. Clin Adv Hematol Oncol. 2020;18(10):647–655.	33201871
Moore KN, et al. *PARP inhibition as frontline therapy in ovarian cancer*. Clin Adv Hematol Oncol. 2020;18 (9):550–556.	33006584
Pujade-Lauraine E, et al. *Management of Platinum-Resistant, Relapsed Epithelial Ovarian Cancer and New Drug Perspectives*. J Clin Oncol. 2019;37 (27):2437–2448.	https://doi.org/10.1200/JCO.19.00194
Pignata S, et al. *Treatment of recurrent ovarian cancer*. Ann Oncol. 2017;28(suppl_8):viii51–viii56.	https://doi.org/10.1093/annonc/mdx441
Keenan TE, et al. *Genomic correlates of response to immune checkpoint blockade*. Nat Med. 2019;25 (3):389–402.	https://doi.org/10.1038/s41591-019-0382-x
Lord CJ, Ashworth A. *BRCAness revisited*. Nat Rev Cancer. 2016;16(2):110–20.	https://doi.org/10.1038/nrc.2015.21
Byrum AK, et al. *Defining and Modulating 'BRCAness'*. Trends Cell Biol. 2019;29(9):740–751.	https://doi.org/10.1016/j.tcb.2019.06.005
Hoppenot C, et al. *Who are the long-term survivors of high grade serous ovarian cancer?* Gynecol Oncol. 2018;148(1):204–212.	https://doi.org/10.1016/j.ygyno.2017.10.032
Chartron E, et al. *Targeting homologous repair deficiency in breast and ovarian cancers: Biological pathways, preclinical and clinical data*. Crit Rev Oncol Hematol. 2019;133:58–73.	https://doi.org/10.1016/j.critrevonc.2018.10.012

Acknowledgment and Conflicts of Interest KE is an editor in Springer Nature Journals and a previous editor for a Springer book (https://link.springer.com/book/10.1007/978-3-030-53821-7). Other authors: none.

Authors' Contribution KE wrote the first draft and coordinated the development of the chapter and shared a preliminary content discussion. OA revised the manuscript and SA supervised the chapter writing. The final draft was reviewed and approved by all the authors. The contents of the chapter reflect the authors' perspectives and not of their institutions of affiliation.

References

Abdel-Rahman O, ElHalawani H, Ahmed H (2016) Doublet BRAF/MEK inhibition versus single-agent BRAF inhibition in the management of BRAF-mutant advanced melanoma, biological rationale and meta-analysis of published data. Clin Transl Oncol 18(8):848–858. https://doi.org/10.1007/s12094-015-1438-0

Abed MN, Abdullah MI, Richardson A (2016) Antagonism of Bcl-XL is necessary for synergy between carboplatin and BH3 mimetics in ovarian cancer cells. J Ovarian Res 9:25. https://doi.org/10.1186/s13048-016-0234-y

Adler E, Mhawech-Fauceglia P, Gayther SA, Lawrenson K (2015) PAX8 expression in ovarian surface epithelial cells. Hum Pathol 46(7):948–956

Aghajanian C, Blank SV, Goff BA, Judson PL, Teneriello MG, Husain A, Sovak MA, Yi J, Nycum LR (2012) OCEANS: a randomized, double-blind, placebo-controlled phase III trial of chemotherapy with or without bevacizumab in patients with platinum-sensitive recurrent epithelial ovarian, primary peritoneal, or fallopian tube cancer. J Clin Oncol 30(17):2039–2045. https://doi.org/10.1200/JCO.2012.42.0505

Aguilera A, García-Muse T (2013) Causes of genome instability. Annu Rev Genet 47:1–32. https://doi.org/10.1146/annurev-genet-111212-133232

Ahmed N, Thompson EW, Quinn MA (2007) Epithelial-mesenchymal interconversions in normal ovarian surface epithelium and ovarian carcinomas: an exception to the norm. J Cell Physiol 213 (3):581–588

Ahn JH, Kim TJ, Lee JH, Choi JH (2017) Mutant p53 stimulates cell invasion through an interaction with Rad21 in human ovarian cancer cells. Sci Rep 7(1):9076. https://doi.org/10.1038/s41598-017-08880-4

Almutairi AR, Alkhatib N, Martin J, Babiker HM, Garland LL, McBride A, Abraham I (2019) Comparative efficacy and safety of immunotherapies targeting the PD-1/PD-L1 pathway for previously treated advanced non-small cell lung cancer: a Bayesian network meta-analysis. Crit Rev Oncol Hematol 142:16–25. https://doi.org/10.1016/j.critrevonc.2019.07.004

Andrade RC, Dos Santos AC, de Aguirre Neto JC et al (2017) TP53 and CDKN1A mutation analysis in families with Li-Fraumeni and Li-Fraumeni like syndromes. Fam Cancer 16 (2):243–248. https://doi.org/10.1007/s10689-016-9935-z

André T, Shiu KK, Kim TW, Jensen BV, Jensen LH, Punt C, Smith D, Garcia-Carbonero R, Benavides M, Gibbs P, de la Fouchardiere C, Rivera F, Elez E, Bendell J, Le DT, Yoshino T, Van Cutsem E, Yang P, Farooqui MZH, Marinello P, Diaz LA Jr, KEYNOTE-177 Investigators (2020) Pembrolizumab in microsatellite-instability-high advanced colorectal cancer. N Engl J Med 383(23):2207–2218. https://doi.org/10.1056/NEJMoa2017699

Apte RS, Chen DS, Ferrara N (2019) VEGF in signaling and disease: beyond discovery and development. Cell 176(6):1248–1264. https://doi.org/10.1016/j.cell.2019.01.021

Armstrong DK, White AJ, Weil SC et al (2013) Farletuzumab (a monoclonal antibody against folate receptor alpha) in relapsed platinum-sensitive ovarian cancer. Gynecol Oncol 129(3):452–458. https://doi.org/10.1016/j.ygyno.2013.03.002

Arteaga CL, Engelman JA (2014) ERBB receptors: from oncogene discovery to basic science to mechanism-based cancer therapeutics. Cancer Cell 25(3):282–303

Ashaie MA, Chowdhury EH (2016) Cadherins: the superfamily critically involved in breast cancer. Curr Pharm Des 22(5):616–638

Ashkenazi A, Fairbrother WJ, Leverson JD, Souers AJ (2017) From basic apoptosis discoveries to advanced selective BCL-2 family inhibitors. Nat Rev Drug Discov 16(4):273–284. https://doi.org/10.1038/nrd.2016.253

Assaraf YG, Leamon CP, Reddy JA (2014) The folate receptor as a rational therapeutic target for personalized cancer treatment. Drug Resist Updat 17(4–6):89–95. https://doi.org/10.1016/j.drup.2014.10.002

Aubrey BJ, Strasser A, Kelly GL (2016) Tumor-suppressor functions of the TP53 pathway. Cold Spring Harb Perspect Med 6(5):a026062. https://doi.org/10.1101/cshperspect.a026062

Au-Yeung G, Lang F, Azar WJ et al (2016) Selective targeting of cyclin E1-amplified high-grade serous ovarian cancer by cyclin-dependent kinase 2 and AKT inhibition. Clin Cancer Res 23 (7):1862–1874

Ayhan A, Kuhn E, Wu RC et al (2017) CCNE1 copy-number gain and overexpression identify ovarian clear cell carcinoma with a poor prognosis. Mod Pathol 30(2):297–303. https://doi.org/10.1038/modpathol.2016.160

Aziz AUR, Farid S, Qin K, Wang H, Liu B (2018a) PIM kinases and their relevance to the PI3K/AKT/mTOR pathway in the regulation of ovarian cancer. Biomolecules 8(1):7. https://doi.org/10.3390/biom8010007

Aziz D, Etemadmoghadam D, Caldon CE et al (2018b) 19q12 amplified and non-amplified subsets of high grade serous ovarian cancer with overexpression of cyclin E1 differ in their molecular drivers and clinical outcomes. Gynecol Oncol 151(2):327–336. https://doi.org/10.1016/j.ygyno.2018.08.039

Bahar-Shany K, Brand H, Sapoznik S et al (2014) Exposure of fallopian tube epithelium to follicular fluid mimics carcinogenic changes in precursor lesions of serous papillary carcinoma. Gynecol Oncol 132(2):322–327. https://doi.org/10.1016/j.ygyno.2013.12.015

Bakkar RM, Xie SS, Urbauer DL et al (2015) Intact PTEN expression by immunohistochemistry is associated with decreased survival in advanced stage ovarian/primary peritoneal high-grade serous carcinoma. Int J Gynecol Pathol 34(6):497–506. https://doi.org/10.1097/PGP.0000000000000205

Bär C, Thum T (2017) Changing direction: from therapeutic telomerase inhibition to activation? Circ Res 120(9):1393–1395. https://doi.org/10.1161/CIRCRESAHA.116.310316

Barbolina MV (2018) Molecular mechanisms regulating organ-specific metastases in epithelial ovarian carcinoma. Cancers (Basel) 10(11):444. https://doi.org/10.3390/cancers10110444

Battista MJ, Cotarelo C, Jakobi S et al (2014) Overexpression of epithelial cell adhesion molecule protein is associated with favorable prognosis in an unselected cohort of ovarian cancer patients. J Cancer Res Clin Oncol 140(7):1097–1102. https://doi.org/10.1007/s00432-014-1672-9

Baumann K, Pfisterer J, Wimberger P et al (2011) Intraperitoneal treatment with the trifunctional bispecific antibody Catumaxomab in patients with platinum-resistant epithelial ovarian cancer: a phase IIa study of the AGO Study Group. Gynecol Oncol 123(1):27–32. https://doi.org/10.1016/j.ygyno.2011.06.004

Bayard Q, Meunier L, Peneau C et al (2018) Cyclin A2/E1 activation defines a hepatocellular carcinoma subclass with a rearrangement signature of replication stress. Nat Commun 9 (1):5235. https://doi.org/10.1038/s41467-018-07552-9

Beck A, Goetsch L, Dumontet C et al (2017) Strategies and challenges for the next generation of antibody-drug conjugates. Nat Rev Drug Discov 16(5):315–337. https://doi.org/10.1038/nrd.2016.268

Bedard PL, Tabernero J, Janku F et al (2015) A phase Ib dose-escalation study of the oral pan-PI3K inhibitor buparlisib (BKM120) in combination with the oral MEK1/2 inhibitor trametinib (GSK1120212) in patients with selected advanced solid tumors. Clin Cancer Res 21 (4):730–738. https://doi.org/10.1158/1078-0432.CCR-14-1814

Behbakht K, Sill MW, Darcy KM et al (2011) Phase II trial of the mTOR inhibitor, temsirolimus and evaluation of circulating tumor cells and tumor biomarkers in persistent and recurrent epithelial ovarian and primary peritoneal malignancies: a Gynecologic Oncology Group study. Gynecol Oncol 123(1):19–26

Bellone S, Siegel ER, Cocco E et al (2009) Overexpression of epithelial cell adhesion molecule in primary, metastatic, and recurrent/chemotherapy-resistant epithelial ovarian cancer: implications for epithelial cell adhesion molecule-specific immunotherapy. Int J Gynecol Cancer 19(5):860–866. https://doi.org/10.1111/IGC.0b013e3181a8331f

Bellone S, Buza N, Choi J, Zammataro L, Gay L, Elvin J, Rimm DL, Liu Y, Ratner ES, Schwartz PE, Santin AD (2018) Exceptional response to pembrolizumab in a metastatic, chemotherapy/radiation-resistant ovarian cancer patient harboring a PD-L1-genetic rearrangement. Clin Cancer Res 24(14):3282–3291. https://doi.org/10.1158/1078-0432.CCR-17-1805

Berek JS, Edwards RP, Parker LP et al (2014) Catumaxomab for the treatment of malignant ascites in patients with chemotherapy-refractory ovarian cancer: a phase II study. Int J Gynecol Cancer 24(9):1583–1589. https://doi.org/10.1097/IGC.0000000000000286

Bergamini A, Ferrero S, Leone Roberti Maggiore U et al (2016) Folate receptor alpha antagonists in preclinical and early stage clinical development for the treatment of epithelial ovarian cancer. Expert Opin Investig Drugs 25(12):1405–1412

Bernardini MQ, Baba T, Lee PS et al (2010) Expression signatures of TP53 mutations in serous ovarian cancers. BMC Cancer 10:237. https://doi.org/10.1186/1471-2407-10-237

Bialucha CU, Collins SD, Li X et al (2017) Discovery and optimization of HKT288, a cadherin-6-targeting ADC for the treatment of ovarian and renal cancers. Cancer Discov 7(9):1030–1045. https://doi.org/10.1158/2159-8290.CD-16-1414

Bielski CM, Zehir A, Penson AV et al (2018) Genome doubling shapes the evolution and prognosis of advanced cancers. Nat Genet 50(8):1189–1195

Bilanges B, Posor Y, Vanhaesebroeck B (2019) PI3K isoforms in cell signalling and vesicle trafficking. Nat Rev Mol Cell Biol 20(9):515–534. https://doi.org/10.1038/s41580-019-0129-z

Boers-Sonderen MJ, de Geus-Oei LF, Desar IM et al (2014) Temsirolimus and pegylated liposomal doxorubicin (PLD) combination therapy in breast, endometrial, and ovarian cancer: phase Ib results and prediction of clinical outcome with FDG-PET/CT. Target Oncol 9(4):339–347. https://doi.org/10.1007/s11523-014-0309-x

Bonnefond ML, Lambert B, Giffard F, Abeilard E, Brotin E, Louis MH, Gueye MS, Gauduchon P, Poulain L, N'Diaye M (2015) Calcium signals inhibition sensitizes ovarian carcinoma cells to anti-Bcl-xL strategies through Mcl-1 down-regulation. Apoptosis 20(4):535–550. https://doi.org/10.1007/s10495-015-1095-3

Bouaoun L, Sonkin D, Ardin M et al (2016) TP53 variations in human cancers: new lessons from the IARC TP53 database and genomics data. Hum Mutat 37(9):865–876. https://doi.org/10.1002/humu.23035

Brachet PE, Fabbro M, Leary A et al (2017) A gineco phase II study of navitoclax (abt 263) in women with platinum resistant/refractory recurrent ovarian cancer (roc). Ann Oncol 28. https://doi.org/10.1093/annonc/mdy285.179

Braem MG, Schouten LJ, Peeters PH et al (2011) Genetic susceptibility to sporadic ovarian cancer: a systematic review. Biochim Biophys Acta 1816(2):132–146. https://doi.org/10.1016/j.bbcan.2011.05.002

Braicu EI, Luketina H, Richter R, Cacsire Castillo-Tong D, Lambrechts S, Mahner S, Concin N, Mentze M, Zeillinger R, Vergote I, Sehouli J (2014) HIF1α is an independent prognostic factor for overall survival in advanced primary epithelial ovarian cancer – a study of the OVCAD Consortium. Onco Targets Ther 7:1563–1569. https://doi.org/10.2147/OTT.S65373

Bregar AJ, Growdon WB (2016) Emerging strategies for targeting PI3K in gynecologic cancer. Gynecol Oncol 140(2):333–344. https://doi.org/10.1016/j.ygyno.2015.09.083

Brosh R, Rotter V (2009) When mutants gain new powers: news from the mutant p53 field. Nat Rev Cancer 9(10):701–713. https://doi.org/10.1038/nrc2693

Brotin E, Meryet-Figuière M, Simonin K, Duval RE, Villedieu M, Leroy-Dudal J, Saison-Behmoaras E, Gauduchon P, Denoyelle C, Poulain L (2010) Bcl-XL and MCL-1 constitute pertinent targets in ovarian carcinoma and their concomitant inhibition is sufficient to induce apoptosis. Int J Cancer 126(4):885–895. https://doi.org/10.1002/ijc.24787

Brüser L, Bogdan S (2017) Adherens junctions on the move-membrane trafficking of e-cadherin. Cold Spring Harb Perspect Biol 9(3):a029140. https://doi.org/10.1101/cshperspect.a029140

Buderath P, Mairinger F, Mairinger E, Böhm K, Mach P, Schmid KW, Kimmig R, Kasimir-Bauer S, Bankfalvi A, Westerwick D, Hager T (2019) Prognostic significance of PD-1 and PD-L1 positive tumor-infiltrating immune cells in ovarian carcinoma. Int J Gynecol Cancer 29 (9):1389–1395. https://doi.org/10.1136/ijgc-2019-000609

Burger RA, Brady MF, Bookman MA, Fleming GF, Monk BJ, Huang H, Mannel RS, Homesley HD, Fowler J, Greer BE, Boente M, Birrer MJ, Liang SX, Gynecologic Oncology Group (2011)

Incorporation of bevacizumab in the primary treatment of ovarian cancer. N Engl J Med 365 (26):2473–2483. https://doi.org/10.1056/NEJMoa1104390
Cai J, Xu L, Tang H et al (2014) The role of the PTEN/PI3K/Akt pathway on prognosis in epithelial ovarian cancer: a meta-analysis. Oncologist 19(5):528–535
Cai L, Michelakos T, Ferrone CR et al (2017) Expression status of folate receptor alpha is a predictor of survival in pancreatic ductal adenocarcinoma. Oncotarget 8(23):37646–37656
Cancer Genome Atlas Research Network (2011) Integrated genomic analyses of ovarian carcinoma. Nature 474(7353):609–615. https://doi.org/10.1038/nature10166
Cantuaria G, Fagotti A, Ferrandina G, Magalhaes A, Nadji M, Angioli R, Penalver M, Mancuso S, Scambia G (2001) GLUT-1 expression in ovarian carcinoma: association with survival and response to chemotherapy. Cancer 92(5):1144–1150. https://doi.org/10.1002/1097-0142(20010901)92:5<1144::aid-cncr1432>3.0.co;2-t
Caramel J, Ligier M, Puisieux A (2018) Pleiotropic roles for ZEB1 in cancer. Cancer Res 78 (1):30–35. https://doi.org/10.1158/0008-5472.CAN-17-2476
Carneiro BA, El-Deiry WS (2020) Targeting apoptosis in cancer therapy. Nat Rev Clin Oncol 17 (7):395–417. https://doi.org/10.1038/s41571-020-0341-y
Castro MP, Whitcomb BP, Zajchowski DA, Coleman RL (2015) Successful use of next generation genomic sequencing (NGS)-directed therapy of clear cell carcinoma of the ovary (CCCO) with trametinib and metformin in a patient with chemotherapy-refractory disease. Gynecol Oncol Res Pract 2:4. https://doi.org/10.1186/s40661-015-0013-2
Chen J, Wang L, Matyunina LV, Hill CG, McDonald JF (2011) Overexpression of miR-429 induces mesenchymal-to-epithelial transition (MET) in metastatic ovarian cancer cells. Gynecol Oncol 121(1):200–205. https://doi.org/10.1016/j.ygyno.2010.12.339
Chen YL, Chang MC, Huang CY et al (2012) Serous ovarian carcinoma patients with high alpha-folate receptor had reducing survival and cytotoxic chemo-response. Mol Oncol 6(3):360–369
Chen C, Li J, Yao G, Chambers SK, Zheng W (2013) Tubal origin of ovarian low-grade serous carcinoma. Am J Clin Exp Obstet Gynecol 1(1):13–36
Chen Y, Wang DD, Wu YP et al (2017) MDM2 promotes epithelial-mesenchymal transition and metastasis of ovarian cancer SKOV3 cells. Br J Cancer 117(8):1192–1201
Chen H, Molberg K, Strickland AL, Castrillon DH, Carrick K, Jiang Q, Niu S, Rivera-Colon G, Gwin K, Hinson S, Lea J, Miller DS, Zheng W, Lucas E (2020) PD-L1 expression and CD8+ tumor-infiltrating lymphocytes in different types of tubo-ovarian carcinoma and their prognostic value in high-grade serous carcinoma. Am J Surg Pathol 44(8):1050–1060. https://doi.org/10.1097/PAS.0000000000001503
Cheung LW, Leung PC, Wong AS (2010) Cadherin switching and activation of p120 catenin signaling are mediators of gonadotropin-releasing hormone to promote tumor cell migration and invasion in ovarian cancer. Oncogene 29(16):2427–2440. https://doi.org/10.1038/onc.2009.523
Chien J, Sicotte H, Fan JB et al (2015) TP53 mutations, tetraploidy and homologous recombination repair defects in early stage high-grade serous ovarian cancer. Nucleic Acids Res 43 (14):6945–6958
Chmelarova M, Baranova I, Ruszova E et al (2018) Importance of cadherins methylation in ovarian cancer: a next generation sequencing approach. Pathol Oncol Res. https://doi.org/10.1007/s12253-018-0500-y
Cho H, Lee YS, Kim J, Chung JY, Kim JH (2013) Overexpression of glucose transporter-1 (GLUT-1) predicts poor prognosis in epithelial ovarian cancer. Cancer Invest 31(9):607–615. https://doi.org/10.3109/07357907.2013.849722
Chui MH, Wang Y, Wu RC et al (2014) Loss of ALDH1A1 expression is an early event in the pathogenesis of ovarian high-grade serous carcinoma. Mod Pathol 28(3):437–445
Cibula D, Zikan M, Dusek L et al (2011) Oral contraceptives and risk of ovarian and breast cancers in BRCA mutation carriers: a meta-analysis. Expert Rev Anticancer Ther 11(8):1197–1207. https://doi.org/10.1586/era.11.38
Coleman RL, Brady MF, Herzog TJ, Sabbatini P, Armstrong DK, Walker JL, Kim BG, Fujiwara K, Tewari KS, O'Malley DM, Davidson SA, Rubin SC, Di Silvestro P, Basen-Engquist K,

Huang H, Chan JK, Spirtos NM, Ashfaq R, Mannel RS (2017a) Bevacizumab and paclitaxel-carboplatin chemotherapy and secondary cytoreduction in recurrent, platinum-sensitive ovarian cancer (NRG Oncology/Gynecologic Oncology Group study GOG-0213): a multicentre, open-label, randomised, phase 3 trial. Lancet Oncol 18(6):779–791. https://doi.org/10.1016/S1470-2045(17)30279-6

Coleman RL, Oza AM, Lorusso D, Aghajanian C, Oaknin A, Dean A, Colombo N, Weberpals JI, Clamp A, Scambia G, Leary A, Holloway RW, Gancedo MA, Fong PC, Goh JC, O'Malley DM, Armstrong DK, Garcia-Donas J, Swisher EM, Floquet A, Konecny GE, McNeish IA, Scott CL, Cameron T, Maloney L, Isaacson J, Goble S, Grace C, Harding TC, Raponi M, Sun J, Lin KK, Giordano H, Ledermann JA, ARIEL3 Investigators (2017b) Rucaparib maintenance treatment for recurrent ovarian carcinoma after response to platinum therapy (ARIEL3): a randomised, double-blind, placebocontrolled, phase 3 trial. Lancet 390(10106):1949–1961. https://doi.org/10.1016/S01406736(17)32440-6. Epub 2017 Sep 12. Erratum in: Lancet. 2017 Oct 28;390(10106):1948

Coleman RL, Fleming GF, Brady MF, Swisher EM, Steffensen KD, Friedlander M, Okamoto A, Moore KN, Efrat Ben-Baruch N, Werner TL, Cloven NG, Oaknin A, Di Silvestro PA, Morgan MA, Nam JH, Leath CA III, Nicum S, Hagemann AR, Littell RD, Cella D, Baron-Hay S, Garcia-Donas J, Mizuno M, Bell-McGuinn K, Sullivan DM, Bach BA, Bhattacharya S, Ratajczak CK, Ansell PJ, Dinh MH, Aghajanian C, Bookman MA (2019) Veliparib with first-line chemotherapy and as maintenance therapy in ovarian cancer. N Engl J Med 381(25):2403–2415. https://doi.org/10.1056/NEJMoa1909707

Collaborative Group on Epidemiological Studies of Ovarian Cancer, Beral V, Doll R, et al. (2008) Ovarian cancer and oral contraceptives: collaborative reanalysis of data from 45 epidemiological studies including 23,257 women with ovarian cancer and 87,303 controls. Lancet 371(9609):303–314. https://doi.org/10.1016/S0140-6736(08)60167-1

Collins C, Nelson WJ (2015) Running with neighbors: coordinating cell migration and cell-cell adhesion. Curr Opin Cell Biol 36:62–70

Colon-Otero G, Weroha SJ, Foster NR et al (2017) Phase 2 trial of everolimus and letrozole in relapsed estrogen receptor-positive high-grade ovarian cancers. Gynecol Oncol 146(1):64–68. https://doi.org/10.1016/j.ygyno.2017.04.020

Cormedi MCV, Van Allen EM, Colli LM (2020) Predicting immunotherapy response through genomics. Curr Opin Genet Dev 66:1–9. https://doi.org/10.1016/j.gde.2020.11.004

Cossa G, Lanzi C, Cassinelli G et al (2014) Differential outcome of MEK1/2 inhibitor-platinum combinations in platinum-sensitive and -resistant ovarian carcinoma cells. Cancer Lett 347(2):212–224. https://doi.org/10.1016/j.canlet.2014.02.016

Cui Y, Qin L, Tian D et al (2018) ZEB1 promotes chemoresistance to cisplatin in ovarian cancer cells by suppressing SLC3A2. Chemotherapy 63(5):262–271. https://doi.org/10.1159/000493864

Damen MPF, van Rheenen J, Scheele CLGJ (2020) Targeting dormant tumor cells to prevent cancer recurrence. FEBS J. https://doi.org/10.1111/febs.15626

De Luca A, Maiello MR, D'Alessio A et al (2012) The RAS/RAF/MEK/ERK and the PI3K/AKT signalling pathways: role in cancer pathogenesis and implications for therapeutic approaches. Expert Opin Ther Targets 16(Suppl 2):S17–S27. https://doi.org/10.1517/14728222.2011.639361

De Palma M, Hanahan D (2012) The biology of personalized cancer medicine: facing individual complexities underlying hallmark capabilities. Mol Oncol 6(2):111–127. https://doi.org/10.1016/j.molonc.2012.01.011

De Picciotto N, Cacheux W, Roth A et al (2016) Ovarian cancer: status of homologous recombination pathway as a predictor of drug response. Crit Rev Oncol 101:50–59. https://doi.org/10.1016/j.critrevonc.2016.02.014

de Wit S, Rossi E, Weber S et al (2019) Single tube liquid biopsy for advanced non-small cell lung cancer. Int J Cancer 144(12):3127–3137. https://doi.org/10.1002/ijc.32056

DeFazio A, Moujaber T, Etemadmoghadam D, Kennedy C, Chiew YE, Balleine RL et al (2016) Abstract A25: brafv600E mutations in serous ovarian cancer and response to the BRAF inhibitor, dabrafenib. Clin Cancer Res 22:a25. https://doi.org/10.1158/1557-3265.OVCA15-A25

Della Pepa C, Tonini G, Santini D et al (2015) Low Grade Serous Ovarian Carcinoma: from the molecular characterization to the best therapeutic strategy. Cancer Treat Rev 41(2):136–143. https://doi.org/10.1016/j.ctrv.2014.12.003

Demir L, Yigit S, Sadullahoglu C et al (2014) Hormone receptor, HER2/NEU and EGFR expression in ovarian carcinoma–is here a prognostic phenotype? Asian Pac J Cancer Prev 15 (22):9739–9745

Deng L, Feng DQ, Ling B (2020) Cyclooxygenase-2 promotes ovarian cancer cell migration and cisplatin resistance via regulating epithelial mesenchymal transition. J Zhejiang Univ Sci B 21 (4):315–326. https://doi.org/10.1631/jzus.B1900445

Despierre E et al (2015) Epidermal growth factor receptor (EGFR) pathway biomarkers in the randomized phase III trial of erlotinib versus observation in ovarian cancer patients with no evidence of disease progression after first-line platinum-based chemotherapy. Target Oncol 10 (4):583–596

Dhillon S (2016) Dabrafenib plus trametinib: a review in advanced melanoma with a BRAF (V600) mutation. Target Oncol 11(3):417–428. https://doi.org/10.1007/s11523-016-0443-8

Di Fiore R, D'Anneo A, Tesoriere G et al (2013) RB1 in cancer: different mechanisms of RB1 inactivation and alterations of pRb pathway in tumorigenesis. J Cell Physiol 228(8):1676–1687. https://doi.org/10.1002/jcp.24329

Diakos CI, Charles KA, McMillan DC et al (2014) Cancer-related inflammation and treatment effectiveness. Lancet Oncol 15(11):e493–e503. https://doi.org/10.1016/S1470-2045(14)70263-3

Dick FA, Rubin SM (2013) Molecular mechanisms underlying RB protein function. Nat Rev Mol Cell Biol 14(5):297–306

Disis ML, Taylor MH, Kelly K et al (2019) Efficacy and safety of avelumab for patients with recurrent or refractory ovarian cancer: phase 1b results from the JAVELIN solid tumor trial. JAMA Oncol 5(3):393–401. https://doi.org/10.1001/jamaoncol.2018.6258

Dong D, Dong Y, Fu J, Lu S, Yuan C, Xia M, Sun L (2020) Bcl2 inhibitor ABT737 reverses the Warburg effect via the Sirt3-HIF1α axis to promote oxidative stress-induced apoptosis in ovarian cancer cells. Life Sci 255:117846. https://doi.org/10.1016/j.lfs.2020.117846

Drew Y, Penson RT, O'Malley DM et al (2020) Phase II study of olaparib (O) plus durvalumab (D) and bevacizumab (B) (MEDIOLA): initial results in patients (pts) with non-germline BRCA-mutated (non-gBRCAm) platinum sensitive relapsed (PSR) ovarian cancer (OC) [ESMO abstract 814MO]. Ann Oncol 31(Suppl 4):S615–S616

du Bois A, Floquet A, Kim JW, Rau J, del Campo JM, Friedlander M, Pignata S, Fujiwara K, Vergote I, Colombo N, Mirza MR, Monk BJ, Kimmig R, Ray-Coquard I, Zang R, Diaz-Padilla I, Baumann KH, Mouret-Reynier MA, Kim JH, Kurzeder C, Lesoin A, Vasey P, Marth C, Canzler U, Scambia G, Shimada M, Calvert P, Pujade-Lauraine E, Kim BG, Herzog TJ, Mitrica I, Schade-Brittinger C, Wang Q, Crescenzo R, Harter P (2014) Incorporation of pazopanib in maintenance therapy of ovarian cancer. J Clin Oncol 32(30):3374–3382. https://doi.org/10.1200/JCO.2014.55.7348

du Bois A, Kristensen G, Ray-Coquard I, Reuss A, Pignata S, Colombo N, Denison U, Vergote I, Del Campo JM, Ottevanger P, Heubner M, Minarik T, Sevin E, de Gregorio N, Bidziński M, Pfisterer J, Malander S, Hilpert F, Mirza MR, Scambia G, Meier W, Nicoletto MO, Bjørge L, Lortholary A, Sailer MO, Merger M, Harter P, AGO Study Group led Gynecologic Cancer Intergroup/European Network of Gynaecologic Oncology Trials Groups Intergroup Consortium (2016) Standard first-line chemotherapy with or without nintedanib for advanced ovarian cancer (AGO-OVAR 12): a randomised, double-blind, placebo-controlled phase 3 trial. Lancet Oncol 17(1):78–89. https://doi.org/10.1016/S1470-2045(15)00366-6

Du J, Sun B, Zhao X, Gu Q, Dong X, Mo J, Sun T, Wang J, Sun R, Liu Y (2014) Hypoxia promotes vasculogenic mimicry formation by inducing epithelial-mesenchymal transition in ovarian carcinoma. Gynecol Oncol 133(3):575–583. https://doi.org/10.1016/j.ygyno.2014.02.034

Du ZH, Bi FF, Wang L, Yang Q (2018) Next-generation sequencing unravels extensive genetic alteration in recurrent ovarian cancer and unique genetic changes in drug-resistant recurrent ovarian cancer. Mol Genet Genomic Med 6(4):638–647. https://doi.org/10.1002/mgg3.414

Duska LR, Krasner CN, O'Malley DM, Hays JL, Modesitt SC, Mathews CA, Moore KN, Thaker PH, Miller A, Purdy C, Zamboni WC, Lucas AT, Supko JG, Schilder RJ (2020) A phase Ib/II and pharmacokinetic study of EP0057 (formerly CRLX101) in combination with weekly paclitaxel in patients with recurrent or persistent epithelial ovarian, fallopian tube, or primary peritoneal cancer. Gynecol Oncol. S0090-8258(20)34228-1. https://doi.org/10.1016/j.ygyno.2020.12.025

Ebnet K, Kummer D, Steinbacher T et al (2018) Regulation of cell polarity by cell adhesion receptors. Semin Cell Dev Biol 81:2–12. https://doi.org/10.1016/j.semcdb.2017.07.032

El Bairi K, Amrani M, Maleb A (2020) Gut microbiota, next-generation sequencing, immune-checkpoint inhibitors, and colorectal cancer: how hot is the link? In: El Bairi K (ed) Illuminating colorectal cancer genomics by next-generation sequencing. Springer, Cham. https://doi.org/10.1007/978-3-030-53821-7_5

El Bairi K, Al Jarroudi O, Afqir S (2021) Revisiting antibody-drug conjugates and their predictive biomarkers in platinum-resistant ovarian cancer. Semin Cancer Biol. S1044-579X(21)00081-X. https://doi.org/10.1016/j.semcancer.2021.03.031

Elyashiv O, Ledermann J, Parmar G, Farrelly L, Counsell N, Feeney A, El-Khouly F, Macdonald I, Neto A, Arthur-Darkwa E, Burnett E, Jayson GC, Mileshkin L, Gourley C, Nicum S (2021) ICON 9-an international phase III randomized study to evaluate the efficacy of maintenance therapy with olaparib and cediranib or olaparib alone in patients with relapsed platinum-sensitive ovarian cancer following a response to platinum-based chemotherapy. Int J Gynecol Cancer 31(1):134–138. https://doi.org/10.1136/ijgc-2020-002073

Emons G, Kurzeder C, Schmalfeldt B et al (2016) Temsirolimus in women with platinum-refractory/resistant ovarian cancer or advanced/recurrent endometrial carcinoma. A phase II study of the AGO-study group (AGO-GYN8). Gynecol Oncol 140(3):450–456. https://doi.org/10.1016/j.ygyno.2015.12.025

Endo H, Inoue M (2019) Dormancy in cancer. Cancer Sci 110(2):474–480. https://doi.org/10.1111/cas.13917

Etemadmoghadam D, de Fazio A, Beroukhim R, Mermel C, George J, Getz G, Tothill R, Okamoto A, Raeder MB, Harnett P, Lade S, Akslen LA, Tinker AV, Locandro B, Alsop K, Chiew YE, Traficante N, Fereday S, Johnson D, Fox S, Sellers W, Urashima M, Salvesen HB, Meyerson M, Bowtell D, AOCS Study Group (2009) Integrated genome-wide DNA copy number and expression analysis identifies distinct mechanisms of primary chemoresistance in ovarian carcinomas. Clin Cancer Res 15(4):1417–1427. https://doi.org/10.1158/1078-0432.CCR-08-1564

Etemadmoghadam D, George J, Cowin PA et al (2010) Amplicon-dependent CCNE1 expression is critical for clonogenic survival after cisplatin treatment and is correlated with 20q11 gain in ovarian cancer. PLoS One 5(11):e15498. https://doi.org/10.1371/journal.pone.0015498

Etemadmoghadam D, Au-Yeung G, Wall M et al (2013a) Resistance to CDK2 inhibitors is associated with selection of polyploid cells in CCNE1-amplified ovarian cancer. Clin Cancer Res 19(21):5960–5971. https://doi.org/10.1158/1078-0432.CCR-13-1337

Etemadmoghadam D, Weir BA, Au-Yeung G et al (2013b) Synthetic lethality between CCNE1 amplification and loss of BRCA1. Proc Natl Acad Sci U S A 110(48):19489–19494

Fardi M, Alivand M, Baradaran B, Farshdousti Hagh M, Solali S (2019) The crucial role of ZEB2: from development to epithelial-to-mesenchymal transition and cancer complexity. J Cell Physiol. https://doi.org/10.1002/jcp.28277

Färkkilä A, Gulhan DC, Casado J et al (2020) Immunogenomic profiling determines responses to combined PARP and PD-1 inhibition in ovarian cancer [published correction appears in Nat

Commun 2020;11(1):2543]. Nat Commun 11(1):1459. https://doi.org/10.1038/s41467-020-15315-8

Farley J, Brady WE, Vathipadiekal V et al (2013) Selumetinib in women with recurrent low-grade serous carcinoma of the ovary or peritoneum: an open-label, single-arm, phase 2 study. Lancet Oncol 14(2):134–140

Fernández ML, DiMattia GE, Dawson A et al (2016) Differences in MEK inhibitor efficacy in molecularly characterized low-grade serous ovarian cancer cell lines. Am J Cancer Res 6 (10):2235–2251

Fernandez ML, Dawson A, Hoenisch J et al (2019) Markers of MEK inhibitor resistance in low-grade serous ovarian cancer: EGFR is a potential therapeutic target. Cancer Cell Int 19:10. https://doi.org/10.1186/s12935-019-0725-1

Ferreira AR, Felgueiras J, Fardilha M (2015) Signaling pathways in anchoring junctions of epithelial cells: cell-to-cell and cell-to-extracellular matrix interactions. J Recept Signal Transduct Res 35(1):67–75. https://doi.org/10.3109/10799893.2014.931426

Flesken-Nikitin A, Hwang CI, Cheng CY, Michurina TV, Enikolopov G, Nikitin AY (2013) Ovarian surface epithelium at the junction area contains a cancer-prone stem cell niche. Nature 495(7440):241–245

Florent R, Weiswald LB, Lambert B, Brotin E, Abeilard E, Louis MH, Babin G, Poulain L, N'Diaye M (2020a) Bim, Puma and Noxa upregulation by Naftopidil sensitizes ovarian cancer to the BH3-mimetic ABT-737 and the MEK inhibitor Trametinib. Cell Death Dis 11(5):380. https://doi.org/10.1038/s41419-020-2588-8

Florent R, Poulain L, N'Diaye M (2020b) Drug repositioning of the α1-adrenergic receptor antagonist naftopidil: a potential new anti-cancer drug? Int J Mol Sci 21(15):5339. https://doi.org/10.3390/ijms21155339

Fortner RT, Poole EM, Wentzensen NA et al (2018) Ovarian cancer risk factors by tumor aggressiveness: an analysis from the Ovarian Cancer Cohort Consortium. Int J Cancer. https://doi.org/10.1002/ijc.32075

Fotiadis D, Kanai Y, Palacín M (2013) The SLC3 and SLC7 families of amino acid transporters. Mol Aspects Med 34(2–3):139–158. https://doi.org/10.1016/j.mam.2012.10.007

Fowler M (2020) Mirvetuximab soravtansine combination yields encouraging response rates in ovarian cancer. Oncology (Williston Park) 34(7):250

Frampton JE (2012) Catumaxomab: in malignant ascites. Drugs 72(10):1399–1410. https://doi.org/10.2165/11209040-000000000-00000

Franzese E, Diana A, Centonze S et al (2020) PARP inhibitors in first-line therapy of ovarian cancer: are there any doubts? Front Oncol 10:782. https://doi.org/10.3389/fonc.2020.00782

Friese C, Harbst K, Borch TH, Westergaard MCW, Pedersen M, Kverneland A, Jönsson G, Donia M, Svane IM, Met Ö (2020) CTLA-4 blockade boosts the expansion of tumor-reactive CD8+ tumor-infiltrating lymphocytes in ovarian cancer. Sci Rep 10(1):3914. https://doi.org/10.1038/s41598-020-60738-4

Fruman DA, Rommel C (2014) PI3K and cancer: lessons, challenges and opportunities. Nat Rev Drug Discov 13(2):140–156

Fu S, Hennessy BT, Ng CS et al (2012) Perifosine plus docetaxel in patients with platinum and taxane resistant or refractory high-grade epithelial ovarian cancer. Gynecol Oncol 126 (1):47–53. https://doi.org/10.1016/j.ygyno.2012.04.006

Fumet JD, Truntzer C, Yarchoan M, Ghiringhelli F (2020) Tumour mutational burden as a biomarker for immunotherapy: current data and emerging concepts. Eur J Cancer 131:40–50. https://doi.org/10.1016/j.ejca.2020.02.038

Galluzzi L, Kepp O, Chan FK, Kroemer G (2017) Necroptosis: mechanisms and relevance to disease. Annu Rev Pathol 12:103–130. https://doi.org/10.1146/annurev-pathol-052016-100247

Galluzzi L, Vitale I, Aaronson SA et al (2018) Molecular mechanisms of cell death: recommendations of the Nomenclature Committee on Cell Death 2018. Cell Death Differ 25 (3):486–541. https://doi.org/10.1038/s41418-017-0012-4

Gao H, Li X, Zhan G et al (2019) Long noncoding RNA MAGI1-IT1 promoted invasion and metastasis of epithelial ovarian cancer via the miR-200a/ZEB axis. Cell Cycle 18 (12):1393–1406. https://doi.org/10.1080/15384101.2019.1618121

Garsed DW, Alsop K, Fereday S et al (2018) Homologous recombination DNA repair pathway disruption and retinoblastoma protein loss are associated with exceptional survival in high-grade serous ovarian cancer. Clin Cancer Res 24(3):569–580. https://doi.org/10.1158/1078-0432.CCR-17-1621

Gershenson DM, Sun CC, Wong KK (2015) Impact of mutational status on survival in low-grade serous carcinoma of the ovary or peritoneum. Br J Cancer 113(9):1254–1258

Gewinner C, Wang ZC, Richardson A et al (2009) Evidence that inositol polyphosphate 4-phosphatase type II is a tumor suppressor that inhibits PI3K signaling. Cancer Cell 16 (2):115–125

Gheldof A, Berx G (2013) Cadherins and epithelial-to-mesenchymal transition. Prog Mol Biol Transl Sci 116:317–336. https://doi.org/10.1016/B978-0-12-394311-8.00014-5

Ghezelayagh TS, Pennington KP, Norquist BM et al (2020) Characterizing TP53 mutations in ovarian carcinomas with and without concurrent BRCA1 or BRCA2 mutations. Gynecol Oncol. https://doi.org/10.1016/j.ygyno.2020.12.007

Ghigo A, Morello F, Perino A et al (2012) Phosphoinositide 3-kinases in health and disease. Subcell Biochem 58:183–213. https://doi.org/10.1007/978-94-007-3012-0_6

Ginter PS, McIntire PJ, Cui X et al (2017) Folate receptor alpha expression is associated with increased risk of recurrence in triple-negative breast cancer. Clin Breast Cancer 17(7):544–549. https://doi.org/10.1016/j.clbc.2017.03.007

Gloushankova NA, Rubtsova SN, Zhitnyak IY (2017) Cadherin-mediated cell-cell interactions in normal and cancer cells. Tissue Barriers 5(3):e1356900

González-Martín A, Pothuri B, Vergote I, DePont Christensen R, Graybill W, Mirza MR, McCormick C, Lorusso D, Hoskins P, Freyer G, Baumann K, Jardon K, Redondo A, Moore RG, Vulsteke C, O'Cearbhaill RE, Lund B, Backes F, Barretina-Ginesta P, Haggerty AF, Rubio-Pérez MJ, Shahin MS, Mangili G, Bradley WH, Bruchim I, Sun K, Malinowska IA, Li Y, Gupta D, Monk BJ, PRIMA/ENGOT-OV26/GOG-3012 Investigators (2019) Niraparib in patients with newly diagnosed advanced ovarian cancer. N Engl J Med 381(25):2391–2402. https://doi.org/10.1056/NEJMoa1910962

González-Martín A, Sanchez Lorenzo L, Colombo N, dePont Christensen R, Heitz F, Meirovitz M, Selle F, van Gorp T, Alvarez N, Sanchez J, Marqués C (2020) A phase III, randomized, double blinded trial of platinum based chemotherapy with or without atezolizumab followed by niraparib maintenance with or without atezolizumab in patients with recurrent ovarian, tubal, or peritoneal cancer and platinum treatment free interval of more than 6 months: engot-Ov41/GEICO 69-O/ANITA Trial. Int J Gynecol Cancer. https://doi.org/10.1136/ijgc-2020-001633

Grisham RN, Iyer G, Garg K et al (2012) BRAF mutation is associated with early stage disease and improved outcome in patients with low-grade serous ovarian cancer. Cancer 119(3):548–554

Grisham RN, Moore KN, Gordon MS et al (2018) Phase Ib study of binimetinib with paclitaxel in patients with platinum-resistant ovarian cancer: final results, potential biomarkers, and extreme responders. Clin Cancer Res 24(22):5525–5533. https://doi.org/10.1158/1078-0432.CCR-18-0494

Grover PK, Cummins AG, Price TJ, Roberts-Thomson IC, Hardingham JE (2014) Circulating tumour cells: the evolving concept and the inadequacy of their enrichment by EpCAM-based methodology for basic and clinical cancer research. Ann Oncol 25(8):1506–1516. https://doi.org/10.1093/annonc/mdu018

Gruosso T, Garnier C, Abelanet S et al (2015) MAP3K8/TPL-2/COT is a potential predictive marker for MEK inhibitor treatment in high-grade serous ovarian carcinomas. Nat Commun 6:8583. https://doi.org/10.1038/ncomms9583

Gugnoni M, Sancisi V, Gandolfi G et al (2017) Cadherin-6 promotes EMT and cancer metastasis by restraining autophagy. Oncogene 36(5):667–677. https://doi.org/10.1038/onc.2016.237

Guha T, Malkin D (2017) Inherited TP53 mutations and the Li-Fraumeni syndrome. Cold Spring Harb Perspect Med 7(4). pii: a026187. https://doi.org/10.1101/cshperspect.a026187

Gupta R, Cristea M, Frankel P, Ruel C, Chen C, Wang Y, Morgan R, Leong L, Chow W, Koczywas M, Koehler S, Lim D, Luu T, Martel C, McNamara M, Somlo G, Twardowski P, Yen Y, Idorenyi A, Raechelle T, Carroll M, Chung V (2019) Randomized trial of oral cyclophosphamide versus oral cyclophosphamide with celecoxib for recurrent epithelial ovarian, fallopian tube, and primary peritoneal cancer. Cancer Treat Res Commun 21:100155. https://doi.org/10.1016/j.ctarc.2019.100155

Hainaut P, Pfeifer GP (2016) Somatic TP53 mutations in the era of genome sequencing. Cold Spring Harb Perspect Med 6(11):a026179. https://doi.org/10.1101/cshperspect.a026179

Hamanishi J, Mandai M, Ikeda T, Minami M, Kawaguchi A, Murayama T, Kanai M, Mori Y, Matsumoto S, Chikuma S, Matsumura N, Abiko K, Baba T, Yamaguchi K, Ueda A, Hosoe Y, Morita S, Yokode M, Shimizu A, Honjo T, Konishi I (2015) Safety and antitumor activity of anti-PD-1 antibody, nivolumab, in patients with platinum-resistant ovarian cancer. J Clin Oncol 33(34):4015–4022. https://doi.org/10.1200/JCO.2015.62.3397

Han C, Bellone S, Zammataro L, Schwartz PE, Santin AD (2018) Binimetinib (MEK162) in recurrent low-grade serous ovarian cancer resistant to chemotherapy and hormonal treatment. Gynecol Oncol Rep 25:41–44. https://doi.org/10.1016/j.gore.2018.05.011

Hanahan D, Coussens LM (2012) Accessories to the crime: functions of cells recruited to the tumor microenvironment. Cancer Cell 21(3):309–322. https://doi.org/10.1016/j.ccr.2012.02.022

Hanahan D, Weinberg RA (2000) The hallmarks of cancer. Cell 100(1):57–70. https://doi.org/10.1016/s0092-8674(00)81683-9

Hanahan D, Weinberg RA (2011) Hallmarks of cancer: the next generation. Cell 14:646–674. https://doi.org/10.1016/j.cell.2011.02.013

Hao J, Yu H, Zhang T, An R, Xue Y (2020) Prognostic impact of tumor-infiltrating lymphocytes in high grade serous ovarian cancer: a systematic review and meta-analysis. Ther Adv Med Oncol 12:1758835920967241. https://doi.org/10.1177/1758835920967241

Hao J, Liu Y, Zhang T, He J, Zhao H, An R, Xue Y (2021) Efficacy and safety of PARP inhibitors in the treatment of advanced ovarian cancer: an updated systematic review and meta-analysis of randomized controlled trials. Crit Rev Oncol Hematol 157:103145. https://doi.org/10.1016/j.critrevonc.2020.103145

Harter P, Pautier P, Van Nieuwenhuysen E, Reuss A, Redondo A, Lindemann K, Kurzeder C, Petru E, Heitz F, Sehouli J, Degregorio N, Wimberger P, Burges A, Cron N, Ledermann J, Lorusso D, Paoletti X, Marme F (2020) Atezolizumab in combination with bevacizumab and chemotherapy versus bevacizumab and chemotherapy in recurrent ovarian cancer – a randomized phase III trial (AGO-OVAR 2.29/ENGOT-ov34). Int J Gynecol Cancer 30 (12):1997–2001. https://doi.org/10.1136/ijgc-2020-001572

Hasegawa K, Kagabu M, Mizuno M et al (2017) Phase II basket trial of perifosine monotherapy for recurrent gynecologic cancer with or without PIK3CA mutations. Invest New Drugs 35 (6):800–812. https://doi.org/10.1007/s10637-017-0504-6

Havrilesky LJ, Moorman PG, Lowery WJ et al (2013) Oral contraceptive pills as primary prevention for ovarian cancer: a systematic review and meta-analysis. Obstet Gynecol 122(1):139–147. https://doi.org/10.1097/AOG.0b013e318291c235

Hazan RB, Qiao R, Keren R, Badano I, Suyama K (2004) Cadherin switch in tumor progression. Ann N Y Acad Sci 1014:155–163. https://doi.org/10.1196/annals.1294.016

Heiss MM, Murawa P, Koralewski P et al (2010) The trifunctional antibody catumaxomab for the treatment of malignant ascites due to epithelial cancer: results of a prospective randomized phase II/III trial. Int J Cancer 127(9):2209–2221. https://doi.org/10.1002/ijc.25423

Herreros-Pomares A, Aguilar-Gallardo C, Calabuig-Fariñas S, Sirera R, Jantus-Lewintre E, Camps C (2018) EpCAM duality becomes this molecule in a new Dr. Jekyll and Mr. Hyde tale. Crit Rev Oncol Hematol 126:52–63. https://doi.org/10.1016/j.critrevonc.2018.03.006

Hew KE, Miller PC, El-Ashry D et al (2015) MAPK activation predicts poor outcome and the MEK inhibitor, selumetinib, reverses antiestrogen resistance in ER-positive high-grade serous ovarian cancer. Clin Cancer Res 22(4):935–947

Høgdall EV, Christensen L, Kjaer SK, Blaakaer J, Christensen IJ, Høgdall CK (2010) Limited prognostic value of tissue protein expression levels of BCl-2 in Danish ovarian cancer patients: from the Danish 'MALOVA' ovarian cancer study. APMIS 118(8):557–564. https://doi.org/10.1111/j.1600-0463.2010.02614.x

Hortobagyi GN, Stemmer SM, Burris HA et al (2016) Ribociclib as first-line therapy for HR-positive, advanced breast cancer. N Engl J Med 375(18):1738–1748

Huang LN, Wang DS, Chen YQ et al (2012) Meta-analysis for cyclin E in lung cancer survival. Clin Chim Acta 413(7-8):663–668. https://doi.org/10.1016/j.cca.2011.12.020

Huang TB, Yan Y, Guo ZF et al (2014a) Aspirin use and the risk of prostate cancer: a metaanalysis of 24 epidemiologic studies. Int Urol Nephrol 46(9):1715–1728. https://doi.org/10.1007/s11255-014-0703-4

Huang HN, Huang WC, Lin CH et al (2014b) Chromosome 20q13.2 ZNF217 locus amplification correlates with decreased E-cadherin expression in ovarian clear cell carcinoma with PI3K-Akt pathway alterations. Hum Pathol 45(11):2318–2325. https://doi.org/10.1016/j.humpath.2014.07.020

Huang HS, Chu SC, Hsu CF et al (2015) Mutagenic, surviving and tumorigenic effects of follicular fluid in the context of p53 loss: initiation of fimbria carcinogenesis. Carcinogenesis 36(11):1419–1428. https://doi.org/10.1093/carcin/bgv132

Hudson LG, Zeineldin R, Stack MS (2008) Phenotypic plasticity of neoplastic ovarian epithelium: unique cadherin profiles in tumor progression. Clin Exp Metastasis 25(6):643–655

Hui G, Meng M (2015) Prognostic value of vascular endothelial growth factor expression in women with ovarian cancer: a meta-analysis. J BUON 20(3):870–878

Hwang WT, Adams SF, Tahirovic E, Hagemann IS, Coukos G (2012) Prognostic significance of tumor-infiltrating T cells in ovarian cancer: a meta-analysis. Gynecol Oncol 124(2):192–198. https://doi.org/10.1016/j.ygyno.2011.09.039

Iavarone C, Zervantonakis IK, Selfors LM, Palakurthi S, Liu JF, Drapkin R, Matulonis UA, Hallberg D, Velculescu VE, Leverson JD, Sampath D, Mills GB, Brugge JS (2019) Combined MEK and BCL-2/XL inhibition is effective in high-grade serous ovarian cancer patient-derived xenograft models and BIM levels are predictive of responsiveness. Mol Cancer Ther 18(3):642–655. https://doi.org/10.1158/1535-7163.MCT-18-0413

Icard P, Shulman S, Farhat D, Steyaert JM, Alifano M, Lincet H (2018) How the Warburg effect supports aggressiveness and drug resistance of cancer cells? Drug Resist Updat 38:1–11. https://doi.org/10.1016/j.drup.2018.03.001

Iyengar M, O'Hayer P, Cole A et al (2018) CDK4/6 inhibition as maintenance and combination therapy for high grade serous ovarian cancer. Oncotarget 9(21):15658–15672. https://doi.org/10.18632/oncotarget.24585

James FR, Jiminez-Linan M, Alsop J, Mack M, Song H, Brenton JD, Pharoah PDP, Ali HR (2017) Association between tumour infiltrating lymphocytes, histotype and clinical outcome in epithelial ovarian cancer. BMC Cancer 17(1):657. https://doi.org/10.1186/s12885-017-3585-x

Jia P, Zhao Z (2019) Characterization of tumor-suppressor gene inactivation events in 33 cancer types. Cell Rep 26(2):496–506.e3. https://doi.org/10.1016/j.celrep.2018.12.066

Jiao S, Xia W, Yamaguchi H, Wei Y, Chen MK, Hsu JM, Hsu JL, Yu WH, Du Y, Lee HH, Li CW, Chou CK, Lim SO, Chang SS, Litton J, Arun B, Hortobagyi GN, Hung MC (2017) PARP inhibitor upregulates PD-L1 expression and enhances cancer-associated immunosuppression. Clin Cancer Res 23(14):3711–3720. https://doi.org/10.1158/1078-0432.CCR-16-3215

Jiménez-Sánchez A, Cybulska P, Mager KL, Koplev S, Cast O, Couturier DL, Memon D, Selenica P, Nikolovski I, Mazaheri Y, Bykov Y, Geyer FC, Macintyre G, Gavarró LM, Drews RM, Gill MB, Papanastasiou AD, Sosa RE, Soslow RA, Walther T, Shen R, Chi DS, Park KJ, Hollmann T, Reis-Filho JS, Markowetz F, Beltrao P, Vargas HA, Zamarin D, Brenton JD, Snyder A, Weigelt B, Sala E, Miller ML (2020) Unraveling tumor-immune heterogeneity in advanced ovarian cancer uncovers immunogenic effect of chemotherapy. Nat Genet 52 (6):582–593. https://doi.org/10.1038/s41588-020-0630-5

Jin Y, Wang H, Liang X, Ma J, Wang Y (2014a) Pathological and prognostic significance of hypoxia-inducible factor 1α expression in epithelial ovarian cancer: a meta-analysis. Tumour Biol 35(8):8149–8159. https://doi.org/10.1007/s13277-014-2059-x

Jin Z, Gu J, Xin X, Li Y, Wang H (2014b) Expression of hexokinase 2 in epithelial ovarian tumors and its clinical significance in serous ovarian cancer. Eur J Gynaecol Oncol 35(5):519–524

Kaldawy A, Segev Y, Lavie O et al (2016) Low-grade serous ovarian cancer: a review. Gynecol Oncol 143(2):433–438. https://doi.org/10.1016/j.ygyno.2016.08.320

Kalli KR, Block MS, Kasi PM et al (2018) Folate receptor alpha peptide vaccine generates immunity in breast and ovarian cancer patients. Clin Cancer Res 24(13):3014–3025. https://doi.org/10.1158/1078-0432.CCR-17-2499

Kang HJ, Chun SM, Kim KR, Sohn I, Sung CO (2013) Clinical relevance of gain-of-function mutations of p53 in high-grade serous ovarian carcinoma. PLoS One 8(8):e72609. https://doi.org/10.1371/journal.pone.0072609

Kanska J, Zakhour M, Taylor-Harding B et al (2016) Cyclin E as a potential therapeutic target in high grade serous ovarian cancer. Gynecol Oncol 143(1):152–158. https://doi.org/10.1016/j.ygyno.2016.07.111

Karnezis AN, Cho KR, Gilks CB et al (2017) The disparate origins of ovarian cancers: pathogenesis and prevention strategies. Nat Rev Cancer 17(1):65–74. https://doi.org/10.1038/nrc.2016.113

Karst AM, Jones PM, Vena N, Ligon AH, Liu JF, Hirsch MS, Etemadmoghadam D, Bowtell DD, Drapkin R (2014) Cyclin E1 deregulation occurs early in secretory cell transformation to promote formation of fallopian tube-derived high-grade serous ovarian cancers. Cancer Res 74(4):1141–1152. https://doi.org/10.1158/0008-5472.CAN-13-2247

Kassem L, Abdel-Rahman O (2016) Targeting mTOR pathway in gynecological malignancies: biological rationale and systematic review of published data. Crit Rev Oncol Hematol 108:1–12. https://doi.org/10.1016/j.critrevonc.2016.10.003

Katagiri A, Nakayama K, Rahman MT et al (2010) MEK inhibition suppresses cell invasion and migration in ovarian cancers with activation of ERK1/2. Exp Ther Med 1(4):591–596

Kato N, Sato Y, Kamataki A et al (2018) PIK3CA hotspot mutations and cyclooxygenase-2-expression in ovarian clear cell carcinomas: a close association with stromal features. Hum Pathol. https://doi.org/10.1016/j.humpath.2018.11.013

Kawanishi S, Ohnishi S, Ma N, Hiraku Y, Murata M (2017) Crosstalk between DNA damage and inflammation in the multiple steps of carcinogenesis. Int J Mol Sci 18(8):1808. https://doi.org/10.3390/ijms18081808

Keenan TE, Burke KP, Van Allen EM (2019) Genomic correlates of response to immune checkpoint blockade. Nat Med 25(3):389–402. https://doi.org/10.1038/s41591-019-0382-x

Kelly RJ (2018) Dabrafenib and trametinib for the treatment of non-small cell lung cancer. Expert Rev Anticancer Ther 18(11):1063–1068. https://doi.org/10.1080/14737140.2018.1521272

Khan AQ, Kuttikrishnan S, Siveen KS et al (2018) RAS-mediated oncogenic signaling pathways in human malignancies. Semin Cancer Biol. pii: s1044-579X(18)30002-6. https://doi.org/10.1016/j.semcancer.2018.03.001

Kim K, Park WY, Kim JY et al (2012) Prognostic relevance of the expression of CA IX, GLUT-1, and VEGF in ovarian epithelial cancers. Korean J Pathol 46(6):532–540. https://doi.org/10.4132/KoreanJPathol.2012.46.6.532

Klezovitch O, Vasioukhin V (2015) Cadherin signaling: keeping cells in touch. F1000Res 4 (F1000ulty Rev):550. https://doi.org/10.12688/f1000research.6445.1

Klotz DM, Wimberger P (2017) Cells of origin of ovarian cancer: ovarian surface epithelium or fallopian tube? Arch Gynecol Obstet 296(6):1055–1062. https://doi.org/10.1007/s00404-017-4529-z

Klymenko Y, Johnson J, Bos B, Lombard R, Campbell L, Loughran E, Stack MS (2017a) Heterogeneous cadherin expression and multicellular aggregate dynamics in ovarian cancer dissemination. Neoplasia 19(7):549–563. https://doi.org/10.1016/j.neo.2017.04.002

Klymenko Y, Kim O, Loughran E, Yang J, Lombard R, Alber M, Stack MS (2017b) Cadherin composition and multicellular aggregate invasion in organotypic models of epithelial ovarian cancer intraperitoneal metastasis. Oncogene 36(42):5840–5851. https://doi.org/10.1038/onc.2017.171

Knödler M, Körfer J, Kunzmann V et al (2018) Randomised phase II trial to investigate catumaxomab (anti-EpCAM × anti-CD3) for treatment of peritoneal carcinomatosis in patients with gastric cancer. Br J Cancer 119(3):296–302. https://doi.org/10.1038/s41416-018-0150-6

Kobayashi H, Ogawa K, Kawahara N et al (2017) Sequential molecular changes and dynamic oxidative stress in high-grade serous ovarian carcinogenesis. Free Radic Res 51(9–10):755–764. https://doi.org/10.1080/10715762.2017.1383605

Köbel M, Kalloger SE, Boyd N et al (2008) Ovarian carcinoma subtypes are different diseases: implications for biomarker studies. PLoS Med 5(12):e232. https://doi.org/10.1371/journal.pmed.0050232

Köbel M, Reuss A, du Bois A et al (2010) The biological and clinical value of p53 expression in pelvic high-grade serous carcinomas. J Pathol 222(2):191–198. https://doi.org/10.1002/path.2744

Koensgen D, Freitag C, Klaman I et al (2010) Expression and localization of E-cadherin in epithelial ovarian cancer. Anticancer Res 30(7):2525–2530

Konstantinopoulos PA, Barry WT, Birrer M, Westin SN, Cadoo KA, Shapiro GI, Mayer EL, O'Cearbhaill RE, Coleman RL, Kochupurakkal B, Whalen C, Curtis J, Farooq S, Luo W, Eismann J, Buss MK, Aghajanian C, Mills GB, Palakurthi S, Kirschmeier P, Liu J, Cantley LC, Kaufmann SH, Swisher EM, D'Andrea AD, Winer E, Wulf GM, Matulonis UA (2019) Olaparib and α-specific PI3K inhibitor alpelisib for patients with epithelial ovarian cancer: a dose-escalation and dose-expansion phase 1b trial. Lancet Oncol 20(4):570–580. https://doi.org/10.1016/S1470-2045(18)30905-7

Kourtidis A, Lu R, Pence LJ, Anastasiadis PZ (2017) A central role for cadherin signaling in cancer. Exp Cell Res 358(1):78–85

Krasner CN, Birrer MJ, Berlin ST, Horowitz NS, Buss MK, Eliasof S et al (2014) Phase II clinical trial evaluating CRLX101 in recurrent ovarian, tubal, and peritoneal cancer. J Clin Oncol 32 (Suppl 5):abstr 5581

Krasner CN, Birrer MJ, Berlin ST et al (2015) Targeting VEGFRi resistance through HIF-1á suppression: phase II clinical trial evaluating CRLX101 as monotherapy and in combination with bevacizumab in recurrent platinum resistant ovarian cancer. J Clin Oncol 33(Suppl 15): abstr 5614. https://doi.org/10.1200/jco.2015.33.15_suppl.tps5614

Krasner C, Birrer M, Peters C et al (2016) Abstract CT090: phase II trial of the NDC CRLX101 in combination with bevacizumab in patients with platinum-resistant ovarian cancer (PROC). Cancer Res 76:CT090. https://doi.org/10.1158/1538-7445.AM2016-CT090

Krebs AM, Mitschke J, Lasierra Losada M et al (2017) The EMT-activator Zeb1 is a key factor for cell plasticity and promotes metastasis in pancreatic cancer. Nat Cell Biol 19(5):518–529. https://doi.org/10.1038/ncb3513

Krishnamurthy A, Jimeno A (2018) Bispecific antibodies for cancer therapy: a review. Pharmacol Ther 185:122–134. https://doi.org/10.1016/j.pharmthera.2017.12.002

Kristeleit R, Davidenko I, Shirinkin V, El-Khouly F, Bondarenko I, Goodheart MJ, Gorbunova V, Penning CA, Shi JG, Liu X, Newton RC, Zhao Y, Maleski J, Leopold L, Schilder RJ (2017) A randomised, open-label, phase 2 study of the IDO1 inhibitor epacadostat (INCB024360) versus tamoxifen as therapy for biochemically recurrent (CA-125 relapse)-only epithelial ovarian cancer, primary peritoneal carcinoma, or fallopian tube cancer. Gynecol Oncol 146 (3):484–490. https://doi.org/10.1016/j.ygyno.2017.07.005

Kroeger PT, Drapkin R (2016) Pathogenesis and heterogeneity of ovarian cancer. Curr Opin Obstet Gynecol 29(1):26–34

Kruk J, Aboul-Enein HY (2017) Reactive oxygen and nitrogen species in carcinogenesis: implications of oxidative stress on the progression and development of several cancer types. Mini Rev Med Chem 17(11):904–919. https://doi.org/10.2174/1389557517666170228115324

Książek K (2020) Where does cellular senescence belong in the pathophysiology of ovarian cancer? Semin Cancer Biol. S1044-579X(20)30260-1. https://doi.org/10.1016/j.semcancer.2020.11.021

Kuhn E, Meeker A, Wang TL, Sehdev AS, Kurman RJ, Shih IM (2010) Shortened telomeres in serous tubal intraepithelial carcinoma: an early event in ovarian high-grade serous carcinogenesis. Am J Surg Pathol 34(6):829–836. https://doi.org/10.1097/PAS.0b013e3181dcede7

Kuhn E, Kurman RJ, Vang R, Sehdev AS, Han G, Soslow R, Wang TL, Shih IM (2012) TP53 mutations in serous tubal intraepithelial carcinoma and concurrent pelvic high-grade serous carcinoma–evidence supporting the clonal relationship of the two lesions. J Pathol 226 (3):421–426. https://doi.org/10.1002/path.3023

Kuhn E, Bahadirli-Talbott A, Shih IM (2014) Frequent CCNE1 amplification in endometrial intraepithelial carcinoma and uterine serous carcinoma. Mod Pathol 27(7):1014–1019. https://doi.org/10.1038/modpathol.2013.209

Kuhn E, Wang TL, Doberstein K et al (2016) CCNE1 amplification and centrosome number abnormality in serous tubal intraepithelial carcinoma: further evidence supporting its role as a precursor of ovarian high-grade serous carcinoma. Mod Pathol 29(10):1254–1261. https://doi.org/10.1038/modpathol.2016.101

Kurtz J, Marth C, Oaknin A, Asselain B, Baumann K, Cibula D et al (2018) ATALANTE (ENGOT-ov29): a randomized, double-blinded, phase III study of atezolizumab versus placebo in patients with late relapse of epithelial ovarian, fallopian tube, or peritoneal cancer treated by platinum-based chemotherapy and bevacizumab. J Clin Oncol 36(Suppl):abstr TPS5607

Kuznetsova AY, Seget K, Moeller GK et al (2015) Chromosomal instability, tolerance of mitotic errors and multidrug resistance are promoted by tetraploidization in human cells. Cell Cycle 14 (17):2810–2820

Kyriakopoulos CE, Braden AM, Kolesar JM et al (2016) A phase I study of tivantinib in combination with temsirolimus in patients with advanced solid tumors. Invest New Drugs 35 (3):290–297

Labidi-Galy SI, Papp E, Hallberg D et al (2017) High grade serous ovarian carcinomas originate in the fallopian tube. Nat Commun 8(1):1093. https://doi.org/10.1038/s41467-017-00962-1

Lam T, Aguirre-Ghiso JA, Geller MA, Aksan A, Azarin SM (2020) Immobilization rapidly selects for chemoresistant ovarian cancer cells with enhanced ability to enter dormancy. Biotechnol Bioeng 117(10):3066–3080. https://doi.org/10.1002/bit.27479

Lambert AW, Pattabiraman DR, Weinberg RA (2017) Emerging biological principles of metastasis. Cell 168(4):670–691. https://doi.org/10.1016/j.cell.2016.11.037

Lampert EJ, Zimmer A, Padget M, Cimino-Mathews A, Nair JR, Liu Y, Swisher EM, Hodge JW, Nixon AB, Nichols E, Bagheri MH, Levy E, Radke MR, Lipkowitz S, Annunziata CM, Taube JM, Steinberg SM, Lee JM (2020) Combination of PARP inhibitor olaparib, and PD-L1 inhibitor durvalumab, in recurrent ovarian cancer: a proof-of-concept phase II study. Clin Cancer Res 26(16):4268–4279. https://doi.org/10.1158/1078-0432.CCR-20-0056

Laplante M, Sabatini DM (2012) mTOR signaling in growth control and disease. Cell 149(2):274–293. https://doi.org/10.1016/j.cell.2012.03.017

Lau MT, So WK, Leung PC (2013) Fibroblast growth factor 2 induces E-cadherin down-regulation via PI3K/Akt/mTOR and MAPK/ERK signaling in ovarian cancer cells. PLoS One 8(3):e59083

Le Page C, Amuzu S, Rahimi K, Gotlieb W, Ragoussis J, Tonin PN (2020) Lessons learned from understanding chemotherapy resistance in epithelial tubo-ovarian carcinoma from BRCA1and BRCA2mutation carriers. Semin Cancer Biol. S1044-579X(20)30177-2. https://doi.org/10.1016/j.semcancer.2020.08.005

Le Saux O, Ray-Coquard I, Labidi-Galy SI (2020) Challenges for immunotherapy for the treatment of platinum resistant ovarian cancer. Semin Cancer Biol. S1044-579X(20)30193-0. https://doi.org/10.1016/j.semcancer.2020.08.017

Leckband DE, de Rooij J (2014) Cadherin adhesion and mechanotransduction. Annu Rev Cell Dev Biol 30:291–315. https://doi.org/10.1146/annurev-cellbio-100913-013212

Ledermann JA, Canevari S, Thigpen T (2015) Targeting the folate receptor: diagnostic and therapeutic approaches to personalize cancer treatments. Ann Oncol 26(10):2034–2043. https://doi.org/10.1093/annonc/mdv250

Ledermann JA, Embleton AC, Raja F, Perren TJ, Jayson GC, GJS R, Kaye SB, Hirte H, Eisenhauer E, Vaughan M, Friedlander M, González-Martín A, Stark D, Clark E, Farrelly L, Swart AM, Cook A, Kaplan RS, MKB P, ICON6 collaborators (2016) Cediranib in patients with relapsed platinum sensitive ovarian cancer (ICON6): a randomised, double-blind, placebocontrolled phase 3 trial. Lancet 387(10023):1066–1074. https://doi.org/10.1016/S0140-6736(15)01167-8. Erratum in: Lancet. 2016 Apr23;387(10029):1722

Ledermann JA, Colombo N, Oza M et al (2020) Avelumab in combination with and/or following chemotherapy vs chemotherapy alone in patients with previously untreated epithelial ovarian cancer: results from the phase 3 javelin ovarian 100 trial. Society of Gynecologic Oncology Annual Meeting on Women's Cancer. LBA 25, Scientific Plenary. https://doi.org/10.1016/j.ygyno.2020.06.025

Lee EK, Matulonis UA (2020) Emerging drugs for the treatment of ovarian cancer: a focused review of PARP inhibitors. Expert Opin Emerg Drugs 25(2):165–188. https://doi.org/10.1080/14728214.2020.1773791

Lee WH, Bookstein R, Hong F et al (1987) Human retinoblastoma susceptibility gene: cloning, identification, and sequence. Science 235(4794):1394–1399

Lee JG, Ahn JH, Jin Kim T, Ho Lee J, Choi JH (2015) Mutant p53 promotes ovarian cancer cell adhesion to mesothelial cells via integrin β4 and Akt signals. Sci Rep 5:12642. https://doi.org/10.1038/srep12642

Lee EK, Xiong N, Cheng SC, Barry WT, Penson RT, Konstantinopoulos PA, Hoffman MA, Horowitz N, Dizon DS, Stover EH, Wright AA, Campos SM, Krasner C, Morrissey S, Whalen C, Quinn R, Matulonis UA, Liu JF (2020) Combined pembrolizumab and pegylated liposomal doxorubicin in platinum resistant ovarian cancer: a phase 2 clinical trial. Gynecol Oncol 159(1):72–78. https://doi.org/10.1016/j.ygyno.2020.07.028

Legge F, Paglia A, D'Asta M et al (2011) Phase II study of the combination carboplatin plus celecoxib in heavily pre-treated recurrent ovarian cancer patients. BMC Cancer 11:214. https://doi.org/10.1186/1471-2407-11-214

Leijen S, van Geel RM, Sonke GS, de Jong D, Rosenberg EH, Marchetti S, Pluim D, van Werkhoven E, Rose S, Lee MA, Freshwater T, Beijnen JH, Schellens JH (2016) Phase II study of WEE1 inhibitor AZD1775s carboplatin in patients with TP53-mutated ovarian cancer refractory or resistant to first-line therapy within 3 months. J Clin Oncol 34(36):4354–4361. https://doi.org/10.1200/JCO.2016.67.5942

Leroy B, Anderson M, Soussi T (2014) TP53 mutations in human cancer: database reassessment and prospects for the next decade. Hum Mutat 35(6):672–688. https://doi.org/10.1002/humu.22552

Lheureux S, N'Diaye M, Blanc-Fournier C, Dugué AE, Clarisse B, Dutoit S, Giffard F, Abeilard E, Briand M, Labiche A, Grellard JM, Crouet H, Martin S, Joly F, Poulain L (2015) Identification of predictive factors of response to the BH3-mimetic molecule ABT-737: an ex vivo experiment in human serous ovarian carcinoma. Int J Cancer 136(5):E340–E350. https://doi.org/10.1002/ijc.29104

Lheureux S, Cristea MC, Bruce JP, Garg S, Cabanero M, Mantia-Smaldone G, Olawaiye AB, Ellard SL, Weberpals JI, Wahner Hendrickson AE, Fleming GF, Welch S, Dhani NC, Stockley T, Rath P, Karakasis K, Jones GN, Jenkins S, Rodriguez-Canales J, Tracy M, Tan Q, Bowering V, Udagani S, Wang L, Kunos CA, Chen E, Pugh TJ, Oza AM (2021) Adavosertib plus gemcitabine for platinum-resistant or platinum-refractory recurrent ovarian cancer: a double-blind, randomised, placebo-controlled, phase 2 trial. Lancet 397 (10271):281–292. https://doi.org/10.1016/S0140-6736(20)32554-X

Li H, Zhang R (2013) Role of EZH2 in epithelial ovarian cancer: from biological insights to therapeutic target. Front Oncol 3:47. https://doi.org/10.3389/fonc.2013.00047

Li SB, Schwartz PE, Lee WH et al (1991) Allele loss at the retinoblastoma locus in human ovarian cancer. J Natl Cancer Inst 83(9):637–640

Li W, Xu XL, Zhang J, Cai JH, Tang YX (2012) Effects of cyclooxygenase inhibitors on survival time in ovarian cancer xenograft-bearing mice. Oncol Lett 4(6):1269–1273. https://doi.org/10.3892/ol.2012.929

Li H, Zeng J, Shen K (2014) PI3K/AKT/mTOR signaling pathway as a therapeutic target for ovarian cancer. Arch Gynecol Obstet 290(6):1067–1078. https://doi.org/10.1007/s00404-014-3377-3

Li C, Bonazzoli E, Bellone S et al (2019a) Mutational landscape of primary, metastatic, and recurrent ovarian cancer reveals c-MYC gains as potential target for BET inhibitors. Proc Natl Acad Sci U S A 116(2):619–624. https://doi.org/10.1073/pnas.1814027116

Li VD, Li KH, Li JT (2019b) TP53 mutations as potential prognostic markers for specific cancers: analysis of data from The Cancer Genome Atlas and the International Agency for Research on Cancer TP53 Database. J Cancer Res Clin Oncol 145(3):625–636. https://doi.org/10.1007/s00432-018-2817-z

Li N, Li H, Wang Y, Cao L, Zhan X (2020) Quantitative proteomics revealed energy metabolism pathway alterations in human epithelial ovarian carcinoma and their regulation by the antiparasite drug ivermectin: data interpretation in the context of 3P medicine. EPMA J 11 (4):661–694. https://doi.org/10.1007/s13167-020-00224-z

Li J, Zou Y, Pei M, Zhang Y, Jiang Y (2021) Berberine inhibits the Warburg effect through TET3/miR-145/HK2 pathways in ovarian cancer cells. J Cancer 12(1):207–216. https://doi.org/10.7150/jca.48896

Lin Q, Liu W, Xu S, Shang H, Li J, Guo Y, Tong J (2021) PARP inhibitors as maintenance therapy in newly diagnosed advanced ovarian cancer: a meta-analysis. BJOG 128(3):485–493. https://doi.org/10.1111/1471-0528.16411

Lincet H, Kafara P, Giffard F, Abeilard-Lemoisson E, Duval M, Louis MH, Poulain L, Icard P (2013) Inhibition of Mcl-1 expression by citrate enhances the effect of Bcl-xL inhibitors on human ovarian carcinoma cells. J Ovarian Res 6(1):72. https://doi.org/10.1186/1757-2215-6-72

Liu F, Yang X, Geng M, Huang M (2018) Targeting ERK, an Achilles' Heel of the MAPK pathway, in cancer therapy. Acta Pharm Sin B 8(4):552–562

Liu JF, Barry WT, Birrer M, Lee JM, Buckanovich RJ, Fleming GF, Rimel BJ, Buss MK, Nattam SR, Hurteau J, Luo W, Curtis J, Whalen C, Kohn EC, Ivy SP, Matulonis UA (2019a) Overall survival and updated progression-free survival outcomes in a randomized phase II study of combination cediranib and olaparib versus olaparib in relapsed platinum-sensitive ovarian cancer. Ann Oncol 30(4):551–557. https://doi.org/10.1093/annonc/mdz018

Liu JF, Gordon M, Veneris J, Braiteh F, Balmanoukian A, Eder JP, Oaknin A, Hamilton E, Wang Y, Sarkar I, Molinero L, Fassò M, O'Hear C, Lin YG, Emens LA (2019b) Safety, clinical activity and biomarker assessments of atezolizumab from a Phase I study in advanced/recurrent ovarian and uterine cancers. Gynecol Oncol 154(2):314–322. https://doi.org/10.1016/j.ygyno.2019.05.021

Liu JF, Herold C, Gray KP et al (2019c) Assessment of combined nivolumab and bevacizumab in relapsed ovarian cancer: a phase 2 clinical trial [published online ahead of print, 2019]. JAMA Oncol 5(12):1731–1738. https://doi.org/10.1001/jamaoncol.2019.3343

Loeian MS, Mehdi Aghaei S, Farhadi F et al (2019) Liquid biopsy using the nanotube-CTC-chip: capture of invasive CTCs with high purity using preferential adherence in breast cancer patients. Lab Chip 19(11):1899–1915. https://doi.org/10.1039/c9lc00274j

Long GV, Hauschild A, Santinami M et al (2017a) Adjuvant dabrafenib plus trametinib in stage III BRAF-mutated melanoma. N Engl J Med 377(19):1813–1823. https://doi.org/10.1056/NEJMoa1708539

Long GV, Flaherty KT, Stroyakovskiy D et al (2017b) Dabrafenib plus trametinib versus dabrafenib monotherapy in patients with metastatic BRAF V600E/K-mutant melanoma: long-term survival and safety analysis of a phase 3 study. Ann Oncol 28(7):1631–1639

Lord CJ, Ashworth A (2012) The DNA damage response and cancer therapy. Nature 481:287. https://doi.org/10.1038/nature10760

LoRusso PM (2016) Inhibition of the PI3K/AKT/mTOR pathway in solid tumors. J Clin Oncol 34 (31):3803–3815. https://doi.org/10.1200/JCO.2014.59.0018

Lu J, Chen H, He F, You Y, Feng Z, Chen W, Li X, Zhao L (2020) Ginsenoside 20(S)-Rg3 upregulates HIF-1α-targeting miR-519a-5p to inhibit the Warburg effect in ovarian cancer cells. Clin Exp Pharmacol Physiol 47(8):1455–1463. https://doi.org/10.1111/1440-1681.13321

Lundgren C, Ahlin C, Holmberg L et al (2015) Cyclin E1 is a strong prognostic marker for death from lymph node negative breast cancer. A population-based case-control study. Acta Oncol 54 (4):538–544. https://doi.org/10.3109/0284186X.2014.965274

Luo H, Xu X, Ye M, Sheng B, Zhu X (2018) The prognostic value of HER2 in ovarian cancer: a meta-analysis of observational studies. PLoS One 13(1):e0191972. https://doi.org/10.1371/journal.pone.0191972

Luther C, Swami U, Zhang J et al (2019) Advanced stage melanoma therapies: detailing the present and exploring the future. Crit Rev Oncol Hematol 133:99–111. https://doi.org/10.1016/j.critrevonc.2018.11.002

Ma Y, Wang W, Idowu MO et al (2018a) Ovarian cancer relies on glucose transporter 1 to fuel glycolysis and growth: anti-tumor activity of BAY-876. Cancers (Basel) 11(1):33. https://doi.org/10.3390/cancers11010033

Ma C, Zhao JZ, Lin RT et al (2018b) Combined overexpression of cadherin 6, cadherin 11 and cluster of differentiation 44 is associated with lymph node metastasis and poor prognosis in oral squamous cell carcinoma. Oncol Lett 15(6):9498–9506

Mabuchi S, Kuroda H, Takahashi R et al (2015) The PI3K/AKT/mTOR pathway as a therapeutic target in ovarian cancer. Gynecol Oncol 137(1):173–179. https://doi.org/10.1016/j.ygyno.2015.02.003

Macpherson AM, Barry SC, Ricciardelli C, Oehler MK (2020) Epithelial ovarian cancer and the immune system: biology, interactions, challenges and potential advances for immunotherapy. J Clin Med 9(9):2967. https://doi.org/10.3390/jcm9092967

Mandilaras V, Garg S, Cabanero M, Tan Q, Pastrello C, Burnier J, Karakasis K, Wang L, Dhani NC, Butler MO, Bedard PL, Siu LL, Clarke B, Shaw PA, Stockley T, Jurisica I, Oza AM, Lheureux S (2019) TP53 mutations in high grade serous ovarian cancer and impact on clinical outcomes: a comparison of next generation sequencing and bioinformatics analyses. Int J Gynecol Cancer. https://doi.org/10.1136/ijgc-2018-000087

Manning AL, Dyson NJ (2012) RB: mitotic implications of a tumour suppressor. Nat Rev Cancer 12(3):220–226. https://doi.org/10.1038/nrc3216

Marth C, Vergote I, Scambia G, Oberaigner W, Clamp A, Berger R, Kurzeder C, Colombo N, Vuylsteke P, Lorusso D, Hall M, Renard V, Pignata S, Kristeleit R, Altintas S, Rustin G, Wenham RM, Mirza MR, Fong PC, Oza A, Monk BJ, Ma H, Vogl FD, Bach BA (2017) ENGOT-ov-6/TRINOVA-2: randomised, double-blind, phase 3 study of pegylated liposomal doxorubicin plus trebananib or placebo in women with recurrent partially platinum-sensitive or resistant ovarian cancer. Eur J Cancer 70:111–121. https://doi.org/10.1016/j.ejca.2016.09.004

Martin de la Fuente L, Westbom-Fremer S, Arildsen NS, Hartman L, Malander S, Kannisto P, Måsbäck A, Hedenfalk I (2020) PD-1/PD-L1 expression and tumor-infiltrating lymphocytes are prognostically favorable in advanced high-grade serous ovarian carcinoma. Virchows Arch 477 (1):83–91. https://doi.org/10.1007/s00428-020-02751-6

Martin LP, Konner JA, Moore KN et al (2017) Characterization of folate receptor alpha (FRα) expression in archival tumor and biopsy samples from relapsed epithelial ovarian cancer patients: a phase I expansion study of the FRα-targeting antibody-drug conjugate mirvetuximab soravtansine. Gynecol Oncol 147(2):402–407. https://doi.org/10.1016/j.ygyno.2017.08.015

Martins FC, Santiago ID, Trinh A et al (2014) Combined image and genomic analysis of high-grade serous ovarian cancer reveals PTEN loss as a common driver event and prognostic classifier. Genome Biol 15(12):526. https://doi.org/10.1186/s13059-014-0526-8

Martowicz A, Spizzo G, Gastl G, Untergasser G (2012) Phenotype-dependent effects of EpCAM expression on growth and invasion of human breast cancer cell lines. BMC Cancer 12:501. https://doi.org/10.1186/1471-2407-12-501

Mattmann ME, Stoops SL, Lindsley CW (2011) Inhibition of Akt with small molecules and biologics: historical perspective and current status of the patent landscape. Expert Opin Ther Pat 21(9):1309–1338

Matulonis UA, Wulf GM, Barry WT et al (2016) Phase I dose escalation study of the PI3kinase pathway inhibitor BKM120 and the oral poly (ADP ribose) polymerase (PARP) inhibitor olaparib for the treatment of high-grade serous ovarian and breast cancer. Ann Oncol 28 (3):512–518

Matulonis UA, Moore KN, Martin LP et al (2018) Mirvetuximab soravtansine, a folate receptor alpha (FRα)-targeting antibody-drug conjugate (ADC), with pembrolizumab in platinum-resistant ovarian cancer (PROC): initial results of an expansion cohort from FORWARD II, a phase Ib study. Ann Oncol 29. https://doi.org/10.1093/annonc/mdy285.157

Matulonis UA, Shapira-Frommer R, Santin AD, Lisyanskaya AS, Pignata S, Vergote I, Raspagliesi F, Sonke GS, Birrer M, Provencher DM, Sehouli J, Colombo N, González-Martín A, Oaknin A, Ottevanger PB, Rudaitis V, Katchar K, Wu H, Keefe S, Ruman J, Ledermann JA (2019) Antitumor activity and safety of pembrolizumab in patients with advanced recurrent ovarian cancer: results from the phase II KEYNOTE-100 study. Ann Oncol 30(7):1080–1087. https://doi.org/10.1093/annonc/mdz135

McAlpine JN, Porter H, Köbel M et al (2012) BRCA1 and BRCA2 mutations correlate with TP53 abnormalities and presence of immune cell infiltrates in ovarian high-grade serous carcinoma. Mod Pathol 25(5):740–750. https://doi.org/10.1038/modpathol.2011.211

McCormick A, Earp E, Leeson C et al (2016) Phosphatase and tensin homolog is a potential target for ovarian cancer sensitization to cytotoxic agents. Int J Gynecol Cancer 26(4):632–639. https://doi.org/10.1097/IGC.0000000000000657

McLachlan J, Gore M, Banerjee S (2016a) Targeting the mitogen-activated protein kinase pathway in low-grade serous carcinoma of the ovary. Pharmacogenomics 17(12):1353–1363. https://doi.org/10.2217/pgs.16.24

McLachlan J, Lima JP, Dumas L, Banerjee S (2016b) Targeted agents and combinations in ovarian cancer: where are we now? Expert Rev Anticancer Ther 16(4):441–454. https://doi.org/10.1586/14737140.2016.1162101

McMullen M, Madariaga A, Lheureux S (2020) New approaches for targeting platinum-resistant ovarian cancer. Semin Cancer Biol. S1044-579X(20)30186-3. https://doi.org/10.1016/j.semcancer.2020.08.013

Mendivil AA, Tung PK, Bohart R, Bechtol K, Goldstein BH (2018) Dramatic clinical response following dabrafenib and trametinib therapy in a heavily pretreated low grade serous ovarian carcinoma patient with a BRAF V600E mutation. Gynecol Oncol Rep 26:41–44. https://doi.org/10.1016/j.gore.2018.09.002

Meng E, Taylor B, Ray A, Shevde LA, Rocconi RP (2012) Targeted inhibition of telomerase activity combined with chemotherapy demonstrates synergy in eliminating ovarian cancer spheroid-forming cells. Gynecol Oncol 124(3):598–605. https://doi.org/10.1016/j.ygyno.2011.11.018

Mesnage SJL, Auguste A, Genestie C, Dunant A, Pain E, Drusch F, Gouy S, Morice P, Bentivegna E, Lhomme C, Pautier P, Michels J, Le Formal A, Cheaib B, Adam J, Leary AF (2017) Neoadjuvant chemotherapy (NACT) increases immune infiltration and programmed death-ligand 1 (PD-L1) expression in epithelial ovarian cancer (EOC). Ann Oncol 28 (3):651–657. https://doi.org/10.1093/annonc/mdw625

Milea A, George SH, Matevski D et al (2014) Retinoblastoma pathway deregulatory mechanisms determine clinical outcome in high-grade serous ovarian carcinoma. Mod Pathol 27 (7):991–1001. https://doi.org/10.1038/modpathol.2013.218

Mirza MR, Monk BJ, Herrstedt J, Oza AM, Mahner S, Redondo A, Fabbro M, Ledermann JA, Lorusso D, Vergote I, Ben-Baruch NE, Marth C, Mądry R, Christensen RD, Berek JS,

Dørum A, Tinker AV, du Bois A, González-Martín A, Follana P, Benigno B, Rosenberg P, Gilbert L, Rimel BJ, Buscema J, Balser JP, Agarwal S, Matulonis UA, ENGOT-OV16/NOVA Investigators (2016) Niraparib maintenance therapy in platinum-sensitive, recurrent ovarian cancer. N Engl J Med 375(22):2154–2164. https://doi.org/10.1056/NEJMoa1611310

Mirza MR, Pignata S, Ledermann JA (2018) Latest clinical evidence and further development of PARP inhibitors in ovarian cancer. Ann Oncol 29(6):1366–1376. https://doi.org/10.1093/annonc/mdy174

Mirza MR, Coleman RL, González-Martín A, Moore KN, Colombo N, Ray-Coquard I, Pignata S (2020) The forefront of ovarian cancer therapy: update on PARP inhibitors. Ann Oncol 31 (9):1148–1159. https://doi.org/10.1016/j.annonc.2020.06.004

Miše BP, Telesmanić VD, Tomić S et al (2015) Correlation between E-cadherin immunoexpression and efficacy of first line platinum-based chemotherapy in advanced high grade serous ovarian cancer. Pathol Oncol Res 21(2):347–356. https://doi.org/10.1007/s12253-014-9827-1

Mitsudomi T, Yatabe Y (2010) Epidermal growth factor receptor in relation to tumor development: EGFR gene and cancer. FEBS J 277(2):301–308. https://doi.org/10.1111/j.1742-4658.2009.07448.x

Mittal K, Donthamsetty S, Kaur R et al (2017) Multinucleated polyploidy drives resistance to Docetaxel chemotherapy in prostate cancer. Br J Cancer 116(9):1186–1194

Moiseeva O, Guillon J, Ferbeyre G (2020) Senescence: a program in the road to cell elimination and cancer. Semin Cancer Biol. S1044-579X(20)30277-7. https://doi.org/10.1016/j.semcancer.2020.12.017

Monk BJ, Poveda A, Vergote I, Raspagliesi F, Fujiwara K, Bae DS, Oaknin A, Ray-Coquard I, Provencher DM, Karlan BY, Lhommé C, Richardson G, Rincón DG, Coleman RL, Herzog TJ, Marth C, Brize A, Fabbro M, Redondo A, Bamias A, Tassoudji M, Navale L, Warner DJ, Oza AM (2014) Anti-angiopoietin therapy with trebananib for recurrent ovarian cancer (TRINOVA-1): a randomised, multicentre, double-blind, placebo-controlled phase 3 trial. Lancet Oncol 15 (8):799–808. https://doi.org/10.1016/S1470-2045(14)70244-X

Monk BJ, Brady MF, Aghajanian C, Lankes HA, Rizack T, Leach J, Fowler JM, Higgins R, Hanjani P, Morgan M, Edwards R, Bradley W, Kolevska T, Foukas P, Swisher EM, Anderson KS, Gottardo R, Bryan JK, Newkirk M, Manjarrez KL, Mannel RS, Hershberg RM, Coukos G (2017) A phase 2, randomized, double-blind, placebo-controlled study of chemo-immunotherapy combination using motolimod with pegylated liposomal doxorubicin in recurrent or persistent ovarian cancer: a Gynecologic Oncology Group partners study. Ann Oncol 28 (5):996–1004. https://doi.org/10.1093/annonc/mdx049

Moore KN, Pignata S (2019) Trials in progress: imagyn050/GOG 3015/ENGOT-OV39. A Phase III, multicenter, randomized study of atezolizumab versus placebo administered in combination with paclitaxel, carboplatin, and bevacizumab to patients with newly-diagnosed stage III or stage IV ovarian, fallopian tube, or primary peritoneal cancer. Int J Gynecol Cancer. https://doi.org/10.1136/ijgc-2018-000071

Moore KN, Borghaei H, O'Malley DM et al (2017) Phase 1 dose-escalation study of mirvetuximab soravtansine (IMGN853), a folate receptor α-targeting antibody-drug conjugate, in patients with solid tumors. Cancer 123(16):3080–3087. https://doi.org/10.1002/cncr.30736

Moore KN, Martin LP, O'Malley DM et al (2018a) A review of mirvetuximab soravtansine in the treatment of platinum-resistant ovarian cancer. Future Oncol 14(2):123–136. https://doi.org/10.2217/fon-2017-0379

Moore KN, O'Malley DM, Vergote I et al (2018b) Safety and activity findings from a phase 1b escalation study of mirvetuximab soravtansine, a folate receptor alpha (FRα)-targeting antibody-drug conjugate (ADC), in combination with carboplatin in patients with platinum-sensitive ovarian cancer. Gynecol Oncol 151(1):46–52. https://doi.org/10.1016/j.ygyno.2018.07.017

Moore K, Colombo N, Scambia G, Kim BG, Oaknin A, Friedlander M, Lisyanskaya A, Floquet A, Leary A, Sonke GS, Gourley C, Banerjee S, Oza A, González-Martín A, Aghajanian C, Bradley W, Mathews C, Liu J, Lowe ES, Bloomfield R, DiSilvestro P (2018c) Maintenance olaparib in patients with newly diagnosed advanced ovarian cancer. N Engl J Med 379 (26):2495–2505. https://doi.org/10.1056/NEJMoa1810858

Moore KN, Secord AA, Geller MA, Miller DS, Cloven N, Fleming GF, Wahner Hendrickson AE, Azodi M, DiSilvestro P, Oza AM, Cristea M, Berek JS, Chan JK, Rimel BJ, Matei DE, Li Y, Sun K, Luptakova K, Matulonis UA, Monk BJ (2019a) Niraparib monotherapy for late-line treatment of ovarian cancer (QUADRA): a multicentre, open-label, single-arm, phase 2 trial. Lancet Oncol 20(5):636–648. https://doi.org/10.1016/S1470-2045(19)30029-4

Moore KN, Oza AM, Colombo N et al (2019b) FORWARD I (GOG 3011): a Phase III study of mirvetuximab soravtansine, a folate receptor alpha (FRa)-targeting antibody-drug conjugate (ADC), versus chemotherapy in patients (pts) with platinum-resistant ovarian cancer (PROC). Ann Oncol 30(Suppl 5):v403–v434. https://doi.org/10.1093/annonc/mdz250

Moore KN, Bookman M, Sehouli J (2020) LBA31 primary results from IMagyn050/GOG 3015/ ENGOT-OV39, a double-blind placebo (pbo)-controlled randomised phase III trial of bevacizumab (bev)-containing therapy ± atezolizumab (atezo) for newly diagnosed stage III/IV ovarian cancer (OC). Ann Oncol. https://doi.org/10.1016/j.annonc.2020.08.2261

Moroney JW, Powderly J, Lieu CH, Bendell JC, Eckhardt SG, Chang CW, Molinero L, Spahn J, Williams P, Lin YG, Hodi FS (2020) Safety and clinical activity of atezolizumab plus bevacizumab in patients with ovarian cancer: a phase Ib study. Clin Cancer Res 26 (21):5631–5637. https://doi.org/10.1158/1078-0432.CCR-20-0477

Morrison J, Thoma C, Goodall RJ et al (2018) Epidermal growth factor receptor blockers for the treatment of ovarian cancer. Cochrane Database Syst Rev 10:CD007927. https://doi.org/10.1002/14651858.CD007927

Morse CB, Toukatly MN, Kilgore MR, Agnew KJ, Bernards SS, Norquist BM, Pennington KP, Garcia RL, Liao JB, Swisher EM (2019) Tumor infiltrating lymphocytes and homologous recombination deficiency are independently associated with improved survival in ovarian carcinoma. Gynecol Oncol 153(2):217–222. https://doi.org/10.1016/j.ygyno.2019.02.011

Moujaber T, Etemadmoghadam D, Kennedy CJ et al (2018) BRAF mutations in low-grade serous ovarian cancer and response to BRAF inhibition. JCO Precis Oncol 2:1–14. https://doi.org/10.1200/PO.17.00221

Mrozik KM, Blaschuk OW, Cheong CM et al (2018) N-cadherin in cancer metastasis, its emerging role in haematological malignancies and potential as a therapeutic target in cancer. BMC Cancer 18:939. https://doi.org/10.1186/s12885-018-4845-0

Murakami R, Matsumura N, Brown JB et al (2017) Exome sequencing landscape analysis in ovarian clear cell carcinoma shed light on key chromosomal regions and mutation gene networks. Am J Pathol 187(10):2246–2258. https://doi.org/10.1016/j.ajpath.2017.06.012

Murakami R, Matsumura N, Michimae H et al (2019) The mesenchymal transition subtype more responsive to dose dense taxane chemotherapy combined with carboplatin than to conventional taxane and carboplatin chemotherapy in high grade serous ovarian carcinoma: a survey of Japanese Gynecologic Oncology Group study (JGOG3016A1). Gynecol Oncol 153 (2):312–319. https://doi.org/10.1016/j.ygyno.2019.02.010

Nadkarni NJ, Geest KD, Neff T et al (2013) Microvessel density and p53 mutations in advanced-stage epithelial ovarian cancer. Cancer Lett 331(1):99–104. https://doi.org/10.1016/j.canlet.2012.12.016

Nakayama N, Nakayama K, Shamima Y et al (2010) Gene amplification CCNE1 is related to poor survival and potential therapeutic target in ovarian cancer. Cancer 116(11):2621–2634. https://doi.org/10.1002/cncr.24987

Naumann RW, Coleman RL, Burger RA et al (2013) PRECEDENT: a randomized phase II trial comparing vintafolide (EC145) and pegylated liposomal doxorubicin (PLD) in combination versus PLD alone in patients with platinum-resistant ovarian cancer. J Clin Oncol 31 (35):4400–4406. https://doi.org/10.1200/JCO.2013.49.7685

O'Malley DM, Matulonis UA, Birrer MJ, Castro CM, Gilbert L, Vergote I, Martin LP, Mantia-Smaldone GM, Martin AG, Bratos R, Penson RT, Malek K, Moore KN (2020) Phase Ib study of mirvetuximab soravtansine, a folate receptor alpha (FRα)-targeting antibody-drug conjugate

(ADC), in combination with bevacizumab in patients with platinum-resistant ovarian cancer. Gynecol Oncol 157(2):379–385. https://doi.org/10.1016/j.ygyno.2020.01.037

Oh J, Barve M, Matthews CM, Koon EC, Heffernan TP, Fine B, Grosen E, Bergman MK, Fleming EL, DeMars LR, West L, Spitz DL, Goodman H, Hancock KC, Wallraven G, Kumar P, Bognar E, Manning L, Pappen BO, Adams N, Senzer N, Nemunaitis J (2016) Phase II study of Vigil® DNA engineered immunotherapy as maintenance in advanced stage ovarian cancer. Gynecol Oncol 143(3):504–510. https://doi.org/10.1016/j.ygyno.2016.09.018

Orbegoso C, Marquina G, George A, Banerjee S (2017) The role of Cediranib in ovarian cancer. Expert Opin Pharmacother 18(15):1637–1648. https://doi.org/10.1080/14656566.2017.1383384

Oza AM, Cook AD, Pfisterer J, Embleton A, Ledermann JA, Pujade-Lauraine E, Kristensen G, Carey MS, Beale P, Cervantes A, Park-Simon TW, Rustin G, Joly F, Mirza MR, Plante M, Quinn M, Poveda A, Jayson GC, Stark D, Swart AM, Farrelly L, Kaplan R, Parmar MK, Perren TJ, ICON7 Trial Investigators (2015a) Standard chemotherapy with or without bevacizumab for women with newly diagnosed ovarian cancer (ICON7): overall survival results of a phase 3 randomised trial. Lancet Oncol 16(8):928–936. https://doi.org/10.1016/S1470-2045(15)00086-8

Oza AM, Vergote IB, Gilbert LG, Lucy P, Ghatage A, Lisyankaya S et al (2015b) A randomized double-blind phase III trial comparing vintafolide (EC145) and pegylated liposomal doxorubicin (PLD/Doxil®/Caelyx®) in combination versus PLD in participants with platinum-resistant ovarian cancer (PROCEED) (NCT01170650). Gynecol Oncol 137:5–6. https://doi.org/10.1016/j.ygyno.2015.01.010

Oza AM, Estevez-Diz M, Grischke EM, Hall M, Marmé F, Provencher D, Uyar D, Weberpals JI, Wenham RM, Laing N, Tracy M, Freshwater T, Lee MA, Liu J, Qiu J, Rose S, Rubin EH, Moore K (2020) A biomarker-enriched, randomized phase II trial of adavosertib (AZD1775) plus paclitaxel and carboplatin for women with platinum-sensitive TP53-mutant ovarian cancer. Clin Cancer Res 26(18):4767–4776. https://doi.org/10.1158/1078-0432.CCR-20-0219

Pal M, Bhattacharya S, Kalyan G et al (2018) Cadherin profiling for therapeutic interventions in Epithelial Mesenchymal Transition (EMT) and tumorigenesis. Exp Cell Res 368(2):137–146. https://doi.org/10.1016/j.yexcr.2018.04.014

Palaia I, Tomao F, Sassu CM, Musacchio L, Benedetti Panici P (2020) Immunotherapy for ovarian cancer: recent advances and combination therapeutic approaches. Onco Targets Ther 13:6109–6129. https://doi.org/10.2147/OTT.S205950

Papa S, Choy PM, Bubici C (2018) The ERK and JNK pathways in the regulation of metabolic reprogramming. Oncogene. https://doi.org/10.1038/s41388-018-0582-8

Pascale RM, Calvisi DF, Simile MM, Feo CF, Feo F (2020) The Warburg effect 97 years after its discovery. Cancers (Basel) 12(10):2819. https://doi.org/10.3390/cancers12102819

Pasquali S, Hadjinicolaou AV, Chiarion Sileni V, Rossi CR, Mocellin S (2018) Systemic treatments for metastatic cutaneous melanoma. Cochrane Database Syst Rev 2(2):CD011123. https://doi.org/10.1002/14651858.CD011123.pub2

Patch AM, Christie EL, Etemadmoghadam D et al (2015) Whole-genome characterization of chemoresistant ovarian cancer. Nature 521(7553):489–494. https://doi.org/10.1038/nature14410

Patel IS, Madan P, Getsios S et al (2003) Cadherin switching in ovarian cancer progression. Int J Cancer 106(2):172–177

Pathak SJ, Mueller JL, Okamoto K et al (2019) EPCAM mutation update: variants associated with congenital tufting enteropathy and Lynch syndrome. Hum Mutat 40(2):142–161. https://doi.org/10.1002/humu.23688

Patriarca C, Macchi RM, Marschner AK, Mellstedt H (2012) Epithelial cell adhesion molecule expression (CD326) in cancer: a short review. Cancer Treat Rev 38(1):68–75. https://doi.org/10.1016/j.ctrv.2011.04.002

Pearce CL, Templeman C, Rossing MA et al (2012) Association between endometriosis and risk of histological subtypes of ovarian cancer: a pooled analysis of case-control studies. Lancet Oncol 13(4):385–394

Peng HL, He L, Zhao X (2012) Association of reduced immunohistochemical expression of E-cadherin with a poor ovarian cancer prognosis--results of a meta-analysis. Asian Pac J Cancer Prev 13(5):2003–2007

Peng DH, Kundu ST, Fradette JJ et al (2019) ZEB1 suppression sensitizes KRAS mutant cancers to MEK inhibition by an IL17RD-dependent mechanism. Sci Transl Med 11(483):eaaq1238. https://doi.org/10.1126/scitranslmed.aaq1238

Penson RT, Valencia RV, Cibula D, Colombo N, Leath CA III, Bidziński M, Kim JW, Nam JH, Madry R, Hernández C, Mora PAR, Ryu SY, Milenkova T, Lowe ES, Barker L, Scambia G (2020) Olaparib versus nonplatinum chemotherapy in patients with platinum-sensitive relapsed ovarian cancer and a germline BRCA1/2 mutation (SOLO3): a randomized phase III trial. J Clin Oncol 38(11):1164–1174. https://doi.org/10.1200/JCO.19.02745

Perren TJ, Swart AM, Pfisterer J, Ledermann JA, Pujade-Lauraine E, Kristensen G, Carey MS, Beale P, Cervantes A, Kurzeder C, du Bois A, Sehouli J, Kimmig R, Stähle A, Collinson F, Essapen S, Gourley C, Lortholary A, Selle F, Mirza MR, Leminen A, Plante M, Stark D, Qian W, Parmar MK, Oza AM, ICON7 Investigators (2011) A phase 3 trial of bevacizumab in ovarian cancer. N Engl J Med 365(26):2484–2496. https://doi.org/10.1056/NEJMoa1103799. Erratum in: N Engl J Med 2012;366(3):284

Petersen S, Wilson AJ, Hirst J, Roby KF, Fadare O, Crispens MA, Beeghly-Fadiel A, Khabele D (2020) CCNE1 and BRD4 co-amplification in high-grade serous ovarian cancer is associated with poor clinical outcomes. Gynecol Oncol 157(2):405–410. https://doi.org/10.1016/j.ygyno.2020.01.038

Pétigny-Lechartier C, Duboc C, Jebahi A et al (2017) The mTORC1/2 inhibitor AZD8055engthens the efficiency of the MEK inhibitor trametinib to reduce the Mcl-1/[Bim and Puma] ratio and to sensitize ovarian carcinoma cells to ABT-737. Mol Cancer Ther 16(1):102–115. https://doi.org/10.1158/1535-7163.MCT-16-0342

Petrillo M et al (2016) Targeting the hallmarks of ovarian cancer: the big picture. Gynecol Oncol 142:176–183

Pham E, Birrer MJ, Eliasof S, Garmey EG, Lazarus D, Lee CR, Man S, Matulonis UA, Peters CG, Xu P, Krasner C, Kerbel RS (2015) Translational impact of nanoparticle-drug conjugate CRLX101 with or without bevacizumab in advanced ovarian cancer. Clin Cancer Res 21 (4):808–818. https://doi.org/10.1158/1078-0432.CCR-14-28102868

Piha-Paul SA, Wheler JJ, Fu S et al (2014) Advanced gynecologic malignancies treated with a combination of the VEGF inhibitor bevacizumab and the mTOR inhibitor temsirolimus. Oncotarget 5(7):1846–1855

Pils D, Bachmayr-Heyda A, Auer K et al (2014) Cyclin E1 (CCNE1) as independent positive prognostic factor in advanced stage serous ovarian cancer patients – a study of the OVCAD consortium. Eur J Cancer 50(1):99–110. https://doi.org/10.1016/j.ejca.2013.09.011

Poveda A, Floquet A, Ledermann JA et al (2020) Final overall survival results from SOLO2/ENGOT-ov21: a phase III trial assessing maintenance olaparib in patients with platinum-sensitive, relapsed ovarian cancer and a BRCA mutation. ASCO20 Virtual Scientific Program. Abstract 6002. Presented at press briefing on May 12, 2020

Pradeep S, Kim SW, Wu SY et al (2014) Hematogenous metastasis of ovarian cancer: rethinking mode of spread. Cancer Cell 26(1):77–91. https://doi.org/10.1016/j.ccr.2014.05.002

Prat J, D'Angelo E, Espinosa I (2018) Ovarian carcinomas: at least five different diseases with distinct histological features and molecular genetics. Hum Pathol 80:11–27. https://doi.org/10.1016/j.humpath.2018.06.018

Prislei S, Martinelli E, Zannoni GF et al (2015) Role and prognostic significance of the epithelial-mesenchymal transition factor ZEB2 in ovarian cancer. Oncotarget 6(22):18966–18979. https://doi.org/10.18632/oncotarget.3943

Pujade-Lauraine E, Hilpert F, Weber B, Reuss A, Poveda A, Kristensen G, Sorio R, Vergote I, Witteveen P, Bamias A, Pereira D, Wimberger P, Oaknin A, Mirza MR, Follana P, Bollag D, Ray-Coquard I (2014) Bevacizumab combined with chemotherapy for platinum-resistant recurrent ovarian cancer: the AURELIA open-label randomized phase III trial. J Clin Oncol 32 (13):1302–1308. https://doi.org/10.1200/JCO.2013.51.4489

Pujade-Lauraine E, Ledermann JA, Selle F, Gebski V, Penson RT, Oza AM, Korach J, Huzarski T, Poveda A, Pignata S, Friedlander M, Colombo N, Harter P, Fujiwara K, Ray-Coquard I, Banerjee S, Liu J, Lowe ES, Bloomfield R, Pautier P, SOLO2/ENGOT-Ov21 Investigators (2017) Olaparib tablets as maintenance therapy in patients with platinum-sensitive, relapsed ovarian cancer and a BRCA1/2 mutation (SOLO2/ENGOT-Ov21): a double-blind, randomised, placebo-controlled, phase 3 trial. Lancet Oncol 18(9):1274–1284. https://doi.org/10.1016/S1470-2045(17)30469-2. Epub 2017. Erratum in: Lancet Oncol 2017;18(9):e510

Pujade-Lauraine E, Fujiwara K, Dychter SS, Devgan G, Monk BJ (2018) Avelumab (anti-PD-L1) in platinum-resistant/refractory ovarian cancer: javelin Ovarian 200 Phase III study design. Future Oncol 14(21):2103–2113. https://doi.org/10.2217/fon-2018-0070

Pujade-Lauraine E, Fujiwara K, Ledermann JAL et al (2019) Avelumab alone or in combination with pegylated liposomal doxorubicin versus pegylated liposomal doxorubicin alone in platinum-resistant or refractory epithelial ovarian cancer: primary and biomarker analysis of the phase III JAVELIN Ovarian 200 trial. Soc Gynecol Oncol Annual Meeting. (LBA1). https://www.sgo50.org/wp-content/uploads/2019/03/SGO-2019-Late-Breaking-Abstracts.pdf. Accessed 16 Jan 2021

Qiao Y, Yang T, Gan Y et al (2018) Associations between aspirin use and the risk of cancers: a meta-analysis of observational studies. BMC Cancer 18(1):288. https://doi.org/10.1186/s12885-018-4156-5

Qiu C, Lu N, Wang X et al (2017) Gene expression profiles of ovarian low-grade serous carcinoma resemble those of fallopian tube epithelium. Gynecol Oncol 147(3):634–641. https://doi.org/10.1016/j.ygyno.2017.09.029

Rafehi S, Ramos Valdes Y, Bertrand M et al (2016) TGFβ signaling regulates epithelial-mesenchymal plasticity in ovarian cancer ascites-derived spheroids. Endocr Relat Cancer 23 (3):147–159. https://doi.org/10.1530/ERC-15-0383

Rahman M, Nakayama K, Rahman MT et al (2012) Clinicopathologic and biological analysis of PIK3CA mutation in ovarian clear cell carcinoma. Hum Pathol 43(12):2197–2206. https://doi.org/10.1016/j.humpath.2012.03.011

Ray-Coquard I, Pautier P, Pignata S, Pérol D, González-Martín A, Berger R, Fujiwara K, Vergote I, Colombo N, Mäenpää J, Selle F, Sehouli J, Lorusso D, Guerra Alía EM, Reinthaller A, Nagao S, Lefeuvre-Plesse C, Canzler U, Scambia G, Lortholary A, Marmé F, Combe P, de Gregorio N, Rodrigues M, Buderath P, Dubot C, Burges A, You B, Pujade-Lauraine E, Harter P, PAOLA-1 Investigators (2019) Olaparib plus Bevacizumab as first-line maintenance in ovarian cancer. N Engl J Med 381(25):2416–2428. https://doi.org/10.1056/NEJMoa1911361

Rechsteiner M, Zimmermann AK, Wild PJ et al (2013) TP53 mutations are common in all subtypes of epithelial ovarian cancer and occur concomitantly with KRAS mutations in the mucinous type. Exp Mol Pathol 95(2):235–241. https://doi.org/10.1016/j.yexmp.2013.08.004

Ren J, Chen Y, Song H, Chen L, Wang R (2013) Inhibition of ZEB1 reverses EMT and chemoresistance in docetaxel-resistant human lung adenocarcinoma cell line. J Cell Biochem 114(6):1395–1403. https://doi.org/10.1002/jcb.24481

Ren YA, Mullany LK, Liu Z, Herron AJ, Wong KK, Richards JS (2016) Mutant p53 promotes epithelial ovarian cancer by regulating tumor differentiation, metastasis, and responsiveness to steroid hormones. Cancer Res 76(8):2206–2218

Reyes HD, Thiel KW, Carlson MJ et al (2014) Comprehensive profiling of EGFR/HER receptors for personalized treatment of gynecologic cancers. Mol Diagn Ther 18(2):137–151. https://doi.org/10.1007/s40291-013-0070-3

Reyners AK, de Munck L, Erdkamp FL et al (2012) A randomized phase II study investigating the addition of the specific COX-2 inhibitor celecoxib to docetaxel plus carboplatin as first-line chemotherapy for stage IC to IV epithelial ovarian cancer, Fallopian tube or primary peritoneal carcinomas: the DoCaCel study. Ann Oncol 23(11):2896–2902. https://doi.org/10.1093/annonc/mds107

Ribas A, Wolchok JD (2018) Cancer immunotherapy using checkpoint blockade. Science 359 (6382):1350–1355. https://doi.org/10.1126/science.aar4060

Rizzo A, Napoli A, Roggiani F, Tomassetti A, Bagnoli M, Mezzanzanica D (2018) One-carbon metabolism: biological players in epithelial ovarian cancer. Int J Mol Sci 19(7):2092. https://doi.org/10.3390/ijms19072092

Roggiani F, Mezzanzanica D, Rea K, Tomassetti A (2016) Guidance of signaling activations by cadherins and integrins in epithelial ovarian cancer cells. Int J Mol Sci 17(9):1387. https://doi.org/10.3390/ijms17091387

Rubinsak LA, Cohen C, Khanna N et al (2018) Folate receptor alpha expression in platinum resistant/refractory ovarian carcinomas and primary endocervical adenocarcinomas. Appl Immunohistochem Mol Morphol 26(8):567–572. https://doi.org/10.1097/PAI.0000000000000476

Ruscito I, Bellati F, Ray-Coquard I, Mirza MR, du Bois A, Gasparri ML, Costanzi F, De Marco MP, Nuti M, Caserta D, Pignata S, Dorigo O, Sehouli J, Braicu EI (2020) Incorporating parp-inhibitors in primary and recurrent ovarian cancer: a meta-analysis of 12 phase II/III randomized controlled trials. Cancer Treat Rev 87:102040. https://doi.org/10.1016/j.ctrv.2020.102040

Russell SE, McCluggage WG (2004) A multistep model for ovarian tumorigenesis: the value of mutation analysis in the KRAS and BRAF genes. J Pathol 203(2):617–619

Russo A, Czarnecki AA, Dean M et al (2018) PTEN loss in the fallopian tube induces hyperplasia and ovarian tumor formation. Oncogene 37(15):1976–1990. https://doi.org/10.1038/s41388-017-0097-8

Sakata J, Kajiyama H, Suzuki S et al (2017) Impact of positive ZEB1 expression in patients with epithelial ovarian carcinoma as an oncologic outcome-predicting indicator. Oncol Lett 14 (4):4287–4293. https://doi.org/10.3892/ol.2017.6658

Saleh T, Carpenter VJ, Bloukh S, Gewirtz DA (2020) Targeting tumor cell senescence and polyploidy as potential therapeutic strategies. Semin Cancer Biol. S1044-579X(20)30270-4. https://doi.org/10.1016/j.semcancer.2020.12.010

Salmena L, Shaw P, Fans I et al (2015) Prognostic value of INPP4B protein immunohistochemistry in ovarian cancer. Eur J Gynaecol Oncol 36(3):260–267

Sarker D, Ang JE, Baird R et al (2014) First-in-human phase I study of pictilisib (GDC-0941), a potent pan-class I phosphatidylinositol-3-kinase (PI3K) inhibitor, in patients with advanced solid tumors. Clin Cancer Res 21(1):77–86

Sato H, Niimi A, Yasuhara T, Permata TBM, Hagiwara Y, Isono M, Nuryadi E, Sekine R, Oike T, Kakoti S, Yoshimoto Y, Held KD, Suzuki Y, Kono K, Miyagawa K, Nakano T, Shibata A (2017) DNA double-strand break repair pathway regulates PD-L1 expression in cancer cells. Nat Commun 8(1):1751. https://doi.org/10.1038/s41467-017-01883-9

Sawada K, Mitra AK, Radjabi AR et al (2008) Loss of E-cadherin promotes ovarian cancer metastasis via alpha 5-integrin, which is a therapeutic target. Cancer Res 68(7):2329–2339

Scaranti M, Cojocaru E, Banerjee S, Banerji U (2020) Exploiting the folate receptor α in oncology. Nat Rev Clin Oncol 17(6):349–359. https://doi.org/10.1038/s41571-020-0339-5

Scheid AD, Beadnell TC, Welch DR (2021) Roles of mitochondria in the hallmarks of metastasis. Br J Cancer 124(1):124–135. https://doi.org/10.1038/s41416-020-01125-8

Schnell U, Cirulli V, Giepmans BN (2013) EpCAM: structure and function in health and disease. Biochim Biophys Acta 1828(8):1989–2001. https://doi.org/10.1016/j.bbamem.2013.04.018

Seagle BL, Yang CP, Eng KH, Dandapani M, Odunsi-Akanji O, Goldberg GL, Odunsi K, Horwitz SB, Shahabi S (2015) TP53 hot spot mutations in ovarian cancer: selective resistance to microtubule stabilizers in vitro and differential survival outcomes from The Cancer Genome Atlas. Gynecol Oncol 138(1):159–164. https://doi.org/10.1016/j.ygyno.2015.04.039

Semaan A, Munkarah AR, Arabi H, Bandyopadhyay S, Seward S, Kumar S, Qazi A, Hussein Y, Morris RT, Ali-Fehmi R (2011) Expression of GLUT-1 in epithelial ovarian carcinoma:

correlation with tumor cell proliferation, angiogenesis, survival and ability to predict optimal cytoreduction. Gynecol Oncol 121(1):181–186. https://doi.org/10.1016/j.ygyno.2010.11.019

Shahbazi MN, Perez-Moreno M (2015) Connections between cadherin-catenin proteins, spindle misorientation, and cancer. Tissue Barriers 3(3):e1045684. https://doi.org/10.1080/21688370.2015.1045684

Shamir ER, Ewald AJ (2015) Adhesion in mammary development: novel roles for E-cadherin in individual and collective cell migration. Curr Top Dev Biol 112:353–382

Shang AQ, Wu J, Bi F et al (2017a) Relationship between HER2 and JAK/STAT-SOCS3 signaling pathway and clinicopathological features and prognosis of ovarian cancer. Cancer Biol Ther 18 (5):314–322

Shang Y, He J, Wang Y, Feng Q, Zhang Y, Guo J, Li J, Li S, Wang Y, Yan G, Ren F, Shi Y, Xu J, Zeps N, Zhai Y, He D, Chang Z (2017b) CHIP/Stub1 regulates the Warburg effect by promoting degradation of PKM2 in ovarian carcinoma. Oncogene 36(29):4191–4200. https://doi.org/10.1038/onc.2017.31

Shen W, Li HL, Liu L, Cheng JX (2017) Expression levels of PTEN, HIF-1α, and VEGF as prognostic factors in ovarian cancer. Eur Rev Med Pharmacol Sci 21(11):2596–2603

Sheppard KE, Cullinane C, Hannan KM et al (2013) Synergistic inhibition of ovarian cancer cell growth by combining selective PI3K/mTOR and RAS/ERK pathway inhibitors. Eur J Cancer 49 (18):3936–3944. https://doi.org/10.1016/j.ejca.2013.08.007

Sherr CJ, McCormick F (2002) The RB and p53 pathways in cancer. Cancer Cell 2(2):103–112

Shibuya Y, Tokunaga H, Saito S et al (2018) Identification of somatic genetic alterations in ovarian clear cell carcinoma with next generation sequencing. Genes Chromosomes Cancer 57 (2):51–60. https://doi.org/10.1002/gcc.22507

Shimogai R, Kigawa J, Itamochi H, Iba T, Kanamori Y, Oishi T, Shimada M, Sato S, Kawaguchi W, Sato S, Terakawa N (2008) Expression of hypoxia-inducible factor 1alpha gene affects the outcome in patients with ovarian cancer. Int J Gynecol Cancer 18 (3):499–505. https://doi.org/10.1111/j.1525-1438.2007.01055.x

Sigismund S, Avanzato D, Lanzetti L (2017) Emerging functions of the EGFR in cancer. Mol Oncol 12(1):3–20

Sikora E, Czarnecka-Herok J, Bojko A, Sunderland P (2020) Therapy-induced polyploidization and senescence: coincidence or interconnection? Semin Cancer Biol. S1044-579X(20)30253-4. https://doi.org/10.1016/j.semcancer.2020.11.015

Silwal-Pandit L, Langerød A, Børresen-Dale AL (2017) TP53 mutations in breast and ovarian cancer. Cold Spring Harb Perspect Med 7(1):a026252. https://doi.org/10.1101/cshperspect.a026252

Simeone P, Trerotola M, Franck J et al (2018) The multiverse nature of epithelial to mesenchymal transition. Semin Cancer Biol. S1044-579X(18)30086-5. https://doi.org/10.1016/j.semcancer.2018.11.004

Simonin K, Brotin E, Dufort S, Dutoit S, Goux D, N'diaye M, Denoyelle C, Gauduchon P, Poulain L (2009) Mcl-1 is an important determinant of the apoptotic response to the BH3-mimetic molecule HA14-1 in cisplatin-resistant ovarian carcinoma cells. Mol Cancer Ther 8 (11):3162–3170. https://doi.org/10.1158/1535-7163.MCT-09-0493

Simpkins F, Jang K, Yoon H et al (2018) Dual Src and MEK inhibition decreases ovarian cancer growth and targets tumor initiating stem-like cells. Clin Cancer Res 24(19):4874–4886. https://doi.org/10.1158/1078-0432.CCR-17-3697

Singer G, Oldt R III, Cohen Y et al (2003) Mutations in BRAF and KRAS characterize the development of low-grade ovarian serous carcinoma. J Natl Cancer Inst 95(6):484–486

Singh R, Letai A, Sarosiek K (2019) Regulation of apoptosis in health and disease: the balancing act of BCL-2 family proteins. Nat Rev Mol Cell Biol 20(3):175–193. https://doi.org/10.1038/s41580-018-0089-8

Skírnisdóttir I, Seidal T (2011) Prognostic impact of concomitant p53 and PTEN on outcome in early stage (FIGO I-II) epithelial ovarian cancer. Int J Gynecol Cancer 21(6):1024–1031. https://doi.org/10.1097/IGC.0b013e31821dc906

Song H, Ramus SJ, Shadforth D et al (2006) Common variants in RB1 gene and risk of invasive ovarian cancer. Cancer Res 66(20):10220–10226
Song H, Kwan SY, Izaguirre DI et al (2013) PAX2 expression in ovarian cancer. Int J Mol Sci 14 (3):6090–6105. https://doi.org/10.3390/ijms14036090
Song N, Liu H, Ma X, Zhang S (2016) Placental growth factor promotes ovarian cancer cell invasion via ZEB2. Cell Physiol Biochem 38(1):351–358. https://doi.org/10.1159/000438635
Sonntag R, Giebeler N, Nevzorova YA et al (2018) Cyclin E1 and cyclin-dependent kinase 2 are critical for initiation, but not for progression of hepatocellular carcinoma. Proc Natl Acad Sci U S A 115(37):9282–9287. https://doi.org/10.1073/pnas.1807155115
Soong TR, Dinulescu DM, Xian W et al (2018) Frontiers in the pathology and pathogenesis of ovarian cancer: cancer precursors and "precursor escape". Hematol Oncol Clin North Am 32 (6):915–928. https://doi.org/10.1016/j.hoc.2018.07.013
Soong TR, Howitt BE, Horowitz N et al (2019) The fallopian tube, "precursor escape" and narrowing the knowledge gap to the origins of high-grade serous carcinoma. Gynecol Oncol 152(2):426–433. https://doi.org/10.1016/j.ygyno.2018.11.033
Soussi T (2010) The history of p53. A perfect example of the drawbacks of scientific paradigms. EMBO Rep 11(11):822–826
Spizzo G, Fong D, Wurm M et al (2011) EpCAM expression in primary tumour tissues and metastases: an immunohistochemical analysis. J Clin Pathol 64(5):415–420. https://doi.org/10.1136/jcp.2011.090274
Spreafico A, Oza AM, Clarke BA et al (2017) Genotype-matched treatment for patients with advanced type I epithelial ovarian cancer (EOC). Gynecol Oncol 144(2):250–255. https://doi.org/10.1016/j.ygyno.2016.12.002
Stamelos VA, Robinson E, Redman CW, Richardson A (2013) Navitoclax augments the activity of carboplatin and paclitaxel combinations in ovarian cancer cells. Gynecol Oncol 128 (2):377–382. https://doi.org/10.1016/j.ygyno.2012.11.019
Stewart D, Cristea M (2019) Antibody-drug conjugates for ovarian cancer: current clinical development. Curr Opin Obstet Gynecol 31(1):18–23. https://doi.org/10.1097/GCO.0000000000000515
Stewart ML, Tamayo P, Wilson AJ et al (2015) KRAS genomic status predicts the sensitivity of ovarian cancer cells to decitabine. Cancer Res 75(14):2897–2906
Stover EH, Howitt B, Lindeman NI et al (2016) Somatic mutations and copy number variations in cancer-associated genes in 695 ovarian cancer patients. [abstract]. In: Proceedings of the 107th Annual Meeting of the American Association for Cancer Research; 2016-20; New Orleans, LA. Philadelphia (PA): aacr. Cancer Res 76(14 Suppl):Abstract nr 95
Stover EH, Baco MB, Cohen O, Li YY, Christie EL, Bagul M, Goodale A, Lee Y, Pantel S, Rees MG, Wei G, Presser AG, Gelbard MK, Zhang W, Zervantonakis IK, Bhola PD, Ryan J, Guerriero JL, Montero J, Liang FJ, Cherniack AD, Piccioni F, Matulonis UA, Bowtell DDL, Sarosiek KA, Letai A, Garraway LA, Johannessen CM, Meyerson M (2019) Pooled genomic screens identify anti-apoptotic genes as targetable mediators of chemotherapy resistance in ovarian cancer. Mol Cancer Res 17(11):2281–2293. https://doi.org/10.1158/1541-7786.MCR-18-1243
Strickland KC, Howitt BE, Shukla SA, Rodig S, Ritterhouse LL, Liu JF, Garber JE, Chowdhury D, Wu CJ, D'Andrea AD, Matulonis UA, Konstantinopoulos PA (2016) Association and prognostic significance of BRCA1/2-mutation status with neoantigen load, number of tumor-infiltrating lymphocytes and expression of PD-1/PD-L1 in high grade serous ovarian cancer. Oncotarget 7 (12):13587–13598. https://doi.org/10.18632/oncotarget.7277
Swisher EM, Lin KK, Oza AM, Scott CL, Giordano H, Sun J, Konecny GE, Coleman RL, Tinker AV, O'Malley DM, Kristeleit RS, Ma L, Bell-McGuinn K, Brenton JD, Cragun JM, Oaknin A, Ray-Coquard I, Harrell MI, Mann E, Kaufmann SH, Floquet A, Leary A, Harding TC, Goble S, Maloney L, Isaacson J, Allen AR, Rolfe L, Yelensky R, Raponi M, McNeish IA (2017) Rucaparib in relapsed, platinum-sensitive high-grade ovarian carcinoma (ARIEL2 Part 1): an

international, multicentre, open-label, phase 2 trial. Lancet Oncol 18(1):75–87. https://doi.org/10.1016/S1470-2045(16)30559-9

Takai M, Terai Y, Kawaguchi H et al (2014) The EMT (epithelial-mesenchymal-transition)-related protein expression indicates the metastatic status and prognosis in patients with ovarian cancer. J Ovarian Res 7:76. https://doi.org/10.1186/1757-2215-7-76

Takekuma M, Wong KK, Coleman RL (2016) A long-term surviving patient with recurrent low-grade serous ovarian carcinoma treated with the MEK1/2 inhibitor, selumetinib. Gynecol Oncol Res Pract 3:5. https://doi.org/10.1186/s40661-016-0026-5

Takenaka M, Saito M, Iwakawa R et al (2015) Profiling of actionable gene alterations in ovarian cancer by targeted deep sequencing. Int J Oncol 46(6):2389–2398. https://doi.org/10.3892/ijo.2015.2951

Tamura R, Tanaka T, Akasaki Y, Murayama Y, Yoshida K, Sasaki H (2019) The role of vascular endothelial growth factor in the hypoxic and immunosuppressive tumor microenvironment: perspectives for therapeutic implications. Med Oncol 37(1):2. https://doi.org/10.1007/s12032-019-1329-2

Tan DS, Agarwal R, Kaye SB (2006) Mechanisms of transcoelomic metastasis in ovarian cancer. Lancet Oncol 7(11):925–934. https://doi.org/10.1016/S1470-2045(06)70939-1

Tang S, Ning Q, Yang L, Mo Z, Tang S (2020) Mechanisms of immune escape in the cancer immune cycle. Int Immunopharmacol 86:106700. https://doi.org/10.1016/j.intimp.2020.106700

Taniguchi K, Karin M (2018) NF-κB, inflammation, immunity and cancer: coming of age. Nat Rev Immunol 18(5):309–324. https://doi.org/10.1038/nri.2017.142

Tayama S, Motohara T, Narantuya D et al (2017) The impact of EpCAM expression on response to chemotherapy and clinical outcomes in patients with epithelial ovarian cancer. Oncotarget 8(27):44312–44325. https://doi.org/10.18632/oncotarget.17871

Telleria CM (2013) Repopulation of ovarian cancer cells after chemotherapy. Cancer Growth Metastasis 6:15–21. https://doi.org/10.4137/CGM.S11333

Temkin SM, Yamada SD, Fleming GF (2010) A phase I study of weekly temsirolimus and topotecan in the treatment of advanced and/or recurrent gynecologic malignancies. Gynecol Oncol 117(3):473–476. https://doi.org/10.1016/j.ygyno.2010.02.022

Teng L, Peng S et al (2015) Conditioned media from human ovarian cancer endothelial progenitor cells induces ovarian cancer cell migration by activating epithelial-to-mesenchymal transition. Cancer Gene Ther 22(11):518–523. https://doi.org/10.1038/cgt.2015.45

Teplinsky E, Muggia F (2015) EGFR and HER2: is there a role in ovarian cancer? Translat Cancer Res 4(1):107–117. https://doi.org/10.3978/j.issn.2218-676X.2015.01.01

Tew WP, Sill MW, Walker JL et al (2018) Randomized phase II trial of bevacizumab plus everolimus versus bevacizumab alone for recurrent or persistent ovarian, fallopian tube or peritoneal carcinoma: an NRG oncology/gynecologic oncology group study. Gynecol Oncol 151(2):257–263. https://doi.org/10.1016/j.ygyno.2018.08.027

Tewari KS, Burger RA, Enserro D, Norquist BM, Swisher EM, Brady MF, Bookman MA, Fleming GF, Huang H, Homesley HD, Fowler JM, Greer BE, Boente M, Liang SX, Ye C, Bais C, Randall LM, Chan JK, Ferriss JS, Coleman RL, Aghajanian C, Herzog TJ, DiSaia PJ, Copeland LJ, Mannel RS, Birrer MJ, Monk BJ (2019) Final overall survival of a randomized trial of bevacizumab for primary treatment of ovarian cancer. J Clin Oncol 37(26):2317–2328. https://doi.org/10.1200/JCO.19.01009

Tomao F, Bardhi E, Di Pinto A, Sassu CM, Biagioli E, Petrella MC, Palaia I, Muzii L, Colombo N, Panici PB (2019) Parp inhibitors as maintenance treatment in platinum sensitive recurrent ovarian cancer: an updated meta-analysis of randomized clinical trials according to BRCA mutational status. Cancer Treat Rev 80:101909. https://doi.org/10.1016/j.ctrv.2019.101909

Topatana W, Juengpanich S, Li S, Cao J, Hu J, Lee J, Suliyanto K, Ma D, Zhang B, Chen M, Cai X (2020) Advances in synthetic lethality for cancer therapy: cellular mechanism and clinical translation. J Hematol Oncol 13(1):118. https://doi.org/10.1186/s13045-020-00956-5

Trabert B, Poole EM, White E et al (2018) Analgesic use and ovarian cancer risk: an analysis in the ovarian cancer cohort consortium. J Natl Cancer Inst. https://doi.org/10.1093/jnci/djy100

Tretter JY, Schorpp K, Luxenburger E et al (2018) A high-content screen for small-molecule regulators of epithelial cell-adhesion molecule (EpCAM) cleavage yields a robust inhibitor. J Biol Chem 293(23):8994–9005. https://doi.org/10.1074/jbc.RA118.002776

Turashvili G, Grisham RN, Chiang S et al (2018) BRAFV600E mutations and immunohistochemical expression of VE1 protein in low-grade serous neoplasms of the ovary. Histopathology 73 (3):438–443. https://doi.org/10.1111/his.13651

Tutlewska K, Lubinski J, Kurzawski G (2013) Germline deletions in the EPCAM gene as a cause of Lynch syndrome – literature review. Hered Cancer Clin Pract 11(1):9. https://doi.org/10.1186/1897-4287-11-9

Urbano AM (2021) Otto Warburg: the journey towards the seminal discovery of tumor cell bioenergetic reprogramming. Biochim Biophys Acta Mol Basis Dis 1867(1):165965. https://doi.org/10.1016/j.bbadis.2020.165965

Usui A, Ko SY, Barengo N, Naora H (2014) P-cadherin promotes ovarian cancer dissemination through tumor cell aggregation and tumor-peritoneum interactions. Mol Cancer Res 12 (4):504–513

van Baal JOAM, van Noorden CJF, Nieuwland R et al (2018) Development of peritoneal carcinomatosis in epithelial ovarian cancer: a review. J Histochem Cytochem 66(2):67–83

Van Berckelaer C, Brouwers AJ, Peeters DJ et al (2016) Current and future role of circulating tumor cells in patients with epithelial ovarian cancer. Eur J Surg Oncol 42(12):1772–1779. https://doi.org/10.1016/j.ejso.2016.05.010

Vanhaesebroeck B, Guillermet-Guibert J, Graupera M et al (2010) The emerging mechanisms of isoform-specific PI3K signalling. Nat Rev Mol Cell Biol 11(5):329–341. https://doi.org/10.1038/nrm2882

Varga A, Piha-Paul S, Ott PA, Mehnert JM, Berton-Rigaud D, Morosky A, Yang P, Ruman J, Matei D (2019) Pembrolizumab in patients with programmed death ligand 1-positive advanced ovarian cancer: analysis of KEYNOTE-028. Gynecol Oncol 152(2):243–250. https://doi.org/10.1016/j.ygyno.2018.11.017

Veneris JT, Matulonis UA, Liu JF, Konstantinopoulos PA (2020) Choosing wisely: selecting PARP inhibitor combinations to promote anti-tumor immune responses beyond BRCA mutations. Gynecol Oncol 156(2):488–497. https://doi.org/10.1016/j.ygyno.2019.09.021

Verdoodt F, Dehlendorff C, Friis S et al (2018) Non-aspirin NSAID use and ovarian cancer mortality. Gynecol Oncol 150(2):331–337. https://doi.org/10.1016/j.ygyno.2018.06.018

Vergote I, Armstrong D, Scambia G et al (2016) A randomized, double-blind, placebo-controlled, phase III study to assess efficacy and safety of weekly farletuzumab in combination with carboplatin and taxane in patients with ovarian cancer in first platinum-sensitive relapse. J Clin Oncol 34(19):2271–2278. https://doi.org/10.1200/JCO.2015.63.2596

Vergote I, du Bois A, Floquet A, Rau J, Kim JW, Del Campo JM, Friedlander M, Pignata S, Fujiwara K, Colombo N, Mirza MR, Monk BJ, Tsibulak I, Calvert PM, Herzog TJ, Hanker LC, Meunier J, Lee JY, Bologna A, Carrasco-Alfonso MJ, Harter P (2019a) Overall survival results of AGO-OVAR16: a phase 3 study of maintenance pazopanib versus placebo in women who have not progressed after first-line chemotherapy for advanced ovarian cancer. Gynecol Oncol 155(2):186–191. https://doi.org/10.1016/j.ygyno.2019.08.024

Vergote I, Scambia G, O'Malley DM, Van Calster B, Park SY, Del Campo JM, Meier W, Bamias A, Colombo N, Wenham RM, Covens A, Marth C, Raza Mirza M, Kroep JR, Ma H, Pickett CA, Monk BJ, TRINOVA-3/ENGOT-ov2/GOG-3001 Investigators (2019b) Trebananib or placebo plus carboplatin and paclitaxel as first-line treatment for advanced ovarian cancer (TRINOVA-3/ENGOT-ov2/GOG-3001): a randomised, double-blind, phase 3 trial. Lancet Oncol 20(6):862–876. https://doi.org/10.1016/S1470-2045(19)30178-0

Verma S, Bartlett CH, Schnell P et al (2016) Palbociclib in combination with fulvestrant in women with hormone receptor-positive/HER2-negative advanced metastatic breast cancer: detailed safety analysis from a multicenter, randomized, placebo-controlled, phase III study (PALOMA-3). Oncologist 21(10):1165–1175

Vieira AF, Paredes J (2015) P-cadherin and the journey to cancer metastasis. Mol Cancer 14:178. https://doi.org/10.1186/s12943-015-0448-4

Vijayakumaran R, Tan KH, Miranda PJ, Haupt S, Haupt Y (2015) Regulation of mutant p53 protein expression. Front Oncol 5:284. https://doi.org/10.3389/fonc.2015.00284

Wakahashi S, Sudo T, Oka N et al (2013) VAV1 represses E-cadherin expression through the transactivation of Snail and Slug: a potential mechanism for aberrant epithelial to mesenchymal transition in human epithelial ovarian cancer. Transl Res 162(3):181–190. https://doi.org/10.1016/j.trsl.2013.06.005

Wang Y, Ma J, Shen H et al (2014) Reactive oxygen species promote ovarian cancer progression via the HIF-1α/LOX/E-cadherin pathway. Oncol Rep 32(5):2150–2158

Wang Y, Zhang FC, Wang YJ (2015) The efficacy and safety of non-steroidal anti-inflammatory drugs in preventing the recurrence of colorectal adenoma: a meta-analysis and systematic review of randomized trials. Colorectal Dis 17(3):188–196. https://doi.org/10.1111/codi.12838

Wang D, Li C, Zhang Y et al (2016a) Combined inhibition of PI3K and PARP is effective in the treatment of ovarian cancer cells with wild-type PIK3CA genes. Gynecol Oncol 142 (3):548–556

Wang Q, Wang B, Zhang YM, Wang W (2016b) The association between CDH1 promoter methylation and patients with ovarian cancer: a systematic meta-analysis. J Ovarian Res 9:23. https://doi.org/10.1186/s13048-016-0231-1

Wang S, Han H, Hu Y et al (2017a) SLC3A2, antigen of mAb 3G9, promotes migration and invasion by upregulating of mucins in gastric cancer. Oncotarget. 8(51):88586–88598. https://doi.org/10.18632/oncotarget.19529

Wang Q, Lou W, Di W, Wu X (2017b) Prognostic value of tumor PD-L1 expression combined with CD8+ tumor infiltrating lymphocytes in high grade serous ovarian cancer. Int Immunopharmacol 52:7–14. https://doi.org/10.1016/j.intimp.2017.08.017

Wang YP, Wang QY, Li CH, Li XW (2018) COX-2 inhibition by celecoxib in epithelial ovarian cancer attenuates E-cadherin suppression through reduced Snail nuclear translocation. Chem Biol Interact 292:24–29. https://doi.org/10.1016/j.cbi.2018.06.020

Wang Y, Wei Z, Pan K, Li J, Chen Q (2020) The function and mechanism of ferroptosis in cancer. Apoptosis 25(11–12):786–798. https://doi.org/10.1007/s10495-020-01638-w

Warburg O (1930) The metabolism of tumours: investigations from the Kaiser Wilhelm Institute for Biology, Berlin-Dahlem. Arnold Constable, London

Warburg O (1956) On respiratory impairment in cancer cells. Science 124(3215):269–270

Webb JR, Milne K, Kroeger DR, Nelson BH (2016) PD-L1 expression is associated with tumor-infiltrating T cells and favorable prognosis in high-grade serous ovarian cancer. Gynecol Oncol 141(2):293–302. https://doi.org/10.1016/j.ygyno.2016.03.008

Welch DR, Hurst DR (2019) Defining the hallmarks of metastasis. Cancer Res 79(12):3011–3027. https://doi.org/10.1158/0008-5472.CAN-19-0458

Wendel JRH, Wang X, Hawkins SM (2018) The endometriotic tumor microenvironment in ovarian cancer. Cancers (Basel) 10(8):261. https://doi.org/10.3390/cancers10080261

Westin SN, Kristeleit RS, Coleman RL et al (2019) Abstract CT158: athena (GOG-3020/ENGOT-ov45): a randomized, double-blind, placebo-controlled, Phase III study of rucaparib + nivolumab following front-line platinum-based chemotherapy in ovarian cancer. Cancer Res 79:CT158

Wojnarowicz PM, Oros KK, Quinn MC et al (2012) The genomic landscape of TP53 and p53 annotated high grade ovarian serous carcinomas from a defined founder population associated with patient outcome. PLoS One 7(9):e45484

Wong KK, Tsang YT, Deavers MT et al (2010) BRAF mutation is rare in advanced-stage low-grade ovarian serous carcinomas. Am J Pathol 177(4):1611–1617

Wong M, Tan N, Zha J, Peale FV, Yue P, Fairbrother WJ, Belmont LD (2012) Navitoclax (ABT-263) reduces Bcl-x(L)-mediated chemoresistance in ovarian cancer models. Mol Cancer Ther 11(4):1026–1035. https://doi.org/10.1158/1535-7163.MCT-11-0693

Wong KK, Izaguirre DI, Kwan SY et al (2013) Poor survival with wild-type TP53 ovarian cancer? Gynecol Oncol 130(3):565–569

Wong SHM, Fang CM, Chuah LH et al (2018) E-cadherin: its dysregulation in carcinogenesis and clinical implications. Crit Rev Oncol Hematol 121:11–22. https://doi.org/10.1016/j.critrevonc.2017.11.010

Wood DJ, Endicott JA (2018) Structural insights into the functional diversity of the CDK-cyclin family. Open Biol 8(9):180112

Woopen H, Pietzner K, Richter R et al (2014) Overexpression of the epithelial cell adhesion molecule is associated with a more favorable prognosis and response to platinum-based chemotherapy in ovarian cancer. J Gynecol Oncol 25(3):221–228. https://doi.org/10.3802/jgo.2014.25.3.221

Wu DI, Liu L, Ren C et al (2016) Epithelial-mesenchymal interconversions and the regulatory function of the ZEB family during the development and progression of ovarian cancer. Oncol Lett 11(2):1463–1468. https://doi.org/10.3892/ol.2016.4092

Wyld L, Bellantuono I, Tchkonia T, Morgan J, Turner O, Foss F, George J, Danson S, Kirkland JL (2020) Senescence and cancer: a review of clinical implications of senescence and senotherapies. Cancers (Basel) 12(8):2134. https://doi.org/10.3390/cancers12082134

Xu Y, Bi R, Xiao Y et al (2017) Low frequency of BRAF and KRAS mutations in Chinese patients with low-grade serous carcinoma of the ovary. Diagn Pathol 12(1):87. https://doi.org/10.1186/s13000-017-0679-3

Xu Y, Zhang Q, Miao C et al (2019) CCNG1 (Cyclin G1) regulation by mutant-P53 via induction of Notch3 expression promotes high-grade serous ovarian cancer (HGSOC) tumorigenesis and progression. Cancer Med 8(1):351–362

Yahyazadeh Mashhadi SM, Kazemimanesh M, Arashkia A et al (2019) Shedding light on the EpCAM: an overview. J Cell Physiol 234(8):12569–12580. https://doi.org/10.1002/jcp.28132

Yan Z, Tian X, Wang R et al (2017) Title prognosis significance of ZEB2 and TGF-β1 as well as other clinical characteristics in epithelial ovarian cancer. Int J Gynecol Cancer 27(7):1343–1349. https://doi.org/10.1097/IGC.0000000000001037

Yang SYC, Lheureux S, Karakasis K et al (2018) Landscape of genomic alterations in high-grade serous ovarian cancer from exceptional long- and short-term survivors. Genome Med 10(1):81. https://doi.org/10.1186/s13073-018-0590-x

Yaswen P, MacKenzie KL, Keith WN, Hentosh P, Rodier F, Zhu J, Firestone GL, Matheu A, Carnero A, Bilsland A, Sundin T, Honoki K, Fujii H, Georgakilas AG, Amedei A, Amin A, Helferich B, Boosani CS, Guha G, Ciriolo MR, Chen S, Mohammed SI, Azmi AS, Bhakta D, Halicka D, Niccolai E, Aquilano K, Ashraf SS, Nowsheen S, Yang X (2015) Therapeutic targeting of replicative immortality. Semin Cancer Biol 35(Suppl):S104–S128. https://doi.org/10.1016/j.semcancer.2015.03.007

Yeh AC, Ramaswamy S (2015) Mechanisms of cancer cell dormancy–another hallmark of cancer? Cancer Res 75(23):5014–5022. https://doi.org/10.1158/0008-5472.CAN-15-1370

Yeku O, Zamarin D, Gallagher J, Aghajanian C, Konner J (2018) A phase II trial of TPIV200 (a polypeptide vaccine against folate receptor alpha) plus durvalumab (anti-PD-L1 antibody) in patients with platinum-resistant ovarian cancer. Gynecol Oncol 149(Suppl):56–57. https://doi.org/10.1016/j.ygyno.2018.04.124

Yeung TL, Leung CS, Yip KP, Au Yeung CL, Wong ST, Mok SC (2015) Cellular and molecular processes in ovarian cancer metastasis. A review in the theme: cell and molecular processes in cancer metastasis. Am J Physiol Cell Physiol 309(7):C444–C456. https://doi.org/10.1152/ajpcell.00188.2015

Yigit S, Demir L, Tarhan MO, Cabuk FK, Ellidokuz H, Erten C, Somali I, Dirican A, Cakalagaoglu F (2012) The clinicopathological significance of Bax and Bcl-2 protein expression with tumor infiltrating lymphocytes in ovarian carcinoma. Neoplasma 59(5):475–485. https://doi.org/10.4149/neo_2012_061

Yokoyama T, Kohn EC, Brill E, Lee JM (2017) Apoptosis is augmented in high-grade serous ovarian cancer by the combined inhibition of Bcl-2/Bcl-xL and PARP. Int J Oncol 50 (4):1064–1074. https://doi.org/10.3892/ijo.2017.3914

Yoshihara K, Tajima A, Komata D et al (2009) Gene expression profiling of advanced-stage serous ovarian cancers distinguishes novel subclasses and implicates ZEB2 in tumor progression and prognosis. Cancer Sci 100(8):1421–1428. https://doi.org/10.1111/j.1349-7006.2009.01204.x

Yu L, Deng L, Li J, Zhang Y, Hu L (2013) The prognostic value of vascular endothelial growth factor in ovarian cancer: a systematic review and meta-analysis. Gynecol Oncol 128 (2):391–396. https://doi.org/10.1016/j.ygyno.2012.11.002

Yu L, Hua X, Yang Y et al (2017) An updated meta-analysis of the prognostic value of decreased E-cadherin expression in ovarian cancer. Oncotarget 8(46):81176–81185. https://doi.org/10.18632/oncotarget.20885

Zamarin D, Walderich S, Holland A, Zhou Q, Iasonos AE, Torrisi JM, Merghoub T, Chesebrough LF, Mcdonnell AS, Gallagher JM, Li Y, Hollmann TJ, Grisham RN, Erskine CL, Block MS, Knutson KL, O'Cearbhaill RE, Aghajanian C, Konner JA (2020a) Safety, immunogenicity, and clinical efficacy of durvalumab in combination with folate receptor alpha vaccine TPIV200 in patients with advanced ovarian cancer: a phase II trial. J Immunother Cancer 8(1):e000829. https://doi.org/10.1136/jitc-2020-000829

Zamarin D, Burger RA, Sill MW, Powell DJ Jr, Lankes HA, Feldman MD, Zivanovic O, Gunderson C, Ko E, Mathews C, Sharma S, Hagemann AR, Khleif S, Aghajanian C (2020b) Randomized phase II trial of nivolumab versus nivolumab and ipilimumab for recurrent or persistent ovarian cancer: an NRG oncology study. J Clin Oncol 38(16):1814–1823. https://doi.org/10.1200/JCO.19.02059

Zannoni GF, Improta G, Chiarello G et al (2014) Mutational status of KRAS, NRAS, and BRAF in primary clear cell ovarian carcinoma. Virchows Arch 465(2):193–198. https://doi.org/10.1007/s00428-014-1599-1

Zannoni GF, Improta G, Pettinato A et al (2016) Molecular status of PI3KCA, KRAS and BRAF in ovarian clear cell carcinoma: an analysis of 63 patients. J Clin Pathol 69(12):1088–1092. https://doi.org/10.1136/jclinpath-2016-203776

Zhang GN, Liu H, Huang JM, Wang L, Zhao JS, Li C, Mi K, Zhu Y, Cheng J, Zha X (2014) TP53 K351N mutation-associated platinum resistance after neoadjuvant chemotherapy in patients with advanced ovarian cancer. Gynecol Oncol 132(3):752–757. https://doi.org/10.1016/j.ygyno.2014.01.028

Zhang D, Bai B, Xi Y et al (2016a) Can aspirin reduce the risk of endometrial cancer? A systematic review and meta-analysis of observational studies. Int J Gynecol Cancer 26(6):1111–1120. https://doi.org/10.1097/IGC.0000000000000731

Zhang X, Liu J, Liang X et al (2016b) History and progression of Fat cadherins in health and disease. Onco Targets Ther 9:7337–7343. https://doi.org/10.2147/OTT.S111176

Zhang M, Zhuang G, Sun X et al (2017) TP53 mutation-mediated genomic instability induces the evolution of chemoresistance and recurrence in epithelial ovarian cancer. Diagn Pathol 12 (1):16. https://doi.org/10.1186/s13000-017-0605-8

Zhang B, Wang L, Zhao X, Wei Y, Zhang Y (2018) Identification of candidate genes associated with chemotherapy resistance in ovarian cancer. Ann Clin Lab Sci 48(5):573–579

Zhang X, Yan K, Deng L, Liang J, Liang H, Feng D, Ling B (2019a) Cyclooxygenase 2 promotes proliferation and invasion in ovarian cancer cells via the PGE2/NF-κB pathway. Cell Transplant 28(1 Suppl):1S–13S. https://doi.org/10.1177/0963689719890597

Zhang Y, Xu L, Li A, Han X (2019b) The roles of ZEB1 in tumorigenic progression and epigenetic modifications. Biomed Pharmacother 110:400–408. https://doi.org/10.1016/j.biopha.2018.11.112

Zhang L, Chen Y, Li F, Bao L, Liu W (2019c) Atezolizumab and bevacizumab attenuate cisplatin resistant ovarian cancer cells progression synergistically via suppressing epithelial-mesenchymal transition. Front Immunol 10:867. https://doi.org/10.3389/fimmu.2019.00867

Zhao R, Diop-Bove N, Visentin M, Goldman ID (2011) Mechanisms of membrane transport of folates into cells and across epithelia. Annu Rev Nutr 31:177–201

Zhao H, Wang J, Zhang Y et al (2018) Prognostic values of CCNE1 amplification and overexpression in cancer patients: a systematic review and meta-analysis. J Cancer 9 (13):2397–2407. https://doi.org/10.7150/jca.24179

Zhou Y, Zheng X, Lu J, Chen W, Li X, Zhao L (2018) Ginsenoside 20(S)-Rg3 inhibits the Warburg effect via modulating DNMT3A/MiR-532-3p/HK2 pathway in ovarian cancer cells. Cell Physiol Biochem 45(6):2548–2559. https://doi.org/10.1159/000488273

Zsiros E, Lynam S, Attwood KM, Wang C, Chilakapati S, Gomez EC, Liu S, Akers S, Lele S, Frederick PJ, Odunsi K (2020) Efficacy and safety of pembrolizumab in combination with bevacizumab and oral metronomic cyclophosphamide in the treatment of recurrent ovarian cancer: a phase 2 nonrandomized clinical trial. JAMA Oncol 7:e205945. https://doi.org/10.1001/jamaoncol.2020.5945

Genetic Alterations in Ovarian Cancer as Prognostic and Predictive Biomarkers of Therapy Response and Surgical Outcomes

4

Khalid El Bairi, Ouissam Al Jarroudi, and Said Afqir

Abstract

The emergence of precision medicine and our latest understanding of the biological characteristics of ovarian cancer (OC) have led to the discovery of drug targets, novel anticancer agents, and their predictive biomarkers. The genetics of OC is an evolving biomarker for predicting outcomes. Several completed and ongoing clinical trials used this concept for better patients' selection and stratification. The exploitation of specific molecular vulnerabilities in OC for drug development such as *BRCA* and *BRCA*ness is a milestone in the current management of this women's cancer. Without a doubt, OC is one of the solid cancers that have benefited from genetic biomarkers for the implementation of targeted agents such as PARP inhibitors in clinical practice. This progress is discussed in this chapter based on recent studies and clinical trials.

Keywords

Genetics · Ovarian cancer · Biomarkers · Survival · Surgery

K. El Bairi (✉) · O. Al Jarroudi · S. Afqir
Department of Medical Oncology, Mohammed VI University Hospital, Oujda, Morocco

Faculty of Medicine and Pharmacy, Mohammed Ist University, Oujda, Morocco
e-mail: k.elbairi@ump.ac.ma

K. El Bairi (ed.), *Ovarian Cancer Biomarkers*,
https://doi.org/10.1007/978-981-16-1873-4_4

4.1 Introduction

Few therapeutic advances were achieved in improving survival outcomes in the first-line therapy of ovarian cancer (OC). However, predictive and prognostic biomarkers have considerably changed outcomes in some settings in women with this aggressive cancer (Le Page et al. 2020a; b; El Bairi et al. 2017a, b; Madariaga et al. 2020). An illustrative example is the important number of clinical trials, prospective studies, and retrospective real-world cohorts that have demonstrated the favorable impact of *BRCA* mutations on therapy response and prognosis in OC (Madariaga et al. 2019; Lorusso et al. 2020). Moreover, *BRCA* mutations and other variants in homologous recombination repair (HRR) genes are now used for OC patients' selection for poly-ADP-ribose polymerase inhibitors (PARPi). *BRCA*, *BRCA*ness, and HRR are associated with genomic instability and synthetic lethality in OC and are potential predictors of pharmacological sensitivity to platinum agents and PARPi (Konstantinopoulos and Matulonis 2018). Remarkably, as a result of the relevant success of cancer genetics in the field of translational oncology, there is an increasing number of clinical trials in OC that use genetic alterations as biomarkers for patient's selection, stratification, and prediction of drug response; particularly using umbrella and basket trial designs (Tsimberidou et al. 2020). As described in the other chapters of this book, some of their results provided considerable information for clinical use and it is not surprising to see other starting and ongoing trials in this highly active research area of OC. The current chapter focuses on the impact of genetic variants on outcomes in OC.

4.2 Ovarian Cancer Genetics as a Biomarker of Response to Chemotherapy and Survival Outcomes

Platinum-based chemotherapy is currently considered the backbone of OC therapy. Carboplatin and cisplatin bind to DNA and induce structural adducts which in turn cause considerable damages to cancer cells, and therefore driving cell cycle arrest and mitochondrial apoptosis (Galluzzi et al. 2012). Enhanced response to these anticancer drugs is observed in patients with mutated *BReast Cancer* 1 and 2 genes (*BRCA1/2*) which confer impairment of DNA repair mechanisms (Quinn et al. 2009; Madariaga et al. 2019). Several preclinical reports have shown that cells harboring *BRCA* variants have superior sensitivity to platinum-based chemotherapy (Madariaga et al. 2019). This loss of function is considered the key driver of responsiveness to these agents and is a well-established predictive biomarker in OC. Clinically, women with both germline and somatic mutated *BRCA* were found to have increased response to platinum-based chemotherapy (Alsop et al. 2012; Gorodnova et al. 2015; Vencken et al. 2011; Pennington et al. 2014; Leunen et al. 2009) (for detailed review, see: Le Page et al. 2020a, b). During a relapse, these improved outcomes were also observed in platinum-resistant OC with *BRCA* mutations (Alsop et al. 2012). Thus, platinum re-challenge is an approach for recurrent OC patients with germline mutated *BRCA* carriers (Madariaga et al.

2019). In addition to high immune infiltrates, increased mutational burden, and loss of heterozygosity, *BRCA* mutations are considered as key determinants of exceptional long-term OC survival (Yang et al. 2018; Hoppenot et al. 2018). This was further confirmed by several meta-analyses of survival outcomes in OC (summarized in Table 4.1). Remarkably, a large study that enrolled 316 high-grade serous OC patients found that *BRCA2*, but not *BRCA1*, was associated with superior

Table 4.1 Summary of recent meta-analyses of the impact of *BRCA* mutations on prognosis and survival

Author/ year	Number of enrolled studies (patients)	Prognostic endpoints	Findings
Huang (2018)	33 (7745)	Overall survival (OS) and progression-free survival (PFS), complete response rate (CRR), partial response rate (PRR), and overall response rate (ORR)	–Mutated *BRCA*1/2 are associated with improved OS (HR: 0.75; 95%; CI: 0.64–0.88) and PFS (HR: 0.80; 95% CI: 0.64–0.99). –Presence of *BRCA*1/2 mutated status is associated with better ORR, higher CRR, and lower PRR but mutated *BRCA1* or *BRCA2* alone were not associated with ORR.
Xu et al. (2017)	34 (18396)	OS and PFS	Mutated *BRCA1* and *BRCA2* demonstrated improved OS and PFS in ovarian cancer patients (HR: 0.73; 95% CI: 0.63–0.86 and HR, 0.57; 95% CI, 0.45–0.73, respectively) and PFS (HR: 0.68; 95% CI: 0.52–0.89 and HR: 0.48; 95% CI: 0.30–0.75, respectively).
Zhong et al. (2014)	14 (9588)	OS and PFS	Ovarian cancer patients with mutated *BRCA1* and *BRCA2* had better OS (HR: 0.76; 95% CI: 0.70–0.83 and HR: 0.58; 95% CI: 0.50–0.66, respectively) and PFS (HR: 0.65; 95% CI: 0.52–0.81 and HR: 0.61; 95% CI: 0.47–0.80, respectively) than non-mutated status
Sun et al. (2014)	35	OS and PFS	Mutated *BRCA* status had a favorable impact on OS (HR: 0.69; 95% CI: 0.61–0.79). Similarly, patients with *BRCA*-mutated had longer PFS (based on 18 studies) (HR: 0.69, 95% CI: 0.63–0.76)

Abbreviations: *BRCA* Breast Cancer gene, *CI* confidence interval, *HR* hazard ratio chemotherapy response and also improved survival outcomes (Yang et al. 2011). Mechanistically, both *BRCA1* and *BRCA2* are important complementary members of the genes involved in DNA damage repair. However, accumulating evidence suggests that the principal function of *BRCA2* is the regulation of RAD51 that has a pivotal role in double-strand break repair (Davies et al. 2001) rather than tumor suppression ensured particularly by *BRCA1*. Functions of BRCA1 encompass cell cycle arrest checkpoint control (Yarden et al. 2002; Sharma et al. 2018), mitotic spindle assembly (Joukov et al. 2006; Xiong et al. 2008), and centrosome duplication (Mullee and Morrison 2016; Kais et al. 2012; Sankaran et al. 2007; Hsu and White 1998) and their failure can predispose to cancer initiation rather than conferring sensitivity to platinum DNA-crosslink agents. Therefore, these fundamental data may explain this difference in survival and drug response in this previous study. Importantly, the "mutator phenotype" hypothesis in OC patients with mutations beyond *BRCA1* is a potential driver of chemotherapy response in this setting as well. Despite these important observations, the acquisition of reversion mutations in *BRCA* genes can restore BRCA proteins expression and induce resistance to platinum-based therapy and also PARPi (Milanesio et al. 2020). Therapeutically, a recent meta-analysis documented that pharmacological blockade of DNA end-joining repair signaling may improve the stability of drug response by preventing the acquisition of reversion *BRCA* mutations (Tobalina et al. 2021). Promisingly, detection of these reversion mutations can be performed using real-time liquid biopsy approaches. Based on massively parallel targeted sequencing, Weigelt et al. showed recently that prospective evaluation of circulating-free DNA has the potential to non-invasively identify putative *BRCA1* or *BRCA2* reversion mutations with restored functions in women with OC and breast cancer (Weigelt et al. 2017). Similarly, two other recent reports confirmed these findings and showed that detected *BRCA* mutations using liquid biopsy in OC patients are associated with acquired resistance to treatments (Christie et al. 2017; Lin et al. 2019). Methylation phenomena in *BRCA1* promoter were also suggested as a biomarker of chemosensitivity in OC (Ignatov et al. 2014). However, a meta-analysis of individual data ($n = 2636$) demonstrated that patients with BRCA1-methylated OC had similar survival outcomes as compared to those with non-BRCA1-methylated tumors (Kalachand et al. 2020). Other mutated genes outside the *BRCA* family (Table 4.2) such as members of the HRR pathway particularly *RAD51,* which are found in approximately 50% of high-grade serous OC, were also found to predict chemosensitivity (Fuh et al. 2020; da Costa et al. 2019). Moreover, this HRR deficiency has also a value for prognostic stratification of OC patients (Takaya et al. 2020; Morse et al. 2019). Patients with this fundamental vulnerability had high infiltration of immune cells particularly tumor-infiltrating lymphocytes (TILs) which correlate with better survival and may make these women highly responsive to immune-checkpoint blockade (Ledermann 2019; Morse et al. 2019; Konstantinopoulos et al. 2015) (*see Chap. 3 for details*). Currently, this biomarker is used for predicting response to PARPi rather than platinum-based

Table 4.2 Other emerging and potential single gene variants or panels with impact on prognosis and survival of ovarian cancer

Genes	Functions/pathways	Clinical impact	References
RAD51B	Repair of DNA double-strand breaks	Acquired chemotherapy resistance	Patch et al. (2015)
RAD51C	Repair of DNA double-strand breaks	Acquired resistance to PARP inhibitors via secondary somatic reversion mutations	Kondrashova et al. (2017)
		Improved overall survival (OS) and sensitivity to platinum	Pennington et al. (2014)
RAD51D	Repair of DNA double-strand breaks	Acquired resistance to PARP inhibitors via secondary somatic reversion mutations	Kondrashova et al. (2017)
TP53	Cell cycle regulation, cell death, and DNA repair	Resistance to platinum- and taxane-based chemotherapy (oncomorphic mutations)	Brachova et al. (2014) (for review, see: Brachova et al. 2013)
		Sensitivity to chemotherapy and improved survival	Wong et al. (2013)
RB1	Cell cycle regulation	Long OS and PFS, and durable response	Garsed et al. (2018)
ADAMTS	Tissue development and maintenance, tumor progression and metastasis (cell migration and angiogenesis)	Significant association with better OS, progression-free survival (PFS), and platinum-free survival	Liu et al. (2015)
CCNE1	Regulation of cell cycle	Poor OS	The Cancer Genome Atlas Research Network, (2011); Nakayama et al. (2010)
CHEK2	Regulation of cell cycle after DNA damage	Poor OS and therapy response	Ow et al. (2014)
KRAS	Proliferative signaling pathways	Resistance to platinum-based therapy	Ratner et al. (2012)
		Sensitivity to decitabine agent	Stewart et al. (2015)
		Improved cancer-specific survival	Nodin et al. (2013)
BRAF	Signal transduction, cell division, and differentiation	Improved OS as compared to *KRAS* mutant or *KRAS*/wild-type *BRAF* tumors	Grisham et al. (2013)
NF1	Regulation of cell cycle	Acquired resistance to chemotherapy	Patch et al. (2015)

(continued)

Table 4.2 (continued)

Genes	Functions/pathways	Clinical impact	References
TAP1	Antigen presentation	Association with OS	Millstein et al. (2020)
ZFHX4	Cell differentiation		
CXCL9	Mediation of T cells recruitment		
FBN1	Extracellular matrix protein		
PTGER3	Receptor of prostaglandin E2		

chemotherapeutics. The European Society for Medical Oncology (ESMO) stated that assays for clinical evaluation of HRR deficiency are useful in predicting the likely magnitude of benefit from PARP inhibition but additional biomarkers with improved accuracy are needed to better stratify patients (Miller et al. 2020).

Research in this area of biomarkers discovery has also provided other perspectives for non-platinum chemotherapy such as the natural compound trabectedin and pegylated liposomal doxorubicin (PLD) (Madariaga et al. 2019; El Bairi et al. 2019). Trabectedin (known as Yondelis®) is a marine compound isolated from the colonial tunicate *Ecteinascidia turbinate* that acts as a cytotoxic alkylating agent and also as a vascular disruptor (El Bairi et al. 2019). It was approved in several countries of the European Union for the treatment of OC as a late-line therapy in combination with PLD for recurrent platinum-sensitive disease. The efficacy of trabectedin was found associated with deficient HRR systems in various clinical trials (El Bairi et al. 2018; Ventriglia et al. 2018). Previously, an exploratory analysis of the randomized phase 3 OVA-301 study that compared the efficacy of trabectedin and PLD versus PLD alone in women with recurrent OC showed that germline *BRCA1* mutant tumors had improved median PFS (13.5 vs. 5.5 months, $p = 0.0002$), OS (23.8 versus 12.5 months, $p = 0.0086$), and higher response rates (49 vs. 28%) (Monk et al. 2015). Moreover, women with *BRCA* wild-type OC had no improvements in median OS (19.1 versus 19.3 months; $p = 0.9377$) (Monk et al. 2015). *BRCA* status and *BRCA*ness were also used for patients' selection in the MITO-15 phase II study that investigated trabectedin in women with recurrent OC (Lorusso et al. 2016). *BRCA* status was not associated with response to trabectedin nor with survival (Lorusso et al. 2016). However, the recent findings of another randomized phase III trial that compared the efficacy of trabectedin combined with PLD in the same previous setting showed significant overall survival (OS) benefits for patients harboring *BRCA* mutations (34.2 vs. 20.9 months; HR: 0.54, 95% CI: 0.33–0.90; $p = 0.016$) (Monk et al. 2020). Similarly, improved outcomes for median PFS were also noticed for patients with *BRCA* mutant tumors (HR: 0.72, 95% CI: 0.48–1.08; $p = 0.039$) (Monk et al. 2020). The DNA damaging agent PLD used in the recurrent setting was also found to be more effective in tumors with *BRCA* mutations. Two previous retrospective studies demonstrated that *BRCA*-associated

OC women had improved sensitivity to PLD, greater PFS (Adams et al. 2011), and also OS (Safra et al. 2014). Regarding taxane chemotherapy which is used in combination with carboplatin in the first-line setting as a standard of care and as a single agent for recurrent platinum-resistant disease; data on *BRCA* as a predictor of response are sparse. In prostate cancer, the correlation between mutated *BRCA* and poor response to docetaxel was noticed (Nientiedt et al. 2017). In addition, mutated *BRCA1*-associated breast cancer was found less sensitive to taxane chemotherapy (Kriege et al. 2012). In OC, the inhibition of endogenous BRCA1 expression was reported to be associated with decreased sensitivity to antimicrotubule agents (Quinn et al. 2007). Moreover, median OS in patients with higher BRCA1-expression was found improved after treatment with taxanes (23 vs. 18.2 months; HR: 0.53; $p = 0.12$) (Quinn et al. 2007). Other emerging genes that might impact drug response and prognosis in OC can be found in Tables 4.2 and 4.3.

4.3 Ovarian Cancer Genetics and Response to PARP Inhibitors

DNA damage response pathway is one of the invested targets in drug discovery for OC. PARP 1 and PARP2 are the principal enzymes of this pathway and are recruited during DNA lesions to orchestrate repair effectors activity (Lord and Ashworth 2017). PARP bound to damaged DNA and transfer poly-ADP-ribose units to various target proteins (PARylation process) required for DNA breaks repair such as topoisomerase and DNA ligase (for review, see: Franzese et al. 2019). Inhibition of PARP mediated DNA repair appeared to be a potential strategy that is widely known as synthetic lethality (Lord et al. 2015; Lord and Ashworth 2017) and has moved successfully into clinical trials several PARPi including rucaparib (Rubraca®), olaparib (Lynparza®), veliparib (ABT-888), niraparib (Zejula®) as well as the next-generation of this category such as talazoparib (Talzenna®). In 2005, two preclinical reports were published in *Nature* by Farmer et al. and Bryant et al. showed that mutant cancer cells with *BRCA* dysfunction are highly sensitive to PARP inhibition (Farmer et al. 2005; Bryant et al. 2005). Based on these substantial findings, this new concept was used as a rationale for developing trial designs of several PARPi for various cancers harboring this signature. In OC, many clinical studies that investigated oral PARPi have achieved their primary objectives and showed positive results from phase II-III trials in the front-line, for recurrent disease, or maintenance settings following platinum-based chemotherapy (Table 4.4).

4.3.1 Olaparib

Olaparib was the first-in-class developed PARPi and approved by the FDA and EMA in 2014 for treating OC (Franzese et al. 2019). Early trials (NCT00516373 and NCT00494442) showed favorable safety and tolerability profile which were represented mainly by reversible fatigue, anemia, and mild gastrointestinal symptoms (Fong et al. 2009, 2010; Audeh et al. 2010). Interestingly, these dose-

Table 4.3 Genetic biomarkers of response to other anticancer drugs used in ovarian cancer therapy

References	Drugs/ regimens	Enrollment	Phase	Biomarkers	Clinical endpoints	Findings
Monk et al. (2017)	Motolimod + pegylated liposomal doxorubicin (PLD)	297 [arm 1: motolimod + PLD ($n = 149$), arm 2: PLD + placebo ($n = 149$)]	Randomized phase II	***TLR8* (SNPs), *BRCA*–Fanconi anemia mutational status**	**PFS and OS**	*TLR8* (SNPs), mutated *BRCA* and did not correlate with PFS or OS
Harter et al. (2016) (AGO-OVAR 16)	Pazopanib	664 (pazopanib, $n = 335$; placebo, $n = 329$)	Randomized phase III (exploratory analysis)	***BRCA1/2***	**Median PFS: Pazopanib arm** –*BRCA*(+): 30.2 months –*BRCA* (−): 17.7 months HR: 0.64; 95% CI: 0.40–1.03; $p = 0.069$ **Median PFS: Placebo arm** –*BRCA*(+): 30.3 months –*BRCA* (−): 14.1 months HR: 0.48; 95% CI: 0.29–0.78; $p = 0.0031$	OC patients with *BRCA1/2* carriers treated with antiangiogenic pazopanib had longer PFS
Monk et al. (2015) (OVA-301) For review, see: Ventriglia et al. (2018)	Trabectedin + PLD	264 [arm 1: trabectedin + PLD ($n = 135$), arm 2: PLD alone ($n = 129$)]	Randomized phase III (exploratory analysis)	***BRCA1*** ***XPG***	**Response rate (RR):** –*BRCA* (+): 49% –*BRCA* (−): 28% ***BRCA* (+):** –**Median PFS:** arm 1: 13.5 vs. 5.5 months for arm	Recurrent OC patients with *BRCA* mutated status treated with trabectedin + PLD had better survival outcomes compared with single-arm PLD

					2, $p = 0.0002$. –**Median OS:** arm 1: 23.8 vs. 12.5 months for arm 2, $p = 0.0086$. ***BRCA* (−):** –**Median PFS:** arm 1: 6.0 vs. 5.4 months for arm 2, $p = 0.2185$ –**Median OS:** arm 1: 19.1 vs. 19.3 months for arm 2, $p = 0.9377$. ***XPG* status:** no significant difference in the two arms	
Hyman et al. (2011)	Topotecan (topoisomerase I inhibitor)	50	Retrospective	***BRCA***	**Median PFS:** –*BRCA* (+): 1.7 months (95% CI: 1.0–2.8) –*BRCA* (−): 2.5 months (95% CI: 1.9–2.8) $p = 0.057$	Topotecan did not demonstrate superiority in platinum-resistant OC patients with *BRCA* positive status

Table 4.4 Landmark completed phase III trials of PARP inhibitors in ovarian cancer

Trial name	Investigated predictive biomarker	Sample size	Anticancer drug	Comparator	Randomization	Setting
NOVA	*BRCA* mutations	553	Niraparib	Placebo	2:1	Maintenance for recurrent platinum-sensitive
SOLO-2	*BRCA* mutations	295	Olaparib	Placebo	2:1	
ARIEL-3	*BRCA* mutations and homologous recombination deficiency (HRD)	564	Rucaparib	Placebo	2:1	
SOLO-1	*BRCA* mutations	391	Olaparib	Placebo	2:1	Maintenance in newly diagnosed
PAOLA-1	*BRCA* mutations and HRD	806	Olaparib	Bevacizumab or placebo	2:1	
VELIA	*BRCA* mutations and HRD	1140	Veliparib	Placebo or carboplatin and paclitaxel	1:1:1	First-line and maintenance
PRIMA	*BRCA* mutations and HRD	733	Niraparib	Placebo	2:1	First-line
SOLO-3	Germline *BRCA* mutations	266	Olaparib	Pegylated liposomal doxorubicin, paclitaxel, gemcitabine, or topotecan	2:1	Recurrent platinum-sensitive

finding trials demonstrated significant antitumor response in OC patients with *BRCA* mutations (Fong et al. 2010; Audeh et al. 2010). In a second interim analysis of OS and a preplanned analysis of data by *BRCA* mutation status of a randomized and double-blind phase II study (NCT00753545) that used olaparib as maintenance treatment for recurrent platinum-sensitive OC, Ledermann et al. found that patients with mutated *BRCA* had significantly longer PFS as compared with wild-type subjects (11.2 vs. 7.4 months) (Ledermann et al. 2014). However, in terms of OS, no significant difference was seen between the two groups (HR: 0.73; 95% CI: 0.45–1.17; $p = 0.19$ for *BRCA* mutated status and (HR: 0.99; 95% CI: 0.63–1.55; $p = 0.96$) for wild-type *BRCA*) (Ledermann et al. 2014). Moving from this immature evidence, the greatest clinical benefit was observed in *BRCA*-mutated recurrent and platinum-sensitive OC patients in another randomized phase II trial (NCT01081951) combining olaparib with standard chemotherapy (Oza et al. 2015). PFS in patients with mutated *BRCA* was significantly improved (HR: 0.21; 95% CI: 0.08–0.55; $p = 0.0015$) (Oza et al. 2015). These data were supported by an updated analysis of OS of NCT00753545 trial and showed that *BRCA*-mutated platinum-sensitive recurrent OC patients appear to have longer OS despite it did not achieve the planned level for statistical significance ($p < 0.0095$) (Ledermann et al. 2016). Confirmatory results from two randomized phase III trials (SOLO-1 and SOLO-2/ENGOT-Ov21) using olaparib as maintenance therapy for OC were reported recently. Pujade-Lauraine et al. conducted a phase III randomized, double-blind and placebo-controlled and multicenter trial to evaluate the efficacy of olaparib as maintenance treatment for platinum-sensitive, relapsed and *BRCA* mutated OC (Pujade-Lauraine et al. 2017). This study (NCT01874353; SOLO-2/ENGOT-Ov21) enrolled 295 patients including 196 in the olaparib arm and showed significantly higher PFS as compared with the placebo arm (19.1 months vs. 5.5 months $p < 0.0001$ respectively) (Pujade-Lauraine et al. 2017). More recently, results from SOLO-1 (NCT01844986) phase III trial that assessed olaparib ($n = 260$) versus placebo ($n = 131$) as maintenance therapy this time for newly diagnosed OC with *BRCA* mutations and after first-line standard chemotherapy demonstrated a gain of 3 years in PFS (despite not reached) in the group who received olaparib after 41 months of follow-up (HR: 0.30; 95% CI: 0.23–0.41; $p < 0.001$) (Moore et al. 2018). Remarkably, a recent meta-analysis that enrolled 8 randomized trials (1957 patients) including SOLO-2 found that patients with *BRCA* carriers exhibited significant survival benefits from olaparib and thus showing decisive additional evidence for this genetic biomarker but with an increased risk of severe anemia which requires regular hematologic surveillance (Guo et al. 2018). Promisingly, further evidence will be released by the ongoing SOLO3 phase III trial that randomizes relapsed OC patients who have received at least 2 prior lines of platinum-based chemotherapy and with *BRCA* carriers to receive olaparib versus standard of care (NCT02282020). Moving beyond *BRCA* biomarkers, it seems that a subset of OC patients with mutations in HRR genes other than traditional *BRCA* may also benefit from olaparib which can expand the use of this drug in the future (Hodgson et al. 2018). Similarly, findings from a comparative molecular analysis of the NCT00753545 trial showed that long-term responders to olaparib maintenance may be multifactorial and related to HRR profile (Lheureux et al. 2017). In the confirmatory SOLO-3 phase III trial, patients with *BRCA* mutated status were randomly assigned to receive olaparib or a non-platinum drug for the platinum-sensitive setting for which objective response rate was the primary endpoint as mandated by the FDA (Penson et al. 2020). The superiority of olaparib was noticed and reached 72.2 as compared to 51.4% in patients treated with standard of care (Penson et al. 2020). The addition of olaparib to bevacizumab for the first-line maintenance therapy was investigated in the PAOLA-1 phase III trial (Ray-Coquard et al. 2019). This study randomized 806 OC patients with mutated *BRCA* to receive olaparib and bevacizumab or bevacizumab + placebo in a 2:1 fashion. A significant hazard ratio of 0.59 resulted in the comparison for PFS. In patients with HRR deficiency, the hazard ratio for progression or death reached a value of 0.33 suggesting the clinical benefits of adding olaparib to anti-angiogenesis in this setting (Ray-Coquard et al. 2019).

4.3.2 Rucaparib

Women with OC who have *BRCA* mutant tumors that were enrolled in the ARIEL-3 randomized and controlled phase III ($n = 564$) for the recurrent platinum-sensitive disease had superior median PFS (HR: 0.23, 95% CI: 0.16–0.34, $p < 0.0001$) (Coleman et al. 2017). Similarly, patients with HRR deficiency had also improved PFS (HR: 0.32, 0.24–0.42, $p < 0.0001$). In the ARIEL-2 phase II trial for the recurrent platinum-sensitive setting that stratified patients into multi-cohorts including those with *BRCA* status, median PFS was also improved in the group treated with rucaparib and having *BRCA* mutations (HR: 0.27, 95% CI: 0.16–0.44, $p < 0.0001$) (Swisher et al. 2017). Notably, *RAD51C* and *RAD51D* genetic variants were found associated with acquired resistance to this PARP inhibitor in OC (Kondrashova et al. 2017). Furthermore, reversion mutations in *BRCA* were also identified in circulating tumor DNA of OC patients with reduced rucaparib PFS as compared to women with no reversion mutations at baseline (median 1.8 vs. 9 months; HR: 0.12; $p < 0.0001$). Thus, combinatorial approaches may be promising to overcome drug resistance to rucaparib (Lin et al. 2019).

4.3.3 Niraparib

To the best of our knowledge, niraparib has been investigated in two randomized phase III trials for OC, NOVA ($n = 553$) and PRIMA ($n = 733$) (*see Chap. 3*). In the NOVA study that explored the efficacy of niraparib in the recurrent platinum-sensitive setting, 203 women had germline mutated *BRCA* and had superior PFS as compared to those treated with placebo (HR: 0.27; 95% CI: 0.17–0.41)

(Mirza et al. 2016). Remarkably, women with HRR deficiency had also improved PFS (HR: 0.38; 95% CI: 0.24–0.59) (Mirza et al. 2016). When niraparib was investigated as a monotherapy in the maintenance setting after response to front line therapy in NOVA study, enrolled women with HRR deficient tumors had clinically and statistically improved PFS (HR: 0.43; 95% CI: 0.31–0.59; $p < 0.001$) (González-Martín et al. 2019). In late lines of recurrent OC therapy, the QUADRA phase II trial explored the efficacy of niraparib in heavily pre-treated patients and showed a clinical activity of this PARPi in women with HRR deficiency including those with or without *BRCA* mutations (Moore et al. 2019).

4.3.4 Veliparib

Veliparib is a new synthetically lethal therapeutic approach for treating OC (Boussios et al. 2020). Previously and based on early signs of efficacy in a phase II trial (Coleman et al. 2015), veliparib as a single agent was studied for platinum-resistant or partially sensitive recurrent OC in a combined phase I/II trial (Steffensen et al. 2017). Veliparib was given to women that have exclusively germline mutated *BRCA* showed clinical activity in this heavily pretreated population including 65% of overall response rate, PFS of 5.6 months, and OS of 13.7 months (Steffensen et al. 2017). VELIA ($n = 1140$) was a landmark three arms phase III trial that explored the efficacy of veliparib in the first-line therapy of OC (Coleman et al. 2019). Women with *BRCA* mutant and HRR deficient tumors treated with veliparib in combination with carboplatin/paclitaxel doublets had favorable outcomes including superior PFS (HR: 0.44 and HR: 0.68 respectively, $p < 0.001$ for both) (Coleman et al. 2019). In a recent biomarker analysis of a phase II study, homeobox A9 (*HOXA9*) promoter methylation in circulating tumor DNA was demonstrated to confer resistance to veliparib (Rusan et al. 2020). Longitudinal monitoring of OC patients based on this liquid biopsy approach showed that methylated *HOXA9* at baseline was significantly correlated with worse outcomes included reduced PFS and OS ($p < 0.0001$ and $p = 0.002$, respectively) (Rusan et al. 2020). Therefore, this may provide perspectives for real-time monitoring using this potential predictive biomarker.

4.4 Ovarian Cancer Genetics and Surgical Outcomes

Usually, cytoreductive debulking surgery is performed for OC patients after primary diagnosis and staging, followed by adjuvant platinum-based chemotherapy or after receiving neoadjuvant chemotherapy (NACT) for women with poor performance status, large tumors, and important volumes of ascites (Vitale et al. 2013). Furthermore, secondary debulking surgery can be performed during recurrences but its role in improving outcomes is still controversial (Lorusso et al. 2012). Resectability and optimal cytoreduction are influenced by several factors such as disease location, the expertise of surgeons as well as probably genetic status such as *BRCA* mutations (Narod 2016; Ponzone 2021). Interestingly, to see whether OC patients with *BRCA* mutations have superior surgical outcomes as compared with those with wild status, some recent reports looked into this matter based on different observational study designs. Earlier in 2012, a retrospective report of 367 stage IIIC-IV high-grade serous OC from the Memorial Sloan Kettering Cancer Center investigated germline *BRCA* mutation status as a predictor of optimal cytoreduction compared to wild-type tumors (Hyman et al. 2012). OC patients with mutated *BRCA* and who underwent surgery had relatively superior rates of optimal debulking as compared with wild-type patients (84.1% vs. 70.1% respectively, $p = 0.02$) (Hyman et al. 2012). However, based on multivariate analysis, this study demonstrated that mutated *BRCA* status is not associated with residual tumor volume (OR: 0.63; 95% CI: 0.31–1.29; $p = 0.21$) suggesting that optimal cytoreduction may be due to surgery alone instead of OC genetics (Hyman et al. 2012). In another retrospective study that enrolled 27 cases with recurrent OC treated with cytoreductive surgery and hyperthermic intraperitoneal chemotherapy (HIPEC) and 84 matched controls treated with systemic chemotherapy alone, women with positive *BRCA* carriers were found to have longer PFS in the HIPEC group as compared with the controls (20.9 vs. 12.6 months, $p = 0.048$) (Safra et al. 2014). Consequently, this confirms the recently published data supporting the impact of the emerging HIPEC in treating OC (van Driel et al. 2018; Spiliotis et al. 2015; Cascales-Campos et al. 2015) especially in patients with *BRCA* mutational status. However, an opposing conclusion from a recent study found that patients with *BRCA1* mutated OC are less likely to achieve no residual disease after debulking surgery than wild-type patients (19% vs. 39%; $p < 0.0001$) (Kotsopoulos et al. 2016). Importantly, the same study found that improved survival outcomes observed in OC patients with mutated *BRCA* status may be due to higher initial sensitivity to platinum-based therapy and, notably, no residual disease at debulking is the strongest predictive factor of long-term survival (Kotsopoulos et al. 2016). Recently, Petrillo et al. evaluated the impact of *BRCA* mutational status on outcomes including optimal debulking in a large multicenter report of women with newly diagnosed high-grade serous OC with stage IIIc and IV disease (Petrillo et al. 2017). Patients with mutated *BRCA* had significantly higher peritoneal tumor load but without having different median PFS when treated with NACT or debulking surgery ($p = 0.268$). Remarkably, patients with wild-type *BRCA* status and who benefited from primary debulking surgery had superior median PFS as compared to those treated with NACT (26 vs. 18 months; $p = 0.003$) (Petrillo et al. 2017). Similarly, Marchetti et al. showed in their recent retrospective cohort that women with *BRCA* wild-type ovarian tumors who underwent complete secondary cytoreductive surgery had superior 5-year post-recurrence survival as compared to those with no surgical intervention (54% vs. 42%; $p = 0.048$) (Marchetti et al. 2018). However, Naumann et al. showed that optimally resected high-grade OC had frequent *BRCA* mutations and dramatically improved median OS (110.4 vs. 67.1 months; HR: 0.28, 95% CI: 0.11–0.73, $p = 0.009$) when treated with HIPEC compared with patients wild type tumors (Naumann et al. 2018). More recently, Gordonova et al. analyzed the medical record of 283 consecutive women who underwent complete or optimal debulking and compared their outcomes based on *BRCA* status (Gorodnova et al. 2019). Again, this study showed that *BRCA* status did not predict outcomes in patients subjected to primary surgery ($p = 0.56$) (Gorodnova et al. 2019). To the best of our knowledge, only one report has prospectively assessed the impact of *BRCA* status on optimal debulking. This was a cohort report that enrolled 107 OC patients including 51.4% of *BRCA* mutated cases (Rudaitis et al. 2014). No significant difference between OC patients harboring *BRCA* mutations and those with wild-type status was seen in terms of optimal debulking surgery (58.2% vs. 53.9%, $p = 0.6994$). However, *BRCA* mutated OC patients had improved median PFS (19 months, 95%; CI: 13–25) compared with wild-type subjects (13 months, 95%; CI: 10–16) ($p = 0.039$) (Rudaitis et al. 2014). In conclusion, it seems that *BRCA* carriers have no impact on optimal debulking for OC patients. However, most of these studies are retrospective in their design and thus, should be commented with caution because of the high risk of biases. Until to date, no definitive answers were provided and most current studies especially clinical trials are investigating *BRCA* as biomarkers for chemotherapy and targeted therapies.

4.5 Conclusion

The genetics of OC is becoming actionable with the arrival of precision medicine in gynecologic oncology. This progress is also supported by the recent development of sequencing technology. To date, several therapies require genetic information of OC patients before their use. Remarkably, this approach has deeply improved outcomes in some settings of this aggressive women's cancer. More research on biomarkers is needed to ensure that patients can achieve maximal clinical benefits from the emerging targeted agents in OC. In this perspective, the currently active clinical trials using *BRCA* status for patients' selection and stratification can improve personalized medicine in the near future (Tables 4.5 and 4.6). For additional reading, see Box 4.1.

Table 4.5 Summary of active clinical trials assessing *BRCA* mutations as prognostic biomarkers in ovarian cancer for patients' selection and stratification

Trial identifier[ǂ]	Objective	Enrollment[@]	Sponsor
NCT02341118	Genomic profiling of *BRCA1/2* mutational status to predict clinical outcomes	2000	University Health Network, Toronto
NCT02321228 (TUBA)[§]	To determine whether an early salpingectomy and a delayed oophorectomy in mutated *BRCA* subjects will improve menopause-related quality of life without increasing OC incidence	510	University Medical Center Nijmegen
NCT00579488	Assessment of clinical outcomes in OC patients with mutated *BRCA*	20,000	Memorial Sloan Kettering Cancer Center in collaboration with Cold Spring Harbor Laboratory
NCT03296826	Identification of clinicopathological features in Japanese women with mutated *BRCA* undergoing RRSO (risk-reducing salpingo-oophorectomy)	600	Translational Research Center for Medical Innovation, Kobe, Hyogo, Japan
NCT03159572 (HITOMI)	Investigation of association between PFS/sensitivity to platinum and germline mutation *BRCA* in breast cancer and OC	700	Translational Research Center for Medical Innovation, Kobe, Hyogo, Japan
NCT03510689 (Gene-HEART study)	Investigation of association between pathogenic *BRCA* mutations in hereditary breast and OC treated with anthracycline-based chemotherapy and the risk to develop cardiovascular disease	150	Abramson Cancer Center of the University of Pennsylvania
NCT01167842	Correlation between molecular findings (*BRCA* mutational status and other mutated genes) with response to treatment, recurrence data and survival	180	University of Washington

[ǂ]Titles of clinical trials were copied as shown by the database (with recruiting or enrolling by invitation studies), [@]Actual or estimated. Data from ClinicalTrials.gov (accessed 12/10/18). [§]Results published, see Harmsen et al.: https://bmccancer.biomedcentral.com/articles/10.1186/s12885-015-1597-y

Table 4.6 Summary of active clinical trials assessing mutated *BRCA* as a predictive biomarker in ovarian cancer for patients' selection and stratification

Trial identifier[‡]	Objective	Phase	Primary endpoints	Status[†]	Enrollment[@]	Sponsor
NCT03117933 (OCTOVA trial)	Comparison of olaparib and cediranib with standard paclitaxel-based chemotherapy in *BRCA* mutated platinum resistant ovarian cancer (OC)	II	Progression-free survival (PFS)	Recruiting	132	University of Oxford in collaboration with AstraZeneca
NCT03402841 (OPINION trial)	Use of olaparib maintenance treatment as monotherapy in platinum sensitive and relapsed OC with non-germline mutated *BRCA*	III	PFS	Recruiting	265	AstraZeneca
NCT03509636	Evaluation of efficacy and safety profile of fluzoparib in *BRCA* mutated and relapsed OC	II	Objective response rate (ORR)	Recruiting	112	Jiangsu HengRui Medicine Co., Ltd.
NCT02203513	Evaluation of LY2606368 (prexasertib, an inhibitor of checkpoint kinase 1 and 2 (Chk1/2) proteins) in *BRCA* mutated OC	II	ORR	Recruiting	153	National Cancer Institute (NCI)
NCT02983799	Assessment of olaparib in platinum-sensitive and relapsed, OC with mutated *BRCA* or aberrations in homologous recombination deficiency (HRD)	II	ORR	Recruiting	260	AstraZeneca
NCT02903004 (MITO23)	Evaluation of safety and efficacy of trabectedin (yondelis) in mutated *BRCA1* and *BRCA2* and BRCAness phenotype advanced OC	III	Overall survival (OS)	Recruiting	244	Fondazione IRCCS Istituto Nazionale dei Tumori, Milano

(continued)

Table 4.6 (continued)

Trial identifier[‡]	Objective	Phase	Primary endpoints	Status[†]	Enrollment[@]	Sponsor
NCT02855944 (ARIEL4)	Assessment of rucaparib versus platinum-based chemotherapy in OC patients harboring mutated *BRCA*	III	PFS	Recruiting	345	Clovis Oncology, Inc. in collaboration with Foundation Medicine
NCT03470805	Study of olaparib in OC patients with BRCA mutations after response to trabectedin and pegylated liposomal doxorubicin	II	PFS	Recruiting	66	Grupo Español de Investigación en Cáncer de Ovario in collaboration with AstraZeneca and Apices Soluciones S.L.
NCT02855697 (MOLTO)	Determination of the feasibility of a second course administration of maintenance olaparib for more than 6 months to recurrent platinum-sensitive and BRCA mutated OC	I	PFS (as secondary outcome measure)	Recruiting	26	Rozalia Lubiatowska, The Christie NHS Foundation Trust
NCT03382574	Comparison of denosumab effects versus not treatment on the fimbrial and fallopian tube tissues of premenopausal *BRCA* mutated OC subjects undergoing risk-reducing salpingo-oophorectomy (RRSO)	I	Ki67 proliferation index after RRSO	Not yet recruiting	60	NCI
NCT02950064	Evaluation of safety, pharmacokinetics, and anticancer activity of BTP-114 in advanced *BRCA* mutated solid tumors including OC	I	Maximum tolerated dose (MTD), PFS, ORR	Recruiting	95	Placon Therapeutics

NCT01989546	Investigation of BMN 673 (talazoparib, a PARP inhibitor) in patients with advanced solid neoplasms including OC and with mutated *BRCA* status	I/II	–	Recruiting	24	NCI
NCT03106987 (OReO trial)	Investigation of safety-efficacy olaparib maintenance re-treatment in patients with relapsed non-mucinous OC based on *BRCA* status as a biomarker	III	PFS	Recruiting	416	AstraZeneca in collaboration with European Network of Gynaecological Oncological Trial Groups (ENGOT)
NCT02489058 (OLALA study)	Assessment of long-term response to olaparib in OC patients based on *BRCA* status and other biomarkers	Observ-ational	–	Recruiting	100	University Health Network, Toronto
NCT03598270 (ANITA)	Double-blinded study of platinum-based chemotherapy +/– atezolizumab followed by niraparib maintenance +/– atezolizumab in subjects with recurrent OC and correlation of *BRCA* mutational status with PFS	III	PFS	Not yet recruiting	414	Grupo Español de Investigación en Cáncer de Ovario in collaboration with Hoffmann-La Roche and Apices Soluciones S.L.
NCT02953457	Evaluation of olaparib combined with durvalumab (Medi4736) and tremelimumab for treating recurrent platinum sensitive or resistant or refractory OC subjects with mutated *BRCA* status	I/II	PFS	Recruiting	39	NCI in collaboration with Roswell Park Cancer Institute

(continued)

Table 4.6 (continued)

Trial identifier[‡]	Objective	Phase	Primary endpoints	Status[†]	Enrollment[@]	Sponsor
NCT03414047	Evaluation of safety/efficacy of prexasertib in women with platinum-resistant or refractory recurrent OC based on *BRCA* mutational status	II	ORR	Recruiting	180	Eli Lilly and Company
NCT03604315	Determination of correlation between *BRCA* mutational status and fluorine F18-fluorthanatrace ([18F] FTT) in OC treated with PARP inhibitors	I	[18F] Fluorthanatrace PET/CT uptake measure	Not yet recruiting	120	M.D. Anderson Cancer Center in collaboration with NCI
NCT03326193	Evaluation of safety/efficacy of niraparib in combination with bevacizumab as maintenance treatment for OC patients based on BRCA status after front-line platinum-based therapy	II	PFS	Recruiting	90	Tesaro, Inc.
NCT03534453 (L-MOCA trial)	Assessment of olaparib as maintenance therapy in *BRCA* mutated status and platinum sensitive relapsed OC patients	III	PFS	Recruiting	300	AstraZeneca
NCT03428802	Evaluation of response rate of pembrolizumab in patients with solid cancers with mutated *BRCA* including OC	II	ORR	Recruiting	40	Rutgers, The State University of New Jersey in collaboration with NCI

NCT03161132 (ROLANDO)	Impact of olaparib combined with pegylated liposomal doxorubicin on PFS in patients with platinum-resistant advanced OC with mutated *BRCA*	II	PFS	Recruiting	32	Grupo Español de Investigación en Cáncer de Ovario in collaboration with AstraZeneca
NCT02567253 (OvIP1 trial)	Assessment of gene expression of selected genes including *BRCA*, *ERCC1* and *CTR1* as predictive biomarkers for intraoperative intraperitoneal chemoperfusion to treat peritoneal minimal residual disease in stage III OC	II	Peritoneal recurrence free survival (PRFS), DFS and OS (as secondary outcome measures)	Recruiting	48	University Hospital, Ghent
NCT03522246 (ATHENA)	Evaluation of rucaparib in combination with nivolumab as maintenance treatment following response to front-line treatment in newly diagnosed OC with a focus on *BRCA* as a predictor of response	III	PFS	Recruiting	1012	Clovis Oncology, Inc.
NCT03552471	Determination of recommended dose, safety and tolerability of mirvetuximab soravtansine combined with rucaparib in patients with endometrial cancer and OC with mutated *BRCA* status	I	PFS and ORR	Recruiting	42	Ohio State University Comprehensive Cancer Center in collaboration with ImmunoGen, Inc. and Clovis Oncology, Inc.

(continued)

Table 4.6 (continued)

Trial identifier[‡]	Objective	Phase	Primary endpoints	Status[†]	Enrollment[@]	Sponsor
NCT03394885 (AdORN trial)	–Study of atezolizumab in combination with neoadjuvant chemotherapy for newly diagnosed and advanced OC –Analysis of association between *BRCA* mutational status and tumor infiltrating lymphocytes (TILs), immune checkpoint receptor, cytokines and PD-L1 expressions and PFS	I/II	OS, PFS and ORR (as secondary outcomes measure)	Recruiting	40	Duke University in collaboration with Johns Hopkins University, Genentech, Inc. and Kaiser Permanente
NCT03586661	Investigation of niraparib in association with copanlisib in treating recurrent endometrial cancer and OC with mutated *BRCA* status	I	PFS (as a secondary outcome measure)	Not yet recruiting	44	M.D. Anderson Cancer Center in collaboration with NCI
NCT02684318	Assessment of predictive capacity and prognostic impact of some selected biomarkers including *BRCA*, *PTEN* and HRD panel in a phase Ib/II evaluating the efficacy and tolerability of PM01183 (lurbinectedin) combined with olaparib for treating advanced tumors including OC	I/II	Dose limiting toxicity (DLT), maximum tolerated dose (MTD) PFS and ORR (as secondary outcomes measure)	Recruiting	100	AstraZeneca and PharmaMar

NCT02734004 (MEDIOLA)	Determination of *BRCA* and *ATM* mutations, and overall mutation burden in a phase I/II evaluating safety/efficacy of MEDI4736 combined with olaparib in advanced cancer patients including OC	I/II	Disease control rate (DCR) and ORR	Recruiting	288	AstraZeneca in collaboration with IQVIA (formerly QuintilesIMS)

[‡]Titles of clinical trials were copied as shown by the database (with recruiting or enrolling by invitation studies), [@]Actual or estimated. Data from ClinicalTrials.gov (accessed 12/10/18). [†] These studies are still ongoing at the time of manuscript writing

Box 4.1 Recommended reading of particular interest

	DOI
Kuroki L, Guntupalli SR. **Treatment of epithelial ovarian cancer**. BMJ. 2020;371:m3773.	10.1136/bmj.m3773
Mirza MR, et al. **The forefront of ovarian cancer therapy: update on PARP inhibitors**. Ann Oncol. 2020;31(9):1148–1159.	10.1016/j.annonc. 2020.06.004
Chan JK, et al. **Selecting new upfront regimens for advanced ovarian cancer with biomarker guidance**. Gynecol Oncol. 2020;159(3):604–606.	10.1016/j.ygyno. 2020.09.017
Haunschild CE, Tewari KS. **The current landscape of molecular profiling in the treatment of epithelial ovarian cancer**. Gynecol Oncol. 2020:S0090-8258(20)33953-6.	10.1016/j.ygyno. 2020.09.043
Byrum AK, et al. **Defining and Modulating 'BRCAness'**. Trends Cell Biol. 2019;29(9):740–751.	10.1016/j.tcb.2019. 06.005
Wakefield MJ, et al. **Diverse mechanisms of PARP inhibitor resistance in ovarian cancer**. Biochim Biophys Acta Rev Cancer. 2019;1872(2):188307.	10.1016/j.bbcan. 2019.08.002
Lord CJ, Ashworth A. **BRCAness revisited**. Nat Rev Cancer. 2016;16(2):110–20.	10.1038/nrc.2015. 21
Lheureux S, et al. **Epithelial ovarian cancer: Evolution of management in the era of precision medicine**. CA Cancer J Clin. 2019;69(4):280–304.	10.3322/caac.21559

Acknowledgment and Conflicts of Interest KE is an editor in Springer Nature Journals and a previous editor for a Springer Book (https://link.springer.com/book/10.1007/978-3-030-53821-7).

Authors' Contribution KE wrote the chapter. OA and SA revised and supervised the chapter writing. The final draft was reviewed and approved by all the authors. The contents of the chapter reflect the authors' perspectives and not of their institutions of affiliation.

References

Adams SF, Marsh EB, Elmasri W, Halberstadt S, Vandecker S, Sammel MD, Bradbury AR, Daly M, Karlan B, Rubin SC (2011) A high response rate to liposomal doxorubicin is seen among women with BRCA mutations treated for recurrent epithelial ovarian cancer. Gynecol Oncol 123(3):486–491. https://doi.org/10.1016/j.ygyno.2011.08.032

Alsop K, Fereday S, Meldrum C, de Fazio A, Emmanuel C, George J, Dobrovic A, Birrer MJ, Webb PM, Stewart C, Friedlander M, Fox S, Bowtell D, Mitchell G (2012) BRCA mutation frequency and patterns of treatment response in BRCA mutation-positive women with ovarian cancer: a report from the Australian Ovarian Cancer Study Group. J Clin Oncol 30(21):2654–2663. https://doi.org/10.1200/JCO.2011.39.8545. Epub 2012 Jun 18. Erratum in: J Clin Oncol. 2012 Nov 20;30(33):4180

Audeh MW, Carmichael J, Penson RT et al (2010) Oral poly(ADP-ribose) polymerase inhibitor olaparib in patients with BRCA1 or BRCA2 mutations and recurrent ovarian cancer: a proof-of-concept trial. Lancet 376(9737):245–251. https://doi.org/10.1016/S0140-6736(10)60893-8

Boussios S, Karihtala P, Moschetta M, Abson C, Karathanasi A, Zakynthinakis-Kyriakou N, Ryan JE, Sheriff M, Rassy E, Pavlidis N (2020) Veliparib in ovarian cancer: a new synthetically lethal therapeutic approach. Investig New Drugs 38(1):181–193. https://doi.org/10.1007/s10637-019-00867-4

Brachova P, Thiel KW, Leslie KK (2013) The consequence of oncomorphic TP53 mutations in ovarian cancer. Int J Mol Sci 14(9):19257–19275. https://doi.org/10.3390/ijms140919257

Brachova P, Mueting SR, Carlson MJ et al (2014) TP53 oncomorphic mutations predict resistance to platinum- and taxane-based standard chemotherapy in patients diagnosed with advanced serous ovarian carcinoma. Int J Oncol 46(2):607–618

Bryant HE, Schultz N, Thomas HD et al (2005) Specific killing of BRCA2-deficient tumours with inhibitors of poly(ADP-ribose) polymerase. Nature 434(7035):913–917

Cancer Genome Atlas Research Network (2011) Integrated genomic analyses of ovarian carcinoma. Nature 474(7353):609–615. https://doi.org/10.1038/nature10166. Erratum in: Nature. 2012 Oct 11;490(7419):298

Cascales Campos P, Gil J, Feliciangeli E et al (2015) HIPEC in ovarian cancer: treatment of a new era or is it the end of the pipeline? Gynecol Oncol 139(2):363–368. https://doi.org/10.1016/j.ygyno.2015.06.012

Christie EL, Fereday S, Doig K, Pattnaik S, Dawson SJ, Bowtell DDL (2017) Reversion of BRCA1/2 germline mutations detected in circulating tumor DNA from patients with high-grade serous ovarian cancer. J Clin Oncol 35(12):1274–1280. https://doi.org/10.1200/JCO.2016.70.4627

Coleman RL, Sill MW, Bell-McGuinn K, Aghajanian C, Gray HJ, Tewari KS, Rubin SC, Rutherford TJ, Chan JK, Chen A, Swisher EM (2015) A phase II evaluation of the potent, highly selective PARP inhibitor veliparib in the treatment of persistent or recurrent epithelial ovarian, fallopian tube, or primary peritoneal cancer in patients who carry a germline BRCA1 or BRCA2 mutation – an NRG Oncology/Gynecologic Oncology Group study. Gynecol Oncol 137(3):386–391. https://doi.org/10.1016/j.ygyno.2015.03.042

Coleman RL, Oza AM, Lorusso D, Aghajanian C, Oaknin A, Dean A, Colombo N, Weberpals JI, Clamp A, Scambia G, Leary A, Holloway RW, Gancedo MA, Fong PC, Goh JC, O'Malley DM, Armstrong DK, Garcia-Donas J, Swisher EM, Floquet A, Konecny GE, IA MN, Scott CL, Cameron T, Maloney L, Isaacson J, Goble S, Grace C, Harding TC, Raponi M, Sun J, Lin KK, Giordano H, Ledermann JA, ARIEL3 Investigators (2017) Rucaparib maintenance treatment for recurrent ovarian carcinoma after response to platinum therapy (ARIEL3): a randomised, double-blind, placebo-controlled, phase 3 trial. Lancet 390(10106):1949–1961. https://doi.org/10.1016/S0140-6736(17)32440-6. Erratum in: Lancet. 2017 Oct 28;390(10106):1948

Coleman RL, Fleming GF, Brady MF, Swisher EM, Steffensen KD, Friedlander M, Okamoto A, Moore KN, Efrat Ben-Baruch N, Werner TL, Cloven NG, Oaknin A, Di Silvestro PA, Morgan MA, Nam JH, Leath CA 3rd, Nicum S, Hagemann AR, Littell RD, Cella D, Baron-Hay S, Garcia-Donas J, Mizuno M, Bell-McGuinn K, Sullivan DM, Bach BA, Bhattacharya S, Ratajczak CK, Ansell PJ, Dinh MH, Aghajanian C, Bookman MA (2019) Veliparib with first-line chemotherapy and as maintenance therapy in ovarian cancer. N Engl J Med 381(25):2403–2415. https://doi.org/10.1056/NEJMoa1909707

da Costa AABA, do Canto LM, Larsen SJ, ARG R, Stecca CE, Petersen AH, Aagaard MM, de Brot L, Baumbach J, Baiocchi G, Achatz MI, Rogatto SR (2019) Genomic profiling in ovarian cancer retreated with platinum based chemotherapy presented homologous recombination deficiency and copy number imbalances of CCNE1 and RB1 genes. BMC Cancer 19(1):422. https://doi.org/10.1186/s12885-019-5622-4

Davies AA, Masson JY, McIlwraith MJ et al (2001) Role of BRCA2 in control of the RAD51 recombination and DNA repair protein. Mol Cell 7(2):273–282

El Bairi K, Amrani M, Kandhro AH, Afqir S (2017a) Prediction of therapy response in ovarian cancer: where are we now? Crit Rev Clin Lab Sci 54(4):233–266. https://doi.org/10.1080/10408363.2017.1313190

El Bairi K, Kandhro AH, Gouri A, Mahfoud W, Louanjli N, Saadani B, Afqir S, Amrani M (2017b) Emerging diagnostic, prognostic and therapeutic biomarkers for ovarian cancer. Cell Oncol (Dordr) 40(2):105–118. https://doi.org/10.1007/s13402-016-0309-1

El Bairi K, Amrani M, Afqir S (2018) Starvation tactics using natural compounds for advanced cancers: pharmacodynamics, clinical efficacy, and predictive biomarkers. Cancer Med 7 (6):2221–2246. https://doi.org/10.1002/cam4.1467

El Bairi K, Atanasov AG, Amrani M, Afqir S (2019) The arrival of predictive biomarkers for monitoring therapy response to natural compounds in cancer drug discovery. Biomed Pharmacother 109:2492–2498. https://doi.org/10.1016/j.biopha.2018.11.097

Farmer H, McCabe N, Lord CJ et al (2005) Targeting the DNA repair defect in BRCA mutant cells as a therapeutic strategy. Nature 434(7035):917–921

Fong PC, Boss DS, Yap TA et al (2009) Inhibition of poly(ADP-ribose) polymerase in tumors from BRCA mutation carriers. N Engl J Med 361(2):123–134. https://doi.org/10.1056/NEJMoa0900212

Fong PC, Yap TA, Boss DS et al (2010) Poly(ADP)-ribose polymerase inhibition: frequent durable responses in BRCA carrier ovarian cancer correlating with platinum-free interval. J Clin Oncol 28(15):2512–2519. https://doi.org/10.1200/JCO.2009.26.9589

Franzese E, Centonze S, Diana A, Carlino F, Guerrera LP, Di Napoli M, De Vita F, Pignata S, Ciardiello F, Orditura M (2019) PARP inhibitors in ovarian cancer. Cancer Treat Rev 73:1–9. https://doi.org/10.1016/j.ctrv.2018.12.002

Fuh K, Mullen M, Blachut B, Stover E, Konstantinopoulos P, Liu J, Matulonis U, Khabele D, Mosammaparast N, Vindigni A (2020) Homologous recombination deficiency real-time clinical assays, ready or not? Gynecol Oncol 159(3):877–886. https://doi.org/10.1016/j.ygyno.2020.08.035

Galluzzi L, Senovilla L, Vitale I, Michels J, Martins I, Kepp O, Castedo M, Kroemer G (2012) Molecular mechanisms of cisplatin resistance. Oncogene 31(15):1869–1883. https://doi.org/10.1038/onc.2011.384

Garsed DW, Alsop K, Fereday S et al (2018) Homologous recombination DNA repair pathway disruption and retinoblastoma protein loss are associated with exceptional survival in high-grade serous ovarian cancer. Clin Cancer Res 24(3):569–580. https://doi.org/10.1158/1078-0432.CCR-17-1621

González-Martín A, Pothuri B, Vergote I, De Pont Christensen R, Graybill W, Mirza MR, McCormick C, Lorusso D, Hoskins P, Freyer G, Baumann K, Jardon K, Redondo A, Moore RG, Vulsteke C, O'Cearbhaill RE, Lund B, Backes F, Barretina-Ginesta P, Haggerty AF, Rubio-Pérez MJ, Shahin MS, Mangili G, Bradley WH, Bruchim I, Sun K, Malinowska IA, Li Y, Gupta D, Monk BJ, PRIMA/ENGOT-OV26/GOG-3012 Investigators (2019) Niraparib in patients with newly diagnosed advanced ovarian cancer. N Engl J Med 381(25):2391–2402. https://doi.org/10.1056/NEJMoa1910962

Gorodnova TV, Sokolenko AP, Ivantsov AO, Iyevleva AG, Suspitsin EN, Aleksakhina SN, Yanus GA, Togo AV, Maximov SY, Imyanitov EN (2015) High response rates to neoadjuvant platinum-based therapy in ovarian cancer patients carrying germ-line BRCA mutation. Cancer Lett 369(2):363–367. https://doi.org/10.1016/j.canlet.2015.08.028

Gorodnova T, Sokolenko A, Ni V, Ivantsov A, Kotiv K, Petrik S, Amelina I, Berlev I, Imyanitov E (2019) BRCA1-associated and sporadic ovarian carcinomas: outcomes of primary cytoreductive surgery or neoadjuvant chemotherapy. Int J Gynecol Cancer 29(4):779–786. https://doi.org/10.1136/ijgc-2018-000175

Grisham RN, Iyer G, Garg K, Delair D, Hyman DM, Zhou Q, Iasonos A, Berger MF, Dao F, Spriggs DR, Levine DA, Aghajanian C, Solit DB (2013) BRAF mutation is associated with early stage disease and improved outcome in patients with low-grade serous ovarian cancer. Cancer 119(3):548–554. https://doi.org/10.1002/cncr.27782

Guo XX, Wu HL, Shi HY, Su L, Zhang X (2018) The efficacy and safety of olaparib in the treatment of cancers: a meta-analysis of randomized controlled trials. Cancer Manag Res 10:2553–2562. https://doi.org/10.2147/CMAR.S169558

Harter P, Johnson T, Berton-Rigaud D, Park SY, Friedlander M, Del Campo JM, Shimada M, Forget F, Mirza MR, Colombo N, Zamagni C, Chan JK, Imhof M, Herzog TJ, O'Donnell D, Heitz F, King K, Stinnett S, Barrett C, Jobanputra M, Xu CF, du Bois A (2016) BRCA1/2 mutations associated with progression-free survival in ovarian cancer patients in the AGO-OVAR 16 study. Gynecol Oncol 140(3):443–449. https://doi.org/10.1016/j.ygyno.2015.12.027

Hodgson DR, Dougherty BA, Lai Z et al (2018) Candidate biomarkers of PARP inhibitor sensitivity in ovarian cancer beyond the BRCA genes. Br J Cancer 119(11):1401–1409. https://doi.org/10.1038/s41416-018-0274-8

Hoppenot C, Eckert MA, Tienda SM, Lengyel E (2018) Who are the long-term survivors of high grade serous ovarian cancer? Gynecol Oncol 148(1):204–212. https://doi.org/10.1016/j.ygyno.2017.10.032

Hsu LC, White RL (1998) BRCA1 is associated with the centrosome during mitosis. Proc Natl Acad Sci U S A 95(22):12983–12988. https://doi.org/10.1073/pnas.95.22.12983

Huang YW (2018) Association of BRCA1/2 mutations with ovarian cancer prognosis: an updated meta-analysis. Medicine (Baltimore) 97(2):e9380. https://doi.org/10.1097/MD.0000000000009380

Hyman DM, Zhou Q, Arnold AG et al (2011) Topotecan in patients with BRCA-associated and sporadic platinum-resistant ovarian, fallopian tube, and primary peritoneal cancers. Gynecol Oncol 123(2):196–199. https://doi.org/10.1016/j.ygyno.2011.07.019

Hyman DM, Long KC, Tanner EJ et al (2012) Outcomes of primary surgical cytoreduction in patients with BRCA-associated high-grade serous ovarian carcinoma. Gynecol Oncol 126(2):224–228. https://doi.org/10.1016/j.ygyno.2012.05.001

Ignatov T, Eggemann H, Costa SD, Roessner A, Kalinski T, Ignatov A (2014) BRCA1 promoter methylation is a marker of better response to platinum-taxane-based therapy in sporadic epithelial ovarian cancer. J Cancer Res Clin Oncol 140(9):1457–1463. https://doi.org/10.1007/s00432-014-1704-5

Joukov V, Groen AC, Prokhorova T, Gerson R, White E, Rodriguez A, Walter JC, Livingston DM (2006) The BRCA1/BARD1 heterodimer modulates ran-dependent mitotic spindle assembly. Cell 127(3):539–552. https://doi.org/10.1016/j.cell.2006.08.053

Kais Z, Chiba N, Ishioka C, Parvin JD (2012) Functional differences among BRCA1 missense mutations in the control of centrosome duplication. Oncogene 31(6):799–804. https://doi.org/10.1038/onc.2011.271

Kalachand RD, Stordal B, Madden S, Chandler B, Cunningham J, Goode EL, Ruscito I, Braicu EI, Sehouli J, Ignatov A, Yu H, Katsaros D, Mills GB, Lu KH, Carey MS, Timms KM, Kupryjanczyk J, Rzepecka IK, Podgorska A, McAlpine JN, Swisher EM, Bernards SS, O'Riain C, O'Toole S, O'Leary JJ, Bowtell DD, Thomas DM, Prieske K, Joosse SA, Woelber L, Chaudhry P, Häfner N, Runnebaum IB, Hennessy BT (2020) BRCA1 promoter methylation and clinical outcomes in ovarian cancer: an individual patient data meta-analysis. J Natl Cancer Inst 112(12):1190–1203. https://doi.org/10.1093/jnci/djaa070

Kondrashova O, Nguyen M, Shield-Artin K, Tinker AV, Teng NNH, Harrell MI, Kuiper MJ, Ho GY, Barker H, Jasin M, Prakash R, Kass EM, Sullivan MR, Brunette GJ, Bernstein KA, Coleman RL, Floquet A, Friedlander M, Kichenadasse G, O'Malley DM, Oza A, Sun J, Robillard L, Maloney L, Bowtell D, Giordano H, Wakefield MJ, Kaufmann SH, Simmons AD, Harding TC, Raponi M, McNeish IA, Swisher EM, Lin KK, Scott CL, AOCS Study Group (2017) Secondary somatic mutations restoring RAD51C and RAD51D associated with acquired resistance to the PARP inhibitor Rucaparib in high-grade ovarian carcinoma. Cancer Discov 7(9):984–998. https://doi.org/10.1158/2159-8290.CD-17-0419

Konstantinopoulos PA, Matulonis UA (2018) Targeting DNA damage response and repair as a therapeutic strategy for ovarian cancer. Hematol Oncol Clin North Am 32(6):997–1010. https://doi.org/10.1016/j.hoc.2018.07.006

Konstantinopoulos PA, Ceccaldi R, Shapiro GI, D'Andrea AD (2015) Homologous recombination deficiency: exploiting the fundamental vulnerability of ovarian cancer. Cancer Discov 5 (11):1137–1154. https://doi.org/10.1158/2159-8290.CD-15-0714

Kotsopoulos J, Rosen B, Fan I et al (2016) Ten-year survival after epithelial ovarian cancer is not associated with BRCA mutation status. Gynecol Oncol 140(1):42–47. https://doi.org/10.1016/j.ygyno.2015.11.009

Kriege M, Jager A, Hooning MJ, Huijskens E, Blom J, van Deurzen CH, Bontenbal M, Collee JM, Menke-Pluijmers MB, Martens JW, Seynaeve C (2012) The efficacy of taxane chemotherapy for metastatic breast cancer in BRCA1 and BRCA2 mutation carriers. Cancer 118(4):899–907. https://doi.org/10.1002/cncr.26351

Le Page C, Amuzu S, Rahimi K, Gotlieb W, Ragoussis J, Tonin PN (2020a) Lessons learned from understanding chemotherapy resistance in epithelial tubo-ovarian carcinoma from BRCA1and BRCA2mutation carriers. Semin Cancer Biol:S1044-579X(20)30177-2. https://doi.org/10.1016/j.semcancer.2020.08.005

Le Page C, Chung J, Rahimi K, Köbel M, Provencher D, Mes-Masson AM (2020b) Exploring the clinical impact of predictive biomarkers in serous ovarian carcinomas. Curr Drug Targets 21 (10):974–995. https://doi.org/10.2174/1389450120666191016143836

Ledermann JA (2019) Do increased tumor infiltrating lymphocytes co-existing with homologous recombination deficiency provide clues to enhance immunotherapy of ovarian cancer? Gynecol Oncol 153(2):213–214. https://doi.org/10.1016/j.ygyno.2019.04.014

Ledermann J, Harter P, Gourley C et al (2014) Olaparib maintenance therapy in patients with platinum-sensitive relapsed serous ovarian cancer: a preplanned retrospective analysis of outcomes by BRCA status in a randomised phase 2 trial. Lancet Oncol 15(8):852–861. https://doi.org/10.1016/S1470-2045(14)70228-1

Ledermann JA, Harter P, Gourley C et al (2016) Overall survival in patients with platinum-sensitive recurrent serous ovarian cancer receiving olaparib maintenance monotherapy: an updated analysis from a randomised, placebo-controlled, double-blind, phase 2 trial. Lancet Oncol 17 (11):1579–1589. https://doi.org/10.1016/S1470-2045(16)30376-X

Leunen K, Cadron I, Van Gorp T, Amant F, Berteloot P, Neven P, Legius E, Vergote I (2009) Does paclitaxel-carboplatin chemotherapy in a dose-dense regimen enhance survival of BRCA-related ovarian cancer patients? Int J Gynecol Cancer 19(9):1501–1504. https://doi.org/10.1111/IGC.0b013e3181bb703f

Lheureux S, Lai Z, Dougherty BA et al (2017) Long-term responders on Olaparib maintenance in high-grade serous ovarian cancer: clinical and molecular characterization. Clin Cancer Res 23 (15):4086–4094. https://doi.org/10.1158/1078-0432.CCR-16-2615

Lin KK, Harrell MI, Oza AM, Oaknin A, Ray-Coquard I, Tinker AV, Helman E, Radke MR, Say C, Vo LT, Mann E, Isaacson JD, Maloney L, O'Malley DM, Chambers SK, Kaufmann SH, Scott CL, Konecny GE, Coleman RL, Sun JX, Giordano H, Brenton JD, Harding TC, McNeish IA, Swisher EM (2019) BRCA reversion mutations in circulating tumor DNA predict primary and acquired resistance to the PARP inhibitor Rucaparib in high-grade ovarian carcinoma. Cancer Discov 9(2):210–219. https://doi.org/10.1158/2159-8290.CD-18-0715

Liu Y, Yasukawa M, Chen K et al (2015) Association of somatic mutations of ADAMTS genes with chemotherapy sensitivity and survival in high-grade serous ovarian carcinoma. JAMA Oncol 1(4):486–494

Lord CJ, Ashworth A (2017) PARP inhibitors: synthetic lethality in the clinic. Science 355 (6330):1152–1158. https://doi.org/10.1126/science.aam7344

Lord CJ, Tutt AN, Ashworth A (2015) Synthetic lethality and cancer therapy: lessons learned from the development of PARP inhibitors. Annu Rev Med 66:455–470. https://doi.org/10.1146/annurev-med-050913-022545

Lorusso D, Mancini M, Di Rocco R et al (2012) The role of secondary surgery in recurrent ovarian cancer. Int J Surg Oncol 2012:613980

Lorusso D, Scambia G, Pignata S, Sorio R, Amadio G, Lepori S, Mosconi A, Pisano C, Mangili G, Maltese G, Sabbatini R, Artioli G, Gamucci T, Di Napoli M, Capoluongo E, Ludovini V,

Raspagliesi F, Ferrandina G (2016) Prospective phase II trial of trabectedin in BRCA-mutated and/or BRCAness phenotype recurrent ovarian cancer patients: the MITO 15 trial. Ann Oncol 27(3):487–493. https://doi.org/10.1093/annonc/mdv608

Lorusso D, Ceni V, Daniele G, Salutari V, Pietragalla A, Muratore M, Nero C, Ciccarone F, Scambia G (2020) Newly diagnosed ovarian cancer: which first-line treatment? Cancer Treat Rev 91:102111. https://doi.org/10.1016/j.ctrv.2020.102111

Madariaga A, Lheureux S, Oza AM (2019) Tailoring ovarian cancer treatment: implications of BRCA1/2 mutations. Cancers (Basel) 11(3):416. https://doi.org/10.3390/cancers11030416

Madariaga A, Bowering V, Ahrari S, Oza AM, Lheureux S (2020) Manage wisely: poly (ADP-ribose) polymerase inhibitor (PARPi) treatment and adverse events. Int J Gynecol Cancer 30(7):903–915. https://doi.org/10.1136/ijgc-2020-001288

Marchetti C, De Leo R, Musella A, D'Indinosante M, Capoluongo E, Minucci A, Benedetti Panici P, Scambia G, Fagotti A (2018) BRCA mutation status to personalize management of recurrent ovarian cancer: a multicenter study. Ann Surg Oncol 25(12):3701–3708. https://doi.org/10.1245/s10434-018-6700-6

Milanesio MC, Giordano S, Valabrega G (2020) Clinical implications of DNA repair defects in high-grade serous ovarian carcinomas. Cancers (Basel) 12(5):1315. https://doi.org/10.3390/cancers12051315

Miller RE, Leary A, Scott CL, Serra V, Lord CJ, Bowtell D, Chang DK, Garsed DW, Jonkers J, Ledermann JA, Nik-Zainal S, Ray-Coquard I, Shah SP, Matias-Guiu X, Swisher EM, Yates LR (2020) ESMO recommendations on predictive biomarker testing for homologous recombination deficiency and PARP inhibitor benefit in ovarian cancer. Ann Oncol 31(12):1606–1622. https://doi.org/10.1016/j.annonc.2020.08.2102

Millstein J, Budden T, Goode EL et al (2020) Prognostic gene expression signature for high-grade serous ovarian cancer. Ann Oncol 31(9):1240–1250. https://doi.org/10.1016/j.annonc.2020.05.019

Mirza MR, Monk BJ, Herrstedt J, Oza AM, Mahner S, Redondo A, Fabbro M, Ledermann JA, Lorusso D, Vergote I, Ben-Baruch NE, Marth C, Mądry R, Christensen RD, Berek JS, Dørum A, Tinker AV, du Bois A, González-Martín A, Follana P, Benigno B, Rosenberg P, Gilbert L, Rimel BJ, Buscema J, Balser JP, Agarwal S, Matulonis UA (2016) ENGOT-OV16/NOVA investigators. Niraparib maintenance therapy in platinum-sensitive, recurrent ovarian cancer. N Engl J Med 375(22):2154–2164. https://doi.org/10.1056/NEJMoa1611310

Monk BJ, Ghatage P, Parekh T, Henitz E, Knoblauch R, Matos-Pita AS, Nieto A, Park YC, Cheng PS, Li W, Favis R, Ricci D, Poveda A (2015) Effect of BRCA1 and XPG mutations on treatment response to trabectedin and pegylated liposomal doxorubicin in patients with advanced ovarian cancer: exploratory analysis of the phase 3 OVA-301 study. Ann Oncol 26(5):914–920. https://doi.org/10.1093/annonc/mdv071

Monk BJ, Brady MF, Aghajanian C et al (2017) A phase 2, randomized, double-blind, placebo-controlled study of chemo-immunotherapy combination using motolimod with pegylated liposomal doxorubicin in recurrent or persistent ovarian cancer: a Gynecologic Oncology Group partners study. Ann Oncol 28(5):996–1004. https://doi.org/10.1093/annonc/mdx049

Monk BJ, Herzog TJ, Wang G, Triantos S, Maul S, Knoblauch R, McGowan T, Shalaby WSW, Coleman RL (2020) A phase 3 randomized, open-label, multicenter trial for safety and efficacy of combined trabectedin and pegylated liposomal doxorubicin therapy for recurrent ovarian cancer. Gynecol Oncol 156(3):535–544. https://doi.org/10.1016/j.ygyno.2019.12.043

Moore K, Colombo N, Scambia G et al (2018) Maintenance Olaparib in patients with newly diagnosed advanced ovarian cancer. N Engl J Med 379(26):2495–2505. https://doi.org/10.1056/NEJMoa1810858

Moore KN, Secord AA, Geller MA, Miller DS, Cloven N, Fleming GF, Wahner Hendrickson AE, Azodi M, DiSilvestro P, Oza AM, Cristea M, Berek JS, Chan JK, Rimel BJ, Matei DE, Li Y, Sun K, Luptakova K, Matulonis UA, Monk BJ (2019) Niraparib monotherapy for late-line treatment of ovarian cancer (QUADRA): a multicentre, open-label, single-arm, phase 2 trial.

Lancet Oncol 20(5):636–648. https://doi.org/10.1016/S1470-2045(19)30029-4. Erratum in: Lancet Oncol. 2019 May;20(5):e242

Morse CB, Toukatly MN, Kilgore MR, Agnew KJ, Bernards SS, Norquist BM, Pennington KP, Garcia RL, Liao JB, Swisher EM (2019) Tumor infiltrating lymphocytes and homologous recombination deficiency are independently associated with improved survival in ovarian carcinoma. Gynecol Oncol 153(2):217–222. https://doi.org/10.1016/j.ygyno.2019.02.011

Mullee LI, Morrison CG (2016) Centrosomes in the DNA damage response--the hub outside the Centre. Chromosom Res 24(1):35–51. https://doi.org/10.1007/s10577-015-9503-7

Nakayama N, Nakayama K, Shamima Y et al (2010) Gene amplification CCNE1 is related to poor survival and potential therapeutic target in ovarian cancer. Cancer 116(11):2621–2634. https://doi.org/10.1002/cncr.24987

Narod S (2016) Can advanced-stage ovarian cancer be cured? Nat Rev Clin Oncol 13(4):255–261. https://doi.org/10.1038/nrclinonc.2015.224

Naumann RW, Morris JC, Tait DL, Higgins RV, Crane EK, Drury LK, Amacker-North L, Templin M, Brown J (2018) Patients with BRCA mutations have superior outcomes after intraperitoneal chemotherapy in optimally resected high grade ovarian cancer. Gynecol Oncol 151(3):477–480. https://doi.org/10.1016/j.ygyno.2018.10.003

Nientiedt C, Heller M, Endris V et al (2017) Mutations in BRCA2 and taxane resistance in prostate cancer. Sci Rep 7(1):4574. https://doi.org/10.1038/s41598-017-04897-x

Nodin B, Zendehrokh N, Sundström M, Jirström K (2013) Clinicopathological correlates and prognostic significance of KRAS mutation status in a pooled prospective cohort of epithelial ovarian cancer. Diagn Pathol 8:106. https://doi.org/10.1186/1746-1596-8-106

Ow GS, Ivshina AV, Fuentes G, Kuznetsov VA (2014) Identification of two poorly prognosed ovarian carcinoma subtypes associated with CHEK2 germ-line mutation and non-CHEK2 somatic mutation gene signatures. Cell Cycle 13(14):2262–2280

Oza AM, Cibula D, Benzaquen AO et al (2015) Olaparib combined with chemotherapy for recurrent platinum-sensitive ovarian cancer: a randomised phase 2 trial. Lancet Oncol 16 (1):87–97. https://doi.org/10.1016/S1470-2045(14)71135-0

Patch AM, Christie EL, Etemadmoghadam D et al (2015) Whole-genome characterization of chemoresistant ovarian cancer. Nature 521(7553):489–494. https://doi.org/10.1038/nature14410

Pennington KP, Walsh T, Harrell MI, Lee MK, Pennil CC, Rendi MH, Thornton A, Norquist BM, Casadei S, Nord AS, Agnew KJ, Pritchard CC, Scroggins S, Garcia RL, King MC, Swisher EM (2014) Germline and somatic mutations in homologous recombination genes predict platinum response and survival in ovarian, fallopian tube, and peritoneal carcinomas. Clin Cancer Res 20 (3):764–775. https://doi.org/10.1158/1078-0432.CCR-13-2287

Penson RT, Valencia RV, Cibula D, Colombo N, Leath CA 3rd, Bidziński M, Kim JW, Nam JH, Madry R, Hernández C, Mora PAR, Ryu SY, Milenkova T, Lowe ES, Barker L, Scambia G (2020) Olaparib versus nonplatinum chemotherapy in patients with platinum-sensitive relapsed ovarian cancer and a germline BRCA1/2 mutation (SOLO3): a randomized phase III trial. J Clin Oncol 38(11):1164–1174. https://doi.org/10.1200/JCO.19.02745

Petrillo M, Marchetti C, De Leo R, Musella A, Capoluongo E, Paris I, Benedetti Panici P, Scambia G, Fagotti A (2017) BRCA mutational status, initial disease presentation, and clinical outcome in high-grade serous advanced ovarian cancer: a multicenter study. Am J Obstet Gynecol 217(3):334.e1–334.e9. https://doi.org/10.1016/j.ajog.2017.05.036

Ponzone R (2021) BRCA1/2 status and chemotherapy response score to tailor ovarian cancer surgery. Crit Rev Oncol Hematol 157:103128. https://doi.org/10.1016/j.critrevonc.2020.103128

Pujade-Lauraine E, Ledermann JA, Selle F et al (2017) Olaparib tablets as maintenance therapy in patients with platinum-sensitive, relapsed ovarian cancer and a BRCA1/2 mutation (SOLO2/ENGOT-Ov21): a double-blind, randomized, placebo-controlled, phase 3 trial. Lancet Oncol 18 (9):1274–1284. https://doi.org/10.1016/S1470-2045(17)30469-2

Quinn JE, James CR, Stewart GE, Mulligan JM, White P, Chang GK, Mullan PB, Johnston PG, Wilson RH, Harkin DP (2007) BRCA1 mRNA expression levels predict for overall survival in ovarian cancer after chemotherapy. Clin Cancer Res 13(24):7413–7420. https://doi.org/10.1158/1078-0432.CCR-07-1083

Quinn JE, Carser JE, James CR et al (2009) BRCA1 and implications for response to chemotherapy in ovarian cancer. Gynecol Oncol 113:134–142. https://doi.org/10.1016/j.ygyno.2008.12.015

Ratner ES, Keane FK, Lindner R, Tassi RA, Paranjape T, Glasgow M, Nallur S, Deng Y, Lu L, Steele L, Sand S, Muller RU, Bignotti E, Bellone S, Boeke M, Yao X, Pecorelli S, Ravaggi A, Katsaros D, Zelterman D, Cristea MC, Yu H, Rutherford TJ, Weitzel JN, Neuhausen SL, Schwartz PE, Slack FJ, Santin AD, Weidhaas JB (2012) A KRAS variant is a biomarker of poor outcome, platinum chemotherapy resistance and a potential target for therapy in ovarian cancer. Oncogene 31(42):4559–4566. https://doi.org/10.1038/onc.2011.539

Ray-Coquard I, Pautier P, Pignata S, Pérol D, González-Martín A, Berger R, Fujiwara K, Vergote I, Colombo N, Mäenpää J, Selle F, Sehouli J, Lorusso D, Guerra Alía EM, Reinthaller A, Nagao S, Lefeuvre-Plesse C, Canzler U, Scambia G, Lortholary A, Marmé F, Combe P, de Gregorio N, Rodrigues M, Buderath P, Dubot C, Burges A, You B, Pujade-Lauraine E, Harter P, PAOLA-1 Investigators (2019) Olaparib plus bevacizumab as first-line maintenance in ovarian cancer. N Engl J Med 381(25):2416–2428. https://doi.org/10.1056/NEJMoa1911361

Rudaitis V, Zvirblis T, Kanopiene D et al (2014) BRCA1/2 mutation status is an independent factor of improved survival for advanced (stage III-IV) ovarian cancer. Int J Gynecol Cancer 24 (8):1395–1400. https://doi.org/10.1097/IGC.0000000000000247

Rusan M, Andersen RF, Jakobsen A, Steffensen KD (2020) Circulating HOXA9-methylated tumour DNA: a novel biomarker of response to poly (ADP-ribose) polymerase inhibition in BRCA-mutated epithelial ovarian cancer. Eur J Cancer 125:121–129. https://doi.org/10.1016/j.ejca.2019.11.012

Safra T, Grisaru D, Inbar M, Abu-Abeid S, Dayan D, Matceyevsky D, Weizman A, Klausner JM (2014) Cytoreduction surgery with hyperthermic intraperitoneal chemotherapy in recurrent ovarian cancer improves progression-free survival, especially in BRCA-positive patients-a case-control study. J Surg Oncol 110(6):661–665. https://doi.org/10.1002/jso.23688

Sankaran S, Crone DE, Palazzo RE, Parvin JD (2007) BRCA1 regulates gamma-tubulin binding to centrosomes. Cancer Biol Ther 6(12):1853–1857. https://doi.org/10.4161/cbt.6.12.5164

Sharma B, Preet Kaur R, Raut S, Munshi A (2018) BRCA1 mutation spectrum, functions, and therapeutic strategies: the story so far. Curr Probl Cancer 42(2):189–207. https://doi.org/10.1016/j.currproblcancer.2018.01.001

Spiliotis J, Halkia E, Lianos E et al (2015) Cytoreductive surgery and HIPEC in recurrent epithelial ovarian cancer: a prospective randomized phase III study. Ann Surg Oncol 22(5):1570–1575. https://doi.org/10.1245/s10434-014-4157-9

Steffensen KD, Adimi P, Jakobsen A (2017) Veliparib monotherapy to patients with BRCA germ line mutation and platinum-resistant or partially platinum-sensitive relapse of epithelial ovarian cancer: a phase I/II study. Int J Gynecol Cancer 27(9):1842–1849. https://doi.org/10.1097/IGC.0000000000001089

Stewart ML, Tamayo P, Wilson AJ, Wang S, Chang YM, Kim JW, Khabele D, Shamji AF, Schreiber SL (2015) KRAS genomic status predicts the sensitivity of ovarian cancer cells to decitabine. Cancer Res 75(14):2897–2906. https://doi.org/10.1158/0008-5472.CAN-14-2860

Sun C, Li N, Ding D, Weng D, Meng L, Chen G, Ma D (2014) The role of BRCA status on the prognosis of patients with epithelial ovarian cancer: a systematic review of the literature with a meta-analysis. PLoS One 9(5):e95285. https://doi.org/10.1371/journal.pone.0095285

Swisher EM, Lin KK, Oza AM, Scott CL, Giordano H, Sun J, Konecny GE, Coleman RL, Tinker AV, O'Malley DM, Kristeleit RS, Ma L, Bell-McGuinn KM, Brenton JD, Cragun JM, Oaknin A, Ray-Coquard I, Harrell MI, Mann E, Kaufmann SH, Floquet A, Leary A, Harding TC, Goble S, Maloney L, Isaacson J, Allen AR, Rolfe L, Yelensky R, Raponi M, McNeish IA (2017) Rucaparib in relapsed, platinum-sensitive high-grade ovarian carcinoma (ARIEL2 part

1): an international, multicentre, open-label, phase 2 trial. Lancet Oncol 18(1):75–87. https://doi.org/10.1016/S1470-2045(16)30559-9
Takaya H, Nakai H, Takamatsu S, Mandai M, Matsumura N (2020) Homologous recombination deficiency status-based classification of high-grade serous ovarian carcinoma. Sci Rep 10 (1):2757. https://doi.org/10.1038/s41598-020-59671-3
Tobalina L, Armenia J, Irving E, O'Connor MJ, Forment JV (2021) A meta-analysis of reversion mutations in BRCA genes identifies signatures of DNA end-joining repair mechanisms driving therapy resistance. Ann Oncol 32(1):103–112. https://doi.org/10.1016/j.annonc.2020.10.470
Tsimberidou AM, Müller P, Ji Y (2020) Innovative trial design in precision oncology. Semin Cancer Biol:S1044-579X(20)30195-4. https://doi.org/10.1016/j.semcancer.2020.09.006
van Driel WJ, Koole SN, Sikorska K et al (2018) Hyperthermic intraperitoneal chemotherapy in ovarian cancer. N Engl J Med 378(3):230–240. https://doi.org/10.1056/NEJMoa1708618
Vencken PMLH, Kriege M, Hoogwerf D, Beugelink S, van der Burg MEL, Hooning MJ, Berns EM, Jager A, Collée M, Burger CW, Seynaeve C (2011) Chemosensitivity and outcome of BRCA1- and BRCA2-associated ovarian cancer patients after first-line chemotherapy compared with sporadic ovarian cancer patients. Ann Oncol 22(6):1346–1352. https://doi.org/10.1093/annonc/mdq628
Ventriglia J, Paciolla I, Cecere SC, Pisano C, Di Napoli M, Arenare L, Setola SV, Losito NS, Califano D, Orditura M, Pignata S (2018) Trabectedin in ovarian cancer: is it now a standard of care? Clin Oncol (R Coll Radiol) 30(8):498–503. https://doi.org/10.1016/j.clon.2018.01.008
Vitale SG, Marilli I, Lodato M et al (2013) The role of cytoreductive surgery in advanced-stage ovarian cancer: a systematic review. Updat Surg 65(4):265–270. https://doi.org/10.1007/s13304-013-0213-4
Weigelt B, Comino-Méndez I, de Bruijn I, Tian L, Meisel JL, García-Murillas I, Fribbens C, Cutts R, Martelotto LG, Ng CKY, Lim RS, Selenica P, Piscuoglio S, Aghajanian C, Norton L, Murali R, Hyman DM, Borsu L, Arcila ME, Konner J, Reis-Filho JS, Greenberg RA, Robson ME, Turner NC (2017) Diverse BRCA1 and BRCA2 reversion mutations in circulating cell-free DNA of therapy-resistant breast or ovarian cancer. Clin Cancer Res 23(21):6708–6720. https://doi.org/10.1158/1078-0432.CCR-17-0544
Wong KK, Izaguirre DI, Kwan SY et al (2013) Poor survival with wild-type TP53 ovarian cancer? Gynecol Oncol 130(3):565–569
Xiong B, Li S, Ai JS, Yin S, Ouyang YC, Sun SC, Chen DY, Sun QY (2008) BRCA1 is required for meiotic spindle assembly and spindle assembly checkpoint activation in mouse oocytes. Biol Reprod 79(4):718–726. https://doi.org/10.1095/biolreprod.108.069641
Xu K, Yang S, Zhao Y (2017) Prognostic significance of BRCA mutations in ovarian cancer: an updated systematic review with meta-analysis. Oncotarget 8(1):285–302. https://doi.org/10.18632/oncotarget.12306
Yang D, Khan S, Sun Y et al (2011) Association of BRCA1 and BRCA2 mutations with survival, chemotherapy sensitivity, and gene mutator phenotype in patients with ovarian cancer [published correction appears in JAMA. 2012 Jan 25;307(4):363]. JAMA 306 (14):1557–1565. https://doi.org/10.1001/jama.2011.1456
Yang SYC, Lheureux S, Karakasis K, Burnier JV, Bruce JP, Clouthier DL, Danesh A, Quevedo R, Dowar M, Hanna Y, Li T, Lu L, Xu W, Clarke BA, Ohashi PS, Shaw PA, Pugh TJ, Oza AM (2018) Landscape of genomic alterations in high-grade serous ovarian cancer from exceptional long- and short-term survivors. Genome Med 10(1):81. https://doi.org/10.1186/s13073-018-0590-x
Yarden RI, Pardo-Reoyo S, Sgagias M, Cowan KH, Brody LC (2002) BRCA1 regulates the G2/M checkpoint by activating Chk1 kinase upon DNA damage. Nat Genet 30(3):285–289. https://doi.org/10.1038/ng837
Zhong Q, Peng HL, Zhao X, Zhang L, Hwang WT (2014) Effects of BRCA1- and BRCA2-related mutations on ovarian and breast cancer survival: a meta-analysis. Clin Cancer Res 21 (1):211–220

The Advent of Circulating Tumor DNA in the Management of Ovarian Cancer

5

Khalid El Bairi, Ouissam Al Jarroudi, Laura Carpenito, Dario Trapani, and Said Afqir

Abstract

Genomically actionable mutations are increasingly used to deliver personalized medical care for patients with ovarian cancer (OC). Liquid biopsy applications encompass the identification and study of circulating tumor DNA (ctDNA), cell-free DNA, circulating tumor cells, and sometimes circulating miRNAs. In the current practice, ctDNA is mostly utilized. The multiple clinical applications of liquid biopsy in oncology have facilitated the implementation of precision medicine in practice. Though not still ready for clinical use in OC daily practice, the use of liquid biopsy in the experimental setting has revolutionized the study of the mechanisms of carcinogenesis and treatment resistance underlying the clinical disease progression. Moreover, as a minimally invasive approach, liquid biopsy can be used to predict response to antineoplastic therapies, including standard platinum-based chemotherapy regimens and PARP inhibitors. In addition, liquid biopsy can also be used in OC to predict recurrence, inform on the prognosis and anticipate clinical progression-free survival events. In this chapter, the clinical relevance and utility of blood-based ctDNA in OC are reviewed.

K. El Bairi (✉) · O. Al Jarroudi · S. Afqir
Department of Medical Oncology, Mohammed VI University Hospital, Oujda, Morocco

Faculty of Medicine and Pharmacy, Mohammed Ist University, Oujda, Morocco
e-mail: k.elbairi@ump.ac.ma

L. Carpenito
Fondazione IRCCS Istituto Nazionale dei Tumori, Milan, Italy

Department of Oncology and Haematology, University of Milan, Milan, Italy

D. Trapani
European Institute of Oncology, IRCCS, Milan, Italy

K. El Bairi (ed.), *Ovarian Cancer Biomarkers*,
https://doi.org/10.1007/978-981-16-1873-4_5

Keywords

Ovarian cancer · Liquid biopsy · Circulating tumor DNA · Outcomes

5.1 Introduction

Ovarian tumor components such as circulating tumor cells (CTCs) (Romero-Laorden et al. 2014), circulating tumor DNA (ctDNA) (Esposito et al. 2014), microRNAs (Wang et al. 2017), and cell–cell communicating exosomes, which are nano-sized vesicles containing nucleic acids and proteins (Li and Wang 2017), can be released into the bloodstream during tumor apoptosis, necrosis, and metastatic spread. Noninvasive quantitative and qualitative assessment of these tumors highly informative "*gold constituents*" may be accomplished with the advent of highly sensitive technologies such as digital polymerase chain reaction (PCR) and next-generation sequencing (NGS) platforms (Zhang et al. 2017) as well as the FDA-approved CellSearch® immuno-magnetic system for CTCs detection and characterization (Sun et al. 2018). This field of oncology is rapidly evolving and has literally experienced an *explosion* of liquid biopsy studies. Ovarian cancer (OC) is a particularly suitable and an ideal candidate for liquid biopsy: first, it sheds a higher quantity of tumor materials in the bloodstream; then, a significant proportion of women can experience a tumor recurrence after the primary treatments and/or tumor progression, after the initial systemic chemotherapy. Therefore, the clinical OC setting recalls the need to identify biomarkers of prognosis, early recurrence and prediction of treatment sensitivity. With the emerging precision oncology, ctDNA-based approaches have provided considerable and actionable data for the development of tools for (a) early detection, (b) real-time and longitudinal monitoring of therapy response, (c) detection of residual disease and recurrence, and (d) study of tumor heterogeneity (Steffensen et al. 2014; Wan et al. 2017; El Bairi et al. 2017a, b; Van Berckelaer et al. 2016) (Fig. 5.1). In this chapter, the advent of ctDNA in OC is reviewed based on several recent developments.

5.2 Circulating Tumor DNA as a Biomarker in Ovarian Cancer

Several recent human trials investigated the clinical value of ctDNA in OC (Table 5.1). Pereira et al. examined the role of ctDNA as a prognostic biomarker in 22 women with OC at the time of surgery and throughout the treatment course, using digital PCR and NGS to identify relevant mutations (Pereira et al. 2015). Notably, this study detected ctDNA in 93.8% of patients comparing it with computed tomography scan findings and CA-125 marker results. Moreover, ctDNA after 6 months of adjuvant treatment was found undetectable and associated with better PFS and OS ($p = 0.0011$ and $p = 0.0194$, respectively) suggesting its potential impact as a prognostic biomarker for disease recurrence and survival rate (Pereira et al. 2015). However, the prognostic value of ctDNA seems to be limited by

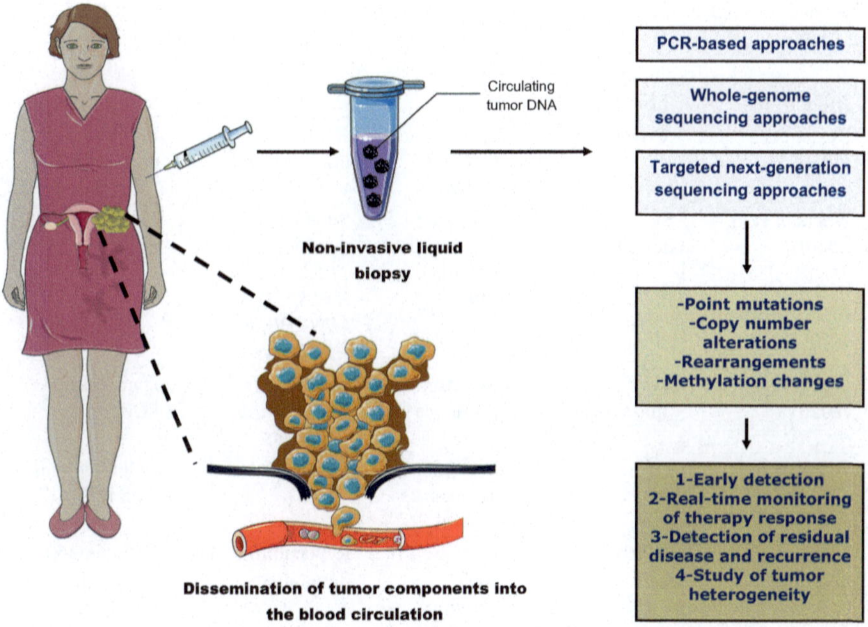

Fig. 5.1 Dissemination of tumor components into the blood circulation

the lack of sufficient data on its correlation with tumor size and stage. The ctDNA based analysis has revealed that mutated *TP53* was the most prevalent gene alteration, followed by low frequent mutations in *PTEN*, *PIK3CA*, *MET*, *KRAS*, *FBXW7*, and *BRAF* genes in patients with high-grade serous tumors (Pereira et al. 2015). To date, the rich source of data regarding initial *TP53* mutations revealed its important driver role in basal-like breast cancers and OC (reviewed elsewhere: Silwal-Pandit et al. 2017). Notably, OC patients with mutated *TP53* appear to have better survival and to be sensitive to chemotherapy (Leijen et al. 2016; Wong et al. 2013). In a retrospective analysis, Parkinson et al. found that decreased *TP53* mutant allele fraction (>6%) in ctDNA is an independent predictive biomarker for time-to-progression endpoint (TTP) (HR: 0.22, 95% CI: 0.07–0.67, $p = 0.008$) in relapsed high-grade serous OC (Parkinson et al. 2016). Furthermore, ctDNA levels were strongly correlated with the total volume of disease ($p < 0.001$) compared to the gold-standard CA-125 biomarker. Likewise, a significant correlation between mutated *TP53* in ctDNA and CA-125 ($p < 0.001$) was reported, thus suggesting its possible use as a highly specific biomarker to predict platinum-based treatment response (Parkinson et al. 2016). Recently, a large study enrolling 121 OC patients demonstrated that the NGS-based detection of somatic and germline *BRCA* mutations in ctDNA is feasible when the standard diagnostic testing is not satisfactory (Ratajska et al. 2017). *BRCA* reversion mutations (also known as *back mutations*) are a mechanism that may explain the acquired resistance to platinum

Table 5.1 Impact of circulating tumor DNA in ovarian cancer management (data from the last 5 years)

Author/year	No. of patients (histology)	Clinical impact	Genetic alteration	Study technique
Rusan et al. (2020)	32 (HGSOC$^{\beta}$)	Response to PARP inhibitors	*HOXA9* methylation	In-house digital droplet PCR
Noguchi et al. (2020)	51 (miscellaneous)	Prediction of progression-free survival (PFS)	Somatic mutations in *TP53, APC, KRAS, EGFR, MET, PIK3CA, NPAP1*, and *ALK*	Illumina NextSeq 500
Ogasawara et al. (2020)	255 (miscellaneous)	Prediction of recurrence	Somatic *PIK3CA* and/or *KRAS* mutations	Digital droplet PCR
Alves et al. (2020)	11 (miscellaneous)	Prediction of disease-free survival	–	Quantitative real-time PCR
Lin et al. (2018)	112 (HGSOC)	Response to PARP inhibitors	Reversion*BRCA1/2* mutations	Guardant360 assay (Illumina HiSeq)
Slavin et al. (2018)	2010	Identification of incidental germline mutations	Variants in 16† genes associated with hereditary cancers	Guardant360 assay (Illumina HiSeq)
Giannopoulou et al. (2018)	50 (HGSOC)$^{¥}$	Prediction of overall survival (OS) and PFS	*ESR1* methylation	Real-time methylation-specific PCR
Christie et al. (2017)	30 (HGSOC)	Therapy response	Reversion *BRCA*1/2 mutations	Targeted sequencing (Illumina MiSeq)
Widschwendter et al. (2017)	151 (miscellaneous)	Early detection and therapy response	DNAme-Marker Panel	Bisulfite sequencing (Illumina MiSeq/HiSeq 2500)
Ratajska et al. (2017)	121 (HGSOC; 72%)	Monitoring of PARP inhibition	*BRCA*1/2	Next-generation sequencing (Illumina)
Parkinson et al. (2016)	40 (HGSOC)	Therapy response	*TP53*	Digital PCR
Harris et al. (2016)	10 (HGSOC)	Therapy response and relapse monitoring	Somatic chromosomal rearrangements	Next-generation sequencing (Illumina HiSeq 2000) and qPCR
Pereira et al. (2015)	22 (21 HGSOC and 1 mixed mesodermal tumor)	Therapy response and survival	*TP53* and other low frequent mutated genes‡	Next-generation sequencing (Illumina HiSeq 2500 and Ion

(continued)

Table 5.1 (continued)

Author/year	No. of patients (histology)	Clinical impact	Genetic alteration	Study technique
				Torrent PGM-Ion AmpliSeq™ Cancer Hotspot Panel v2) and digital PCR

[β]including four patients with non-serous tumors. [†]APC, ATM, BRCA1, BRCA2, CDKN2A, KIT, MLH1, NF1, PTEN, RB1, RET, SMAD4, STK11, TP53, TSC1, and VHL. [ǂ]PTEN, PIK3CA, MET, KRAS, FBXW7, and BRAF. Abbreviations: *ALK* anaplastic lymphoma kinase, *APC* adenomatous polyposis coli, *BRCA* breast cancer gene, *DNA* deoxyribonucleic acid, *EGFR* epidermal growth factor receptor, *ESR1* estrogen receptor 1, *HGSOC* high-grade serous ovarian cancer, *HOXA9* homebox A9, *KRAS* Kirsten rat sarcoma, *MET* mesenchymal–epithelial transition factor, *NPAP1* nuclear protein-associated protein 1, *PARP* poly-ADP ribose polymerase, *PIK3CA* phosphatidylinositol-4,5-bisphosphate 3-kinase, *TP53* tumor protein 53, *PCR* polymerase chain reaction, *qPCR* quantitative polymerase chain reaction. [¥]53 primary tumors and 50 corresponding plasma samples

and PARP inhibition-based chemotherapy in OC and leading to the restoration of wild-type functions of this gene (Sakai et al. 2008; Norquist et al. 2011). These secondary mutations can take place in germline or somatic mutated *BRCA* alleles (Carneiro et al. 2018) and usually alter the structure of the primary frameshift into an in-frame internal deletion and leads to partly functional BRCA proteins (Ganesan 2018). As demonstrated by the previous study, detection of secondary reversion *BRCA* mutations in ctDNA allows the selection of patients that can benefit from PARP inhibition therapy which has recently shown a potential clinical response in OC (Ratajska et al. 2017; Ledermann 2016). Furthermore, in another study that recruited 30 patients with recurrent high-grade serous OC with known germline *BRCA1* or *BRCA2* status, reversion mutations detected in ctDNA based on targeted NGS assay were found to drive poor response to PARP inhibition and platinum-based treatments (Christie et al. 2017). However, despite reversion *BRCA* mutations were identified in ctDNA in an unbiased manner, this approach is limited by the fact that wild-type *BRCA* alleles-based DNA may be abundantly released in the blood from normal cells which will possibly influence the sensitivity of these NSG assays (Christie et al. 2017). More recently, 10,888 unselected patients with advanced cancers (stage III/IV), including OC patients ($n = 210$, 2%), were enrolled in a large cohort to identify incidental germline mutations in 16 actionable genes based on the Guardant 360™ NGS-based assay (Slavin et al. 2018). Variants in clinically targetable genes, such as *BRCA* in ctDNA, were found to be the highest among patients with OC compared with other advanced cancers (8.13% vs. 3.46%, 3.34%, and 2.2% for prostate, pancreatic, and breast tumors respectively) (Slavin et al. 2018). Similarly, Lin et al., in a study ($n = 112$) that used Guardant-360assay, has recently shown that patients with OC, without *BRCA* reversion mutations, had longer median PFS than those with reversion mutations identified in ctDNA before PARP inhibitors-based treatments (9.0 vs. 1.8 months; HR: 0.12; $p < 0.0001$) (Lin et al. 2018). Moreover, baseline ctDNA in OC at the time of diagnosis has also a value for predicting recurrence. In this regard, a large retrospective cohort of 255 patients with epithelial OC demonstrated that the presence of detectable ctDNA is an independent biomarker for recurrence (HR: 0.38, 95% CI: 0.18–0.79; $p = 0.01$) (Ogasawara et al. 2020). This suggests that tumor seeding can occur in localized OC. Moreover, other pilot studies confirmed the feasibility of this noninvasive approach in predicting outcomes in patients with OC (Alves et al. 2020; Noguchi et al. 2020). Taken together, these preliminary findings can establish prognostic value and efficient real-time monitoring of anticancer treatments, if validated in large cohorts using standardized assays such as companion diagnostics. Remarkably, concordance between genomic alterations in ctDNA and primary tumors was also noticed suggesting an added value of this approach as a diagnostic tool (reviewed elsewhere: Cheng et al. 2017). Moreover, the combination of cell-free DNA with CA125 and the emerging biomarker HE4 may improve the accuracy of OC detection as supported by an earlier report (Shao et al. 2015). Therefore, multimarker panels are supposed to improve the sensitivity and specificity of this liquid biopsy-based approach.

Another application of liquid biopsy is the ability to assess gene methylation and other epigenetic changes as biomarkers for early detection and prognostication purposes (El Bairi et al. 2018; Tomasetti et al. 2017). In OC, the clinical significance of methylation patterns in ctDNA has been examined by Widschwendter et al. in 151 patients with various histologies, based on a multi-marker panel (three methylated regions *COL23A1*, *C2CD4D*, and *WNT6* genes) using bisulfite sequencing; the pretreatment of DNA samples before the sequencing is one standard procedure to study the DNA methylation pattern (Widschwendter et al. 2017). This methylation panel has demonstrated to discriminate patients with OC from healthy women or patients with a benign pelvic mass, with specificity and sensitivity of 90.7% (95%, CI: 84.3–94.8%) and 41.4% (95% CI: 24.1–60.9%) respectively (Widschwendter et al. 2017). Remarkably, this panel showed superiority in predicting chemotherapy response compared with CA-125 (78% of responders and 86% of non-responders ($p = 0.04$) vs. 20% and 75% respectively) (Widschwendter et al. 2017). Correlation between changes in methylation in primary tumors and ctDNA based on real-time methylation PCR (mPCR) and its association with clinical outcomes was also reported in a recent study enrolling 50 patients with high-grade OC (Giannopoulou et al. 2018). Methylated *ESR1* in ctDNA, a gene encoding for the estrogen receptor, was found to be significantly associated with primary tumors ($p = 0.004$) (Giannopoulou et al. 2018). Importantly, methylated *ESR1* was also found to predict better overall survival ($p = 0.027$) and progression-free survival ($p = 0.041$) (Giannopoulou et al. 2018). More recently, homeobox A9 (*HOXA9*) promoter methylation in ctDNA was found to predict response to PARP inhibitors (Rusan et al. 2020). The findings of this cohort ($n = 32$) of a phase II trial that investigated veliparib for platinum-resistant OC patients with *BRCA* mutations demonstrated that detectable methylated *HOXA9* at baseline and before each treatment cycle was associated with worse outcomes. Patients that were positive for this biomarker had a reduced PFS (5.1 vs 8.3 months; $p < 0.0001$) and OS (9.5 vs

19.4 months; $p = 0.002$). This longitudinal monitoring also showed that patients that were positive at baseline and that had undetectable methylated *HOXA9* ctDNA showed improved outcomes on multivariate analysis (Rusan et al. 2020).

In addition to point mutations and DNA methylation, chromosomal rearrangements in ctDNA were also investigated based on whole-genome sequencing technology and appear to have greater tumor specificity in OC (Harris et al. 2016). Aberrant chromosomal junctions were identified in ctDNA of OC patients ($n = 8$) before cytoreductive surgery in which five subjects had undetectable post-surgical ctDNA and therefore, supporting its possible use for monitoring therapeutic interventions (Harris et al. 2016). Still, results from these proof-of-principle studies remain immature in these small populations of OC patients. Also, these studies have been conducted based on relatively small samples and different methodologies and technologies which require meta-analytic approaches to combine their data. In this perspective, only one previous meta-analysis was performed by Zhou et al. and it has pooled the results of nine studies (462 patients and 407 controls) to assess the diagnostic value of circulating cell-free DNA (cfDNA) in OC (Zhou et al. 2016). Pooled sensitivity of cfDNA (0.70; 95% CI: 0.65–0.74) was found poor but its specificity (0.90; 95% CI: 0.87–0.93) reached an acceptable value for OC diagnosis (Zhou et al. 2016). As expected, subgroup analysis indicated that studies with large sample sizes detected OC accurately compared with small sample ones. In the case of specimen types, plasma-based assays were found to have high sensitivity but low specificity (0.72 and 0.89, respectively) in comparison with serum-based tests (0.65 and 0.93, respectively) (Zhou et al. 2016). When compared with the most recent meta-analysis by Dayyani et al. that investigated the diagnostic value of the standard CA-125 showing an area under the curve (AUC) of 0.883 (95%; CI: 0.771–0.950) (Dayyani et al. 2016), the AUC of cfDNA was relatively greater [0.89 (95%; CI: 0.83–0.95)], thus demonstrating a better accuracy (Zhou et al. 2016). In this meta-analysis, significant heterogeneity (sensitivity: $I^2 = 85.2\%$ and specificity: $I^2 = 78.5\%$) was observed among enrolled studies (Zhou et al. 2016). Meta-regression was utilized to identify the source of this heterogeneity and accordingly, no covariates such as study design, sample type, location, etc. were found to influence it and therefore the source of this heterogeneity could not be detected (Zhou et al. 2016). Furthermore, potential bias and quality appraisal of methodological quality of selected studies for the meta-analysis was assessed using QUADAS-2 (Whiting et al. 2011). This tool indicated that the study design did not considerably involve the accuracy of cfDNA as a diagnostic biomarker for OC (Zhou et al. 2016). As this field is rapidly evolving, future meta-analyses will provide sizable evidence when additional studies are available.

5.3 Perspectives: Ongoing Clinical Trials Investigating ctDNA for Ovarian Cancer

Clinical trials on this topic (Table 5.2) have the potential to provide accurate findings by increasing power and providing well-designed biomarker cohorts. The design of clinical trials for several interventions across the cancer continuum embraces

Table 5.2 Summary of ongoing clinical trials assessing ctDNA as a biomarker for diagnosis, prognosis and therapy response prediction in ovarian cancer

Trial identifier	Purposes/Objectives	Study design	Enrollment[a]	Sponsor
NCT03614689	Study of correlation between ctDNA, OC recurrence, mutational status, therapy response, and characteristics of immune repertoire before and after therapy	Prospective	100	Geneplus-Beijing Co. Ltd. in collaboration with Peking Union Medical College Hospital
NCT03155451	Detection of ctDNA in plasma for OC diagnosis	Prospective case-control	43	RenJi Hospital
NCT03691012	Application of ctDNA in peripheral blood as a biomarker for recurrence of stage I-IV epithelial OC after debulking surgery or following adjuvant chemotherapy	Prospective and multicenter	100	Walter and Eliza Hall Institute of Medical in collaboration with Johns Hopkins University
NCT03302884 (CIDOC)	Exploration of ctDNA dynamics as a biomarker for early OC recurrence and treatment efficacy after front-line treatments	Prospective and multicenter	150	Institut Paoli-Calmettes in collaboration with AstraZeneca
NCT02822157 (CLIO)	Assessment of ctDNA for monitoring olaparib-based treatment in OC	Randomized phase II trial (crossover assignment)	160	Universitaire Ziekenhuizen Leuven in collaboration with AstraZeneca
NCT03622983 (PELVIMASS2)	Collection of biological samples including ctDNA and detailed clinical data for future personalized medical interventions such as prediction of treatment response in patients with pelvic cancers	Prospective	500 (pelvic neoplasms including OC)	Centre Hospitalier Intercommunal Creteil
NCT03017573 (SCANDARE)	Correlation between ctDNA levels, de novo mutations, and immune response	Prospective	500 (ovarian, breast, head, and neck cancers)	Institut Curie

NCT02489058 (OLALA)	Study of ctDNA for monitoring therapy response to olaparib	Retrospective/prospective	100	University Health Network, Toronto
NCT03783949 (EUDARIO)	Study of ctDNA as a biomarker in a 3-arm phase II trial assessing safety/efficacy of ganetespib combined with carboplatin followed by niraparib vs. ganetespib+ carboplatin followed by ganetespib and niraparib vs. carboplatin + standard chemotherapy followed by niraparib maintenance in platinum-sensitive OC (as an additional outcome measure)	Randomized multicenter phase II study (parallel assignment)	120	Universitaire Ziekenhuizen Leuven in collaboration with European Commission
NCT03277209	Study of changes in ctDNA dynamics before and after a treatment based on continuous intravenous administration of plerixafor (a CXCR4 antagonist) and its impact on immune microenvironment in pancreatic, ovarian, and colorectal carcinomas patients(as an additional outcome measure)	Interventional phase I trial	–	Weill Medical College of Cornell University in collaboration with Cambridge University Hospitals NHS Foundation Trust
NCT02644369 (INSPIRE)	Study of changes in ctDNA as a genomic biomarker for therapy response to pembrolizumab in advanced solid cancers including epithelial OC (as a secondary outcome measure)	Interventional phase II trial	100	University Health Network, Toronto in collaboration with Merck Sharp & Dohme Corp.
NCT02797977	Assessment of ctDNA as a predictive biomarker for Chk1 inhibition in advanced cancers including high-grade OC	Nonrandomized phase I/II trial	140	Sierra Oncology, Inc.

(continued)

Table 5.2 (continued)

Trial identifier	Purposes/Objectives	Study design	Enrollment[a]	Sponsor
NCT01350908	Quantification of ctDNA in blood samples of OC patients and comparison of related detection techniques (PAP pyrophosphorolysis activated polymerization), BEAMing, and NGS)	–	25	Institut Curie
NCT02811224	Determination of sensitivity of a detecting assay of ctDNA in OC	Prospective case control	50	Scripps Translational Science Institute

[a]estimated sample size

innovative technologies to boost cancer care advancements and validate the clinical utility, safety, and effectiveness. Research questions, in fact, shall find validations only in the context of controlled studies. The use of liquid biopsy in clinical trials has been initially developed to study the treatment response. However, while liquid biopsy applications have found room in the clinical care of some patients with selected tumor types, mostly as plasma-based assays for non-small cell lung cancer, several clinical trials are assessing their utility in a spectrum of diseases (Snow et al. 2019).

The presence of tumor ctDNA has been historically identified in healthy subjects (Mandel and Metais 1948), and in patients with cancer, suggesting ab initio a role for both the early diagnosis and treatment of human cancers. In OC, the identification of ctDNA in healthy subjects has prompted the applications for the screening of solid tumors, providing the high capacity of DNA shedding into the plasma of some cancers (Alharbi et al. 2018). The lack of effective screening mechanisms based on plasma markers and imaging for OC has illuminated an important unmet need, for the deadliest women's pelvic tumor (Jacobs et al. 2016). The first clinical studies of the screening of OC have provided quite variegated results: essentially, sensitivity is interestingly elevated with ctDNA but diagnostic specificity still too low for screening purposes (Vanderstichele et al. 2017). Whole-genome sequencing, targeted gene sequencing by quantitative PCR, and DNA methylation pattern studies have been utilized in clinical trials for OC screening (Pereira et al. 2015); however, the definition of an exact role and clinical position is still a matter of research. To date, no cancer screening has been successfully implemented on liquid biopsy, though highly promising (Lo and Lam 2020). Presently, one clinical trial led by Shanghai Jiao Tong University in China and based on the study of the ctDNA methylation levels by deep sequencing-Sequencing is ongoing for screening purposes (NCT03155451). The incorporation of the information from ctDNA will aid in the definition of effective early detection interventions for patients at average or increased risk of OC, alone or in the context of more complex decisional algorithms. Possibly, high-performing ctDNA-based strategies will help reduce the incidence of advanced disease, inform on the appropriate timing of prophylactic surgeries in high-risk patients and enhance the family screening, for selected pedigrees.

Levels of ctDNA are influenced also by the disease burden and affected in the quantity and quality by the carcinogenesis dynamics of clone selection-turnover and treatment responses. The concept of earlier treatment in OC, based on the use of plasma biomarkers of relapse (e.g., CA125), has never been truly supported in women receiving and completing primary treatments (Krell et al. 2017). The CA125-triggered treatment has not been demonstrated to improve the outcome in women with no macroscopic OC recurrence (Krell et al. 2017). However, CA125 is an imperfect biomarker, and susceptible to a number of non-oncogenic phenomena, including inflammatory processes (Kim et al. 2016). So far, the definition of the most meaningful prognostic determinants in OC patients is based on the clinical and radiological findings, e.g., platinum sensitivity (Krell et al. 2017). Therefore, clinical implementation of plasma-based markers that better predict the true cancer relapse events are highly warranted, to understand if the therapeutic exposure of the initial clones driving the recurrence in the preclinical stage can improve cancer survival. Based on these assumptions, prospective clinical trials have been designed and are ongoing to identify and validate ctDNA-based biomarkers for recurrence of stage I-IV epithelial OC after debulking surgery or following adjuvant chemotherapy (NCT03691012) and explore the ctDNA dynamics (NCT03302884/CIDOC).

In addition, several trials are also exploring the opportunity to study the variations in the ctDNA during treatment or the identification of resistance-driving clones. The phase 2 clinical trial ARIEL2 enrolled patients to receive the anti-PARP rucaparib; a subset of patients performed a liquid biopsy, to understand how the quantitative changes in the ctDNA could predict treatment response. None of the patients with persistently elevated ctDNA experienced a radiological tumor response, while 80% of patients with a demonstrated reduction of ctDNA (i.e., decreased level of 50% or more after a single treatment cycle) experienced a radiological tumor response, suggesting a possible predictive role (Piskorz et al. 2016). Therefore, prospective clinical trials have been designed to understand how ctDNA quantitative dynamics can affect the prognosis and serve as clinically useful and valid predictive biomarkers (NCT03302884/CIDOC). Also, ctDNA quantitative evaluations can be useful to understand the on-target mechanisms of resistance, as discussed above for the intragenic reversion mutations of *BRCA1/2*, linked to acquired resistance to PARP inhibitors (Christie et al. 2017). The ongoing prospective clinical trials aim to confirm the clinical value of longitudinal mutational evaluations with ctDNA during treatments for PARP inhibitors (NCT02822157/CLIO, NCT02489058/OLALA) and/or other targeted agents (NCT03622983/PELVIMASS2, NCT03783949/EUDARIO, NCT02797977).

Moreover, experimental evidence has demonstrated a possible role of liquid biopsy in the monitoring of response to immunotherapeutic agents (IO). The assessment of tumor response in patients receiving IO has been sometimes challenging, especially for patients experiencing an initial tumor progression followed by a durable cancer response (i.e., pseudo-progression). Accordingly, ctDNA-based assays that correlate with the true cancer burden may be desirable. Indeed, one study confirmed the prognostic value of ctDNA reduction in patients receiving IO, including a cohort of women with high-grade serous ovarian cancer (Bratman et al. 2020). This recapitulates the findings with chemotherapy and targeted agents. Consistently, ctDNA applications in IO treatment response monitoring have been implemented in ongoing clinical studies (NCT03017573/SCANDARE, NCT03277209, NCT02644369/INSPIRE). The possibility to collect samples during routine clinical procedures for standard clinical assessments of patients with OC is a major favoring characteristic for the clinical implementation of liquid biopsy, as its noninvasive nature. While the utility, reproducibility, and value of ctDNA assays in the clinical practice are still investigational, the OC biology and the preliminary exploratory findings from small cohorts suggest a promising role in the clinical practice, across the spectrum of cancer continuum.

5.4 Feasibility, Availability, and Accessibility of Liquid Biopsy-based Methodologies for Clinical Applications: Addressing Barriers, Framing Solutions for Cancer Resilient Health Systems

The implementation of innovative medical technologies developed in resource-rich settings can often encounter barriers in different health system contextures (Lustberg et al. 2018). For the approved indications, the role of assays based on liquid biopsy is complementary, and not entirely intended to replace tissue-based diagnostics; they are used mostly to characterize predictive and prognostic biomarkers (Goodsaid 2019). As a result, a number of regulators and decision-makers have questioned the true clinical utility of ctDNA assays outside clinical trials, thus they have not supported the coverage by the national health insurance schemes (Lustberg et al. 2018). The liquid biopsy technologies are sophisticated and costly, therefore demanding elevated financial resources and skilled health personnel.

In low- and middle-income countries, the implementation of effective cancer control programs is challenged by the scarcity of resources, often weakened by non-resilient health systems, unprepared to face the rapidly increasing cancer burden (Wambalaba et al. 2019). Accordingly, the selection and prioritization of cancer interventions are critical to assure the delivery of quality cancer interventions to a large proportion of the population, pursuing for a universal health care. Nevertheless, some authors have reported possible benefits in the implementation of ctDNA techniques in low- and middle-income countries. The possibility to collect blood samples virtually anywhere, stored in local laboratories, and then analyzed in reference centers is one of the advantages (Temilola et al. 2019). For many patients, in fact, the first and most important barrier to cancer care is to have a diagnosis of the malignancy, to seek medical care, and to perform the diagnostic tissue biopsy—representing one of the most significant reasons for delays in cancer treatments and advanced cancer presentations (Brand et al. 2019; Trapani et al. 2021). However, evidence to support a complete replacement of tissue biopsy with liquid biopsy for diagnostic purposes is not entirely supported, as the role of ctDNA assays is mostly complementary, and not intended to make the diagnosis of cancer (Adeola et al. 2017). Therefore, no implementation should be endorsed in the absence of good prospective clinical data, and validations in the ethnic subgroups of interest. For example, only a minority of the patients enrolled in the clinical studies of liquid biopsy belong to African ancestry, and African-based studies are only a small number. One research showed that the majority of African-based studies were done in Egypt, with a few other studies from Northern Africa and South Africa (Temilola et al. 2019). Advocating for inclusiveness in clinical trials and evaluating the local utility of new medical technologies have emerged as health imperatives, ensuring valuable investments with measurable population health and economic gains (Dilla et al. 2015).

The implementation of innovative health interventions like liquid biopsy with no cognition of the utility, health gains, budgetary impact, and reimbursement decisions are common sources of inefficiency in the health investments. For example, three African countries (Kenya, Tunisia, and South Africa) have made available to the public some liquid biopsy kits (Kinyua 2018); however, these interventions have soon become prerogative of only a minority of the populations, as they are de facto unaffordable to the greatest proportion of the patients. The financial barriers and the lack of consistent data on effectiveness and cost-effectiveness can prevent all the good narratives to develop implementation research of liquid biopsy in low- and middle-income countries, including serving the most remote areas and disadvantaged populations. In addition, the risk to increase the health care gap is large, including through an elevated exposure to catastrophic health expenditure.

Nowadays, it is imperative to expand the options of cancer services in low- and middle-income countries through a phased approach. The safety, feasibility, sustainability, and cost-effectiveness of new technologies must be viewed in a context-appropriate cancer planning perspective, and not as a mere race for the most innovative devices. Therefore, research investments must be oriented to boost the local capacities through international and national efforts, including regulated agreements with the private sector, and always developed in alignment with the goals of the national cancer control planning (Jamison et al. 2018).

The use of liquid biopsy could also help in the promotion of the best treatment practices, in the context of clinical trials. Whether liquid biopsy should be implemented in the clinical practice for women with OC in low- and middle-income countries nowadays is unlikely to be realistic. However, the strengthening of clinical research is the imperative of the cancer agenda, including with the use of new technologies—when intended to enforce the local evidence-based practices, scale-up the workforce, and develop training programs—resulting in a health system benefit of the cancer research, therefore translated in a population benefit with societal gains. Major advancements in cancer care will be stated only under a goal-oriented research agenda, making sure that priority investments are not distracted by more appealing but not presently useful interventions. It is necessary to work for population-based cancer care that is affordable, accessible, and designed to respond to local health needs through global health tools and technologies.

5.5 Conclusions

Liquid biopsy is a novel noninvasive approach that can provide a more accurate prognostic evaluation and prediction of therapeutic response. Moreover, its potential role in the early detection of the disease and in cancer screening needs to be further investigated. To date, OC represents the fifth cause of death from cancer in the women population and it has the worst prognosis among gynecological tumors (Giannopoulou et al. 2019). This aggressive cancer is still diagnosed at an advanced stage despite general improvements made in the management of the disease. The lack of clearly defined biomarkers for early detection plays an important role that has to be addressed. Liquid biopsy may represent a new promising tool in the management of OC, offering improvements in monitoring the disease course, treatment response, and prediction of resistance to anticancer therapies. It may be useful to develop more personalized and evidence-based therapy for this aggressive disease.

There is still much to do for an optimal management and a better therapeutic outcome for women with OC. The available data are based on pilot exploratory studies. Improved and standardized techniques, reproducibility of results, large OC patients sampling, and longer follow-up are mandatory before implementing ctDNA approach in clinical practice. Additional data and further reading are detailed in prior reviews (Box 5.1).

Box 5.1 Recommended reading of particular interest

	DOI
Keller L, et al. **Clinical relevance of blood-based ctDNA analysis: mutation detection and beyond**. Br J Cancer. 2020.	10.1038/s41416-020-01047-5
Pantel K, Alix-Panabières C. **Liquid biopsy and minimal residual disease - latest advances and implications for cure.** Nat Rev Clin Oncol. 2019;16(7):409–424.	10.1038/s41571-019-0187-3
Cescon DW et al. **Circulating tumor DNA and liquid biopsy in oncology**. Nat Cancer. 2020, 1, 276–290.	10.3390/cancers12102880
Cheng ML, et al. **Circulating tumor DNA in advanced solid tumors: Clinical relevance and future directions**. CA Cancer J Clin. 2020.	10.3322/caac.21650
Pessoa LS, et al. **ctDNA as a cancer biomarker: A broad overview**. Crit Rev Oncol Hematol. 2020;155:103109.	10.1016/j.critrevonc.2020.103109
Davidson B. **Circulating tumor cells and cell-free nucleic acids in patients with gynecological malignancies**. Virchows Arch. 2018;473(4):395–403.	10.1007/s00428-018-2447-5
Zheng X, et al. **Extracellular vesicle-based liquid biopsy holds great promise for the management of ovarian cancer.** Biochim Biophys Acta Rev Cancer. 2020;1874(1):188395.	10.1016/j.bbcan.2020.188395
Asante DB, et al. **Liquid biopsy in ovarian cancer using circulating tumor DNA and cells: Ready for prime time?** Cancer Lett. 2020;468:59–71.	10.1016/j.canlet.2019.10.014

Acknowledgment and Conflicts of Interest KE is an editor in Springer Nature Journals and a previous editor for a Springer Book (https://link.springer.com/book/10.1007/978-3-030-53821-7). Other authors: none.

Authors' Contribution KE reviewed the literature and wrote the manuscript. LC and DT wrote the perspectives section and revised the chapter content. OA and SA revised and supervised the chapter writing. The final draft was reviewed and approved by all the authors. The contents of the chapter reflect the authors' perspectives and not of their institutions of affiliation.

References

Adeola HA, Blackburn JM, Rebbeck TR, Zerbini LF (2017) Emerging proteomics biomarkers and prostate cancer burden in Africa. Oncotarget 8(23):37991–38007. https://doi.org/10.18632/oncotarget.16568

Alharbi M, Zuñiga F, Elfeky O et al (2018) The potential role of miRNAs and exosomes in chemotherapy in ovarian cancer. Endocr Relat Cancer 25(12):R663–R685

Alves MC, Fonseca FLA, Yamada AMTD, Barros LADR, Lopes A, Silva LCFF, Luz AS, Melo Cruz FJS, Del Giglio A (2020) Increased circulating tumor DNA as a noninvasive biomarker of early treatment response in patients with metastatic ovarian carcinoma: a pilot study. Tumour Biol 42(5):1010428320919198. https://doi.org/10.1177/1010428320919198

Brand NR, Qu LG, Chao A, Ilbawi AM (2019) Delays and barriers to cancer care in low- and middle-income countries: a systematic review. Oncologist 24(12):e1371–e1380. https://doi.org/10.1634/theoncologist.2019-0057

Bratman SV, Yang YC, Iafolla MAJ et al (2020) Personalized circulating tumor DNA analysis as a predictive biomarker in solid tumor patients treated with pembrolizumab. Nat Cancer 1(9):873–881. https://doi.org/10.1038/s43018-020-0096-5

Carneiro BA, Collier KA, Nagy RJ et al (2018) Acquired resistance to the PARP inhibitor olaparib in BRCA2-associated prostate cancer due to biallelic BRCA2 reversion mutations restoring both germline and somatic loss of function mutations. JCO Precis Oncol 2:1–8. https://doi.org/10.1200/PO.17.00176

Cheng X, Zhang L, Chen Y, Qing C (2017) Circulating cell-free DNA and circulating tumor cells, the "liquid biopsies" in ovarian cancer. J Ovarian Res 10(1):75. https://doi.org/10.1186/s13048-017-0369-5

Christie EL, Fereday S, Doig K et al (2017) Reversion of BRCA1/2 germline mutations detected in circulating tumor DNA from patients with high-grade serous ovarian cancer. J Clin Oncol 35(12):1274–1280. https://doi.org/10.1200/JCO.2016.70.4627

Dayyani F, Uhlig S, Colson B et al (2016) Diagnostic performance of risk of ovarian malignancy algorithm against CA125 and HE4 in connection with ovarian cancer: a meta-analysis. Int J Gynecol Cancer 26(9):1586–1593

Dilla T, Lizan L, Paz S et al (2015) Do new cancer drugs offer good value for money? The perspectives of oncologists, health care policy makers, patients, and the general population. Patient Prefer Adherence 10:1–7. https://doi.org/10.2147/PPA.S93760

El Bairi K et al (2017a) Prediction of therapy response in ovarian cancer: where are we now? Crit Rev Clin Lab Sci 54:233–266

El Bairi K et al (2017b) Emerging diagnostic, prognostic and therapeutic biomarkers for ovarian cancer. Cell Oncol 40:105–118

El Bairi K, Tariq K, Himri I et al (2018) Decoding colorectal cancer epigenomics. Cancer Genet 220:49–76. https://doi.org/10.1016/j.cancergen.2017.11.001

Esposito A, Bardelli A, Criscitiello C et al (2014) Monitoring tumor-derived cell-free DNA in patients with solid tumors: clinical perspectives and research opportunities. Cancer Treat Rev 40(5):648–655. https://doi.org/10.1016/j.ctrv.2013.10.003

Ganesan S (2018) Tumor suppressor tolerance: reversion mutations in BRCA1 and BRCA2 and resistance to PARP inhibitors and platinum. JCO Precis Oncol 2:1–4. https://doi.org/10.1200/PO.18.00001

Giannopoulou L, Mastoraki S, Buderath P et al (2018) ESR1 methylation in primary tumors and paired circulating tumor DNA of patients with high-grade serous ovarian cancer. Gynecol Oncol 150(2):355–360. https://doi.org/10.1016/j.ygyno.2018.05.026

Giannopoulou L, Zavridou M, Kasimir-Bauer S, Lianidou ES (2019) Liquid biopsy in ovarian cancer: the potential of circulating miRNAs and exosomes. Transl Res 205:77–91. https://doi.org/10.1016/j.trsl.2018.10.003. Epub 2018 Oct 12

Goodsaid FM (2019) The labyrinth of product development and regulatory approvals in liquid biopsy diagnostics. Clin Transl Sci 12(5):431–439. https://doi.org/10.1111/cts.12657

Harris FR, Kovtun IV, Smadbeck J et al (2016) Quantification of somatic chromosomal rearrangements in circulating cell-free DNA from ovarian cancers. Sci Rep 6:29831. https://doi.org/10.1038/srep29831

Jacobs IJ, Menon U, Ryan A et al (2016) Ovarian cancer screening and mortality in the UK collaborative trial of ovarian cancer screening (UKCTOCS): a randomised controlled trial. Lancet 387(10022):945–956

Jamison DT, Alwan A, Mock CN et al (2018) Universal health coverage and intersectoral action for health: key messages from disease control priorities, 3rd edition. Lancet 391 (10125):1108–1120. https://doi.org/10.1016/S0140-6736(17)32906-9

Kim HS, Choi HY, Lee M et al (2016) Systemic inflammatory response markers and CA-125 levels in ovarian clear cell carcinoma: a two center cohort study. Cancer Res Treat 48(1):250–258. https://doi.org/10.4143/crt.2014.324

Kinyua P (2018) Kenya-third African country to use blood-based tests to detect cancer. Jamhuri News, 21 May 2018

Krell D, Said Battistino F, Benafif S et al (2017) Audit of CA125 follow-up after first-line therapy for ovarian Cancer. Int J Gynecol Cancer 27(6):1118–1122. https://doi.org/10.1097/IGC.0000000000000956

Ledermann JA (2016) PARP inhibitors in ovarian cancer. Ann Oncol 27(Suppl1):i40–i44. https://doi.org/10.1093/annonc/mdw094

Leijen S, van Geel RM, Sonke GS et al (2016) Phase II study of WEE1 inhibitor AZD1775 plus carboplatin in patients with TP53-mutated ovarian cancer refractory or resistant to first-line therapy within 3 months. J Clin Oncol 34(36):4354–4361

Li X, Wang X (2017) The emerging roles and therapeutic potential of exosomes in epithelial ovarian cancer. Mol Cancer 16(1):92. https://doi.org/10.1186/s12943-017-0659-y

Lin KK, Harrell MI, Oza AM et al (2018) BRCA reversion mutations in circulating tumor DNA predict primary and acquired resistance to the PARP inhibitor Rucaparib in high-grade ovarian carcinoma. Cancer Discov 9(2):210–219. pii: CD-18-0715. https://doi.org/10.1158/2159-8290.CD-18-0715

Lo YMD, Lam WKJ (2020) Towards multi-cancer screening using liquid biopsies. Nat Rev Clin Oncol 2020(17):525–526. https://doi.org/10.1038/s41571-020-0404-0

Lustberg MB, Stover DG, Chalmers JJ (2018) Implementing liquid biopsies in clinical trials: state of affairs, opportunities, and challenges. Cancer J 24(2):61–64. https://doi.org/10.1097/PPO.0000000000000309

Mandel P, Metais P (1948) Les acides nucléiques du plasma sanguin chez l'Homme. C R Seances Soc Biol Fil 142:241–243

Noguchi T, Iwahashi N, Sakai K, Matsuda K, Matsukawa H, Toujima S, Nishio K, Ino K (2020) Comprehensive gene mutation profiling of circulating tumor DNA in ovarian Cancer: its pathological and prognostic impact. Cancers (Basel) 12(11):3382. https://doi.org/10.3390/cancers12113382

Norquist B, Wurz KA, Pennil CC et al (2011) Secondary somatic mutations restoring BRCA1/2 predict chemotherapy resistance in hereditary ovarian carcinomas. J Clin Oncol 29 (22):3008–3015

Ogasawara A, Hihara T, Shintani D, Yabuno A, Ikeda Y, Tai K, Fujiwara K, Watanabe K, Hasegawa K (2020) Evaluation of circulating tumor DNA in patients with ovarian cancer harboring somatic PIK3CA or KRAS mutations. Cancer Res Treat 52(4):1219–1228. https://doi.org/10.4143/crt.2019.688

Parkinson CA, Gale D, Piskorz AM et al (2016) Exploratory analysis of TP53 mutations in circulating tumour DNA as biomarkers of treatment response for patients with relapsed high-grade serous ovarian carcinoma: a retrospective study. PLoS Med 13(12):e1002198. https://doi.org/10.1371/journal.pmed.1002198

Pereira E, Camacho-Vanegas O, Anand S et al (2015) Personalized circulating tumor DNA biomarkers dynamically predict treatment response and survival in gynecologic cancers. PLoS One 10(12):e0145754. https://doi.org/10.1371/journal.pone.0145754

Piskorz AM, Lin KK, Morris JA et al (2016) Feasibility of monitoring response to PARP inhibitor rucaparib with targeted deep sequencing of circulating tumor DNA in women with high-grade serous carcinoma on the ARIEL2 trial. J Clin Oncol 34:5549. https://doi.org/10.1200/JCO.2016.34.15_suppl.5549

Ratajska M, Koczkowska M, Żuk M et al (2017) Detection of BRCA1/2 mutations in circulating tumor DNA from patients with ovarian cancer. Oncotarget 8(60):101325–101332. https://doi.org/10.18632/oncotarget.20722

Romero-Laorden N, Olmos D, Fehm T et al (2014) Circulating and disseminated tumor cells in ovarian cancer: a systematic review. Gynecol Oncol 133(3):632–639. https://doi.org/10.1016/j.ygyno.2014.03.016

Rusan M, Andersen RF, Jakobsen A, Steffensen KD (2020) Circulating HOXA9-methylated tumour DNA: a novel biomarker of response to poly (ADP-ribose) polymerase inhibition in BRCA-mutated epithelial ovarian cancer. Eur J Cancer 125:121–129. https://doi.org/10.1016/j.ejca.2019.11.012

Sakai W, Swisher EM, Karlan BY et al (2008) Secondary mutations as a mechanism of cisplatin resistance in BRCA2-mutated cancers. Nature 451(7182):1116–1120

Shao X, He Y, Ji M, Chen X, Qi J, Shi W et al (2015) Quantitative analysis of cell-free DNA in ovarian cancer. Oncol Lett 10(6):3478–3482

Silwal-Pandit L, Langerød A, Børresen-Dale AL (2017) TP53 mutations in breast and ovarian cancer. Cold Spring Harb Perspect Med 7(1):a026252. https://doi.org/10.1101/cshperspect.a026252

Slavin TP, Banks KC, Chudova D et al (2018) Identification of incidental germline mutations in patients with advanced solid tumors who underwent cell-free circulating tumor DNA sequencing. J Clin Oncol 36:JCO1800328. https://doi.org/10.1200/JCO.18.00328

Snow A, Chen D, Lang JE (2019) The current status of the clinical utility of liquid biopsies in cancer. Expert Rev Mol Diagn 19(11):1031–1041. https://doi.org/10.1080/14737159.2019.1664290

Steffensen KD, Madsen CV, Andersen RF, Waldstrøm M, Adimi P, Jakobsen A (2014) Prognostic importance of cell-free DNA in chemotherapy resistant ovarian cancer treated with bevacizumab. Eur J Cancer 50(15):2611–2618. https://doi.org/10.1016/j.ejca.2014.06.022

Sun Y, Haglund TA, Rogers AJ et al (2018) Review: microfluidics technologies for blood-based cancer liquid biopsies. Anal Chim Acta 1012:10–29. https://doi.org/10.1016/j.aca.2017.12.050

Temilola DO, Wium M, Coulidiati TH et al (2019) The prospect and challenges to the flow of liquid biopsy in Africa. Cell 8(8):862. https://doi.org/10.3390/cells8080862

Tomasetti M, Amati M, Neuzil J et al (2017) Circulating epigenetic biomarkers in lung malignancies: from early diagnosis to therapy. Lung Cancer 107:65–72. https://doi.org/10.1016/j.lungcan.2016.05.023

Trapani D, Lengyel CG, Habeeb BS et al (2021) The global landscape of availability, accessibility and affordability of essential diagnostics and therapeutics for the management of HER2-positive breast cancer: the ONCOLLEGE-001 survey. J Cancer Policy 28:100285. https://doi.org/10.1016/j.jcpo.2021.100285

Van Berckelaer C, Brouwers AJ, Peeters DJ et al (2016) Current and future role of circulating tumor cells in patients with epithelial ovarian cancer. Eur J Surg Oncol 42(12):1772–1779. https://doi.org/10.1016/j.ejso.2016.05.010

Vanderstichele A, Busschaert P, Smeets D et al (2017) Chromosomal instability in cell-free DNA as a highly specific biomarker for detection of ovarian cancer in women with adnexal masses. Clin Cancer Res 23:2223–2231. https://doi.org/10.1158/1078-0432.CCR-16-1078

Wambalaba FW, Son B, Wambalaba AE et al (2019) Prevalence and capacity of cancer diagnostics and treatment: a demand and supply survey of health-care facilities in Kenya. Cancer Control 26(1):1073274819886930. https://doi.org/10.1177/1073274819886930

Wan JCM, Massie C, Garcia-Corbacho J et al (2017) Liquid biopsies come of age: towards implementation of circulating tumour DNA. Nat Rev Cancer 17(4):223–238. https://doi.org/10.1038/nrc.2017.7

Wang X, Ivan M, Hawkins SM (2017) The role of MicroRNA molecules and MicroRNA-regulating machinery in the pathogenesis and progression of epithelial ovarian cancer. Gynecol Oncol 147(2):481–487

Whiting PF, Rutjes AW, Westwood ME et al (2011) QUADAS-2: a revised tool for the quality assessment of diagnostic accuracy studies. Ann Intern Med 155(8):529–536. https://doi.org/10.7326/0003-4819-155-8-201110180-00009

Widschwendter M, Zikan M, Wahl B et al (2017) The potential of circulating tumor DNA methylation analysis for the early detection and management of ovarian cancer. Genome Med 9(1):116. https://doi.org/10.1186/s13073-017-0500-7

Wong KK, Izaguirre DI, Kwan SY et al (2013) Poor survival with wild-type TP53 ovarian cancer? Gynecol Oncol 130(3):565–569

Zhang YC, Zhou Q, Wu YL (2017) The emerging roles of NGS-based liquid biopsy in non-small cell lung cancer. J Hematol Oncol 10(1):167. https://doi.org/10.1186/s13045-017-0536-6

Zhou Q, Li W, Leng B et al (2016) Circulating cell free DNA as the diagnostic marker for ovarian cancer: a systematic review and meta-analysis. PLoS One 11(6):e0155495. https://doi.org/10.1371/journal.pone.0155495

Proteomic Biomarkers for Early Detection and Patients' Stratification in Ovarian Cancer: A Brief Overview

6

Marco Petrillo, Carlo Ronsini, Davide Calandra, Margherita Dessole, and Salvatore Dessole

Abstract

Quantitative proteomic profiling is progressively emerging as a reliable strategy to achieve early diagnosis, and prognostic stratification in epithelial ovarian cancer (OC). In particular, specific proteomic profiles of tumor-derived circulating proteins involved in regulating apoptosis, epithelial-to-mesenchymal transition, and cellular motility seem to show promising performances in early disease identification and prognostic stratification. Furthermore, proteomic characterization of ascites and pleural effusions will significantly improve the accuracy of predicting outcomes and selecting OC patients to benefit from the current therapies. Cancer tissues, pleural effusions, and ascitic fluids should be considered as the best biological samples for proteomic profiling to achieve the optimal use of biomarkers. On the other hand, plasma circulating-free proteins, or tumor-derived extracellular vesicles-embedded proteins are considered as the most appropriate source of data for early disease identification in OC patients. In the next decade, proteomic profiling will certainly be introduced in the clinical algorithms of the management of OC.

M. Petrillo (✉) · S. Dessole
PhD School in Biomedical Sciences, University of Sassari, Sassari, Italy

Obstetrics and Gynecology Clinic, University of Sassari, Sassari, Italy

C. Ronsini
Department of Woman and Child Health, IRCCS Fondazione Policlinico Agostino Gemelli, Rome, Italy

D. Calandra
Obstetrics and Gynecology Clinic, University of Chieti, Chieti, Italy

M. Dessole
PhD School in Biomedical Sciences, University of Sassari, Sassari, Italy

K. El Bairi (ed.), *Ovarian Cancer Biomarkers*,
https://doi.org/10.1007/978-981-16-1873-4_6

Keywords

Ovarian cancer · Biomarkers · Proteomics · Extracellular vesicles

6.1 Introduction

Epithelial ovarian cancer (OC) is a leading cause of cancer-related deaths in the female population (Sung et al. 2021). Due to the lack of early symptoms, patients with OC are often diagnosed with an advanced stage of disease. In fact, approximately 60% of women have stage IIIC–IV disease at diagnosis, which is associated with a 5-year survival below 30% (Elstrand et al. 2012). The most relevant issue to achieve early detection of the disease is the absence of related symptoms before the occurrence of diffuse peritoneal carcinomatosis. Only two biomarkers, cancer antigen 125 (CA-125) and human epididymis 4 (HE4) are currently used in clinical practice as reliable serological tests for diagnosis and disease monitoring of OC (El Bairi et al. 2017, 2020). In this perspective, several studies have demonstrated that the serum dosage of both HE4 and CA-125 has the highest sensitivity in the detection of OC and in particular when combined (Moore et al. 2008; Leung et al. 2016; Montagnana et al. 2009). Several clinical algorithms based on the combined assessment of CA-125 serum levels, and ultrasound pelvic examination have been developed as screening approaches in women with ovarian mass. However, overall discriminating performances in terms of sensitivity and specificity appeared to be disappointing; therefore, nowadays, despite initial promising findings, there is no validated screening algorithm able to accurately detect OC earlier. Furthermore, with the advent of personalized medicine, there is a growing awareness in the scientific community that OC does not represent a unique disease, but a complex, and heterogeneous biological entity (Petrillo et al. 2016). Therefore, emphasizing the need to completely change our point of view, moving from the traditional clinical approach that one fits for all, to the evidence-based strategy that every clinical strategy should be tailored to the patients' specific disease. In this context, it is expected that the proteomic strategies support the genomic-based approach for disease profiling. As previously mentioned, the lack of effective clinical strategies in achieving early diagnosis has created an increasing interest in proteomic approaches. In particular, genomic-based profiling is certainly useful to characterize the pattern of gene expression in cancer cells, but the functional role of a specific gene product can be definitely assessed only by focusing on the proteins level. For these reasons, there is a great expectation on the potential benefits in terms of accurate disease characterization that can be achieved with the advent of the proteomic era. In this context, proteomic analysis includes several different strategies, including protein structural identification, quantification of protein levels, description of protein–protein interaction, posttranslational modifications, and functional analysis. Proteomics has greatly advanced from initial gel-based procedures (one- and two-dimensional sodium dodecyl sulfate-polyacrylamide gel electrophoresis) to mass spectrometry-based (MS) methods. In particular, innovative approaches such as electrospray ionization-MS and matrix-assisted laser desorption/ ionization (MALDI)-MS are emerging as reliable strategies to achieve an accurate and reliable protein profiling in oncology. The availability of quantitative methods that are able to identify deregulated protein expression represents a further step toward future use of proteomic platforms for disease characterization in patients with OC. The aim of this chapter is to briefly give an overview of the current knowledge on investigated proteomic biomarkers in OC.

6.2 Proteomics and Ovarian Cancer

6.2.1 Ovarian Cancer Cell Lines and Tumor Tissues

OC cell lines traditionally represent the first step of preclinical cancer research. These experimental models enable the investigation of biological mechanisms sustaining proliferation and development of metastatic potential as well as the characterization of gene and protein expression. On the other hand, recent evidence has clearly demonstrated that several OC cell lines are characterized by a hypermutated genotype, which is frequently very different from OC tissues retrieved from tumor biopsies (Domcke et al. 2013). For these reasons, the results obtained from preclinical in vitro models should be always considered with great caution, and in vivo validation is mandatory. Focusing on proteomic profiling of OC cell lines, several interesting data have been published suggesting that specific protein panels may be involved in driving drug resistance (Agarwal and Kaye 2003; Li et al. 2010; Chappell et al. 2012; Chen et al. 2014). In particular, a study conducted by Li et al. identified a panel of 28 proteins in several cancer cell lines involved in the development of cisplatin resistance (Li et al. 2010). These potential biomarkers were classified into eight functional groups: calcium-binding proteins, chaperones, extracellular matrix, DNA damage repair complex, mitochondrial proteins, transcription factor, cytoskeletal proteins, and signaling transducing factors (Li et al. 2010). Unfortunately, these interesting preliminary data were not validated in patients' samples. The complete proteomic profiling of tumor tissues is certainly a very. However, it is well known that formalin tissue fixation produces cross-links among proteins on cancer tissues; thus, masking epitopes in proteomic characterization. Furthermore, surgical contamination and tumor disease heterogeneity are also other potential pitfalls. On the other hand, the availability of novel techniques for protein extraction, together with improvement of quantitative proteomic strategies allow a reliable proteomic characterization even on formalin-fixed embedded protein (FFPE) blocks. Few studies that investigated the differences in terms of proteomic profiles in OC tumor histotypes have been published. A specific proteomic profile has been suggested for high-grade serous histology (An et al. 2006). Notably, the most relevant findings have been reported by Wiegand et al. which identified 50 proteins differentially expressed in clear cell and endometrioid OC as compared with high-grade serous histology (Wiegand et al. 2014). In particular, this study found a specific biological mechanism at a proteomic level that is probably involved in tumor development for both clear-cell and endometrioid OC. In fact, the authors detected increased levels of phosphorylated AKT protein in tumor tissues, together with a reduced expression of BAF250a; this protein acts as tumor suppressor promoting apoptotic cascade. It can be hypothesized that in the process of endometrioid and clear-cell carcinogenesis, phosphorylation of AKT protein occurs as an early event, and in turn suppresses BAF250a expression at the genomic level (Wiegand et al. 2014). Awaiting further experimental confirmations, these data represent a relevant contribution of proteomic tissue characterization for early diagnosis and disease profiling of OC (Wiegand et al. 2014). Furthermore, the experimental evidence showing a relevant biological role of phosphorylated AKT protein in OC introduced another crucial point of proteomic tissue characterization which is represented by the identification of posttranscriptional modifications. In fact, it is well known that the biological processes such as glycosylation or phosphorylation may produce activation, or silencing of a protein function, and these relevant biological mechanisms can be detected only through proteomic analysis, and not using a traditional genomic approach. A plethora of studies have been published and showed the relevance of phosphorylated protein isoforms in driving tumor angiogenesis, apoptosis blockade, epithelial-to-mesenchymal transition, and chemoresistance through the activation of several pathways including NFκB, mitogen-activated protein kinase (MAPK), Src, and PI3K (Elzek and Rodland 2015). Unfortunately, despite the important amount of literature suggesting, and clearly demonstrating the role of these phosphorylated proteins in cancer development, none of these molecules have successfully entered into clinical practice as diagnostic biomarkers. One of the potential reasons to explain this contrasting scenario is the lack of proteomic data confirming at the protein level the above-mentioned findings that have been identified only at the genomic level.

6.2.2 Proteomic Plasma Analysis

Serum derived from cancer patients certainly represents the most appropriate sample to be used for proteomic characterization. Compared with tumor tissues, serological samples can be easily achieved, and during sampling, it can avoid contamination using an appropriate protocol for collection and early processing (Fig. 6.1). Furthermore, compared with FFPE blocks, no fixation is required, and tumor tissue is not manipulated; thus, avoiding cross-links between proteins. On the other hand, the number of tumor-derived proteins released in the blood is very low. Therefore, it is not surprising that only with the availability of innovative quantitatively spectroscopic techniques such as SELDI-TOF that we were able to correctly identify tumor-derived circulating proteins.

In OC, a relevant proteomic serological profiling has been conducted by Zhang et al. that showed that a panel of circulating proteins has been found to be differentially expressed in OC patients as compared with healthy subjects, thus, allowing the earliest proteomic-based strategy for early diagnosis (Zhang et al. 2004). These results have been further evaluated to develop a five proteins algorithm, called

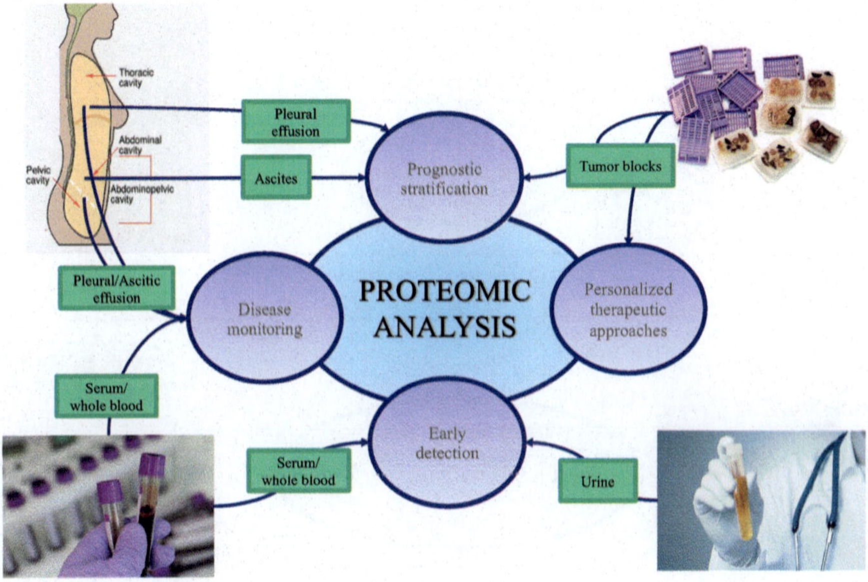

Fig. 6.1 The proteomic approach in ovarian cancer

OVA1 test, based on the combined dosage of apolipoprotein A1, prealbumin, transferrin, β-2 microglobulin, and CA-125 (Ueland et al. 2011). The OVA1 assay also received class II FDA approval to be used in combination with ultrasound evaluation for the triage of suspicious pelvic mass. Unfortunately, premarketing approval is still needed despite these interesting data. Definitive clinical data are still omitted, but these results, for the first time, opened the route for serological proteomic profiling that is able to increase the diagnostic performance of CA-125 alone in the detection and stratification of OC patients (Fig. 6.2). Based on proteomic profiling of TCGA samples, Yang et al. showed a high-throughput protein profiling which allowed the identification of an algorithm of nine proteins called PROVAR which is able to predict disease progression in OC (Yang et al. 2013). Again, also for the PROVAR test, a clinical validation has not been performed, thus not allowing a safe translation from laboratory to clinical practice. Another experimental approach for proteomic profiling of OC patients is represented by the combined evaluation of blood and tumor samples. This strategy is of great value to correctly identify tumor-derived proteins that may be involved not only in carcinogenesis, but also in the development of drug resistance. An interesting study based on this approach showed a statistically significant lower expression of APOA1 and serotransferrin in both serum and cancer tissue samples of OC patients compared with healthy subjects (Wegdam et al. 2014), thus providing a partial confirmation of the Zhang's findings (Zhang et al. 2004). Another emerging scientific field is represented by the so-called circulating *secretomes* or secretomics which analyzes the secreted extracellular proteins in the blood (Madden et al. 2020). Circulating extracellular proteins in the

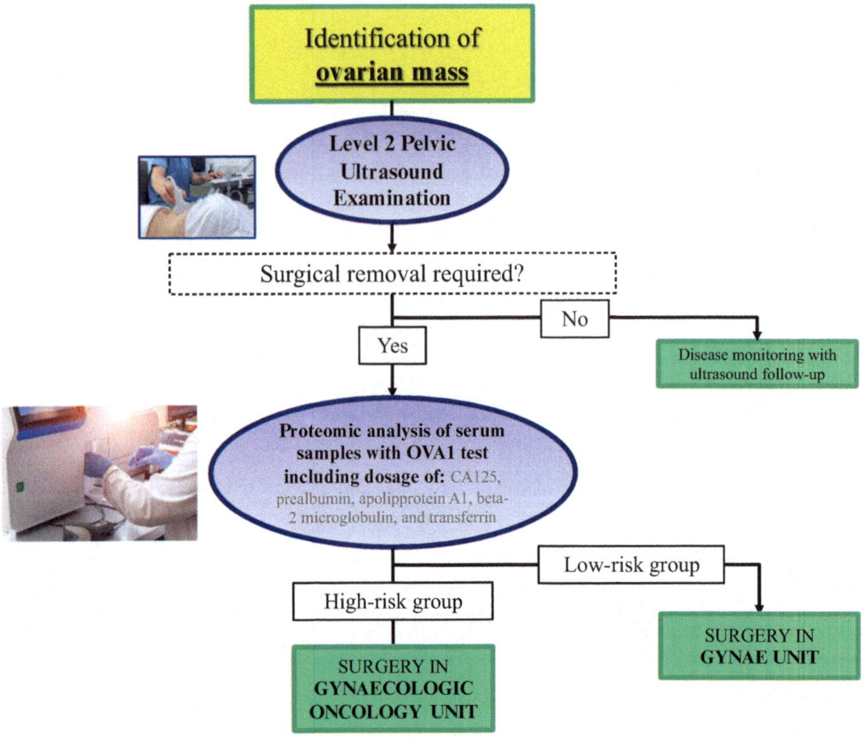

Fig. 6.2 Integration of proteomics in the diagnostic algorithms for early identification of epithelial ovarian cancer

blood are glycosylated which makes them suitable for proteomic biomarker discovery. Interestingly, several previous studies used this approach (Tian et al. 2011; Pan et al. 2011; Faca et al. 2008; Gunawardana et al. 2009). In conclusion, the profiling of circulating proteins appears as a promising field for the identification of biomarkers for the diagnosis and stratification of OC patients.

6.2.3 Proteomic Analysis of Ascitic and Pleural Effusions

The vast majority of OC patients develop ascites along with their disease natural history. Unfortunately, this event is related to peritoneal cancer spread, and it is obviously associated with late FIGO stages. Therefore, ascitic fluids are certainly a relevant source for biomarkers development and their proteomic profiling may be of great value to study the mechanisms of disease spread, and patients' prognostic stratification. However, ascitic samples cannot be used for early disease detection. Interestingly, a complete proteomic profiling of ascites from OC patients revealed a panel of 50 differentially expressed proteins (Gortzak-Uzan et al. 2008; Kuk et al. 2009). However, as described in Table 6.1, these studies do not have a potential

Table 6.1 Proteomic analysis in ovarian cancer patients: Comparison of different biological sources

	Biological source		
	Tumor tissue	Plasma	Ascitic and pleural effusions
Samples collection	• Need of invasive procedure • High risks of contamination	• Easy • Low risks of contamination	• Need of invasive procedure • Low risks of contamination
Technical aspects	• High amount of tumor-derived proteins • Need of accurate microdissection to reduce contaminations bias • Epitopes masking: potential concerns in detecting specific protein profiles due to formalin fixation	• Low amount of tumor-derived proteins: need of high sensitivity proteomic strategies	• High amount of tumor-derived proteins
Clinical role and implications	*Early disease diagnosis* • Limited value *Disease stratification* • Potentially relevant value	*Early disease diagnosis* • Great value *Disease stratification* • Great value, particularly when combined with tumor, and ascitic fluids evaluation	*Early disease diagnosis* • No value *Disease stratification* • Potentially relevant value
Scientific evidence	*Early disease diagnosis* • Limited evidences for clinical translation *Disease stratification* • Limited evidences for clinical translation	*Early disease diagnosis* • FDA approved panel to be further validated in a clinical scenario • Relevant evidences on circulating extracellular vesicles ready to be validated in clinical scenarios *Disease stratification* • Limited evidences for clinical translation	*Early disease diagnosis* • Limited evidences for clinical translation *Disease stratification* • Limited evidences for clinical translation

clinical horizon as this approach has no clinical value for performing proteomic profiling of ascitic fluids to achieve early disease detection. On the other hand, the role of proteomic profiling of pleural effusion in the prognostic stratification of OC patients seems to be promising (Davidson et al. 2006; reviewed elsewhere: El Bairi et al. 2017; Carvalho et al. 2019). Reduced survival was seen in patients with increased levels of AKT, and JNK proteins; thus, another opportunity for further clinical validation of these biomarkers for prognostic disease stratification (Davidson et al. 2006).

6.3 Proteomics and Extracellular Vesicles: A Promising Approach in Ovarian Cancer

In the last decade, the role of extracellular vesicles and their cargoes as diagnostic, prognostic, and predictive biomarkers have been widely studied in cancer (Srivastava et al. 2021; Amintas et al. 2021). Extracellular vesicles (EVs) are divided into three types based on their size: exosomes (30–100 nm), microvesicles (100 nm–1 μm), and apoptotic bodies (500 nm–3 μm). Regarding their functional features, exosomes seem to play a crucial role in regulating several biological mechanisms involved in cancer growth, and metastatic development, acting as mediators of cellular crosstalk in cancer tissue (Elewaily and Elsergany 2021). Exosomes can contain a complex cargo of materials, including microRNAs and occasionally genomic DNA. The vast majority of miRNAs circulates in body fluids of patients as cell-free RNAs, and for these reasons, they have been considered for several years as potential biomarkers to be used in liquid biopsy approaches. However, circulating miRNAs are quickly removed by enzymatic RNAse activity. Therefore, these biomarkers do not appear as easily manageable diagnostic tools to be used in screening diagnostic tools. On the other hand, circulating miRNAs embedded in tumor-derived EVs are certainly more stable, and easier to be used in diagnostic algorithms, particularly considering that some specific miRNAs panels are differentially expressed in OC patients compared to healthy women (Mahdian-Shakib et al. 2016; Montagnana et al. 2017). Finally, EVs are easily identifiable in various body fluids, such as blood, serum, and urine, making them reliable markers that are easy to find and potentially very useful in clinical practice. Recently, Barnabas et al. conducted a proteomic analysis of EVs-related proteins in utero-tubal lavage from healthy women, and OC patients and showed a panel of nine proteins (SERPINB5, S100A14. MYH11, CLCA4, S100A2, IVL, CD109, NNMT, ENPP3) that were differentially expressed in the two groups, and involved in regulating kinase activity, cellular motility, and apoptosis modulating p53 pathway (Barnabas et al. 2019). Unfortunately, the diagnostic performance of these proteomic biomarkers in the early detection of OC was around 75%, being therefore promising, but still not adequate for clinical use (Barnabas et al. 2019). Furthermore, as previously mentioned, proteomic profiling of ascites and pleural effusion may be certainly regarded as a potentially useful tool to achieve final diagnosis. In particular, the evaluation of EVs embedded miRNAs, and proteins may be certainly regarded as a very interesting approach with a panel of proteins (NANOG, SPINT2, and ZEB2), and miRNAs (miR-29a, miR-30d, and miR-205) differentially expressed in OC patients and healthy women (Yamamoto et al. 2018). However, this experimental approach appears very questionable, since ascitic fluids, which appear in women with late-stage disease, do not represent a useful biological sample to be used for early diagnosis. For, these reasons, the studies comparing the proteomic profile of ascitic fluids in OC patients and healthy controls do not have the appropriate design to provide clinically useful insights. Interestingly, a previous report failed to identify differences in terms of proteomic profile between OC patients and healthy subjects (Zhao et al. 2014). However, when focusing only on women with an advanced stage of disease, a higher level of circulating HSP27-related EVs in patients with peritoneal carcinomatosis was noticed (Zhao et al. 2014). Thus, again highlighting the need to focus scientific efforts on specific subgroups of OC patients in future biomarker research. Another crucial point is represented by the potential role of EVs proteomic profiling for early identification of chemoresistance. A recently published study by Guerra et al. showed a correlation between reduced circulating levels of EVs-embedded RAB7A protein and the development of cisplatin resistance (Guerra et al. 2019). Furthermore, poor drug response is related to several complex biological mechanisms involving also epithelial-to-mesenchymal transition which is principally based on cytoskeletal and extracellular matrix modifications. Therefore, it is not surprising that the recently published data showed increased levels of EVs-embedded matrix metalloproteinase 1 (MMP1) in peritoneal lesions with intrinsic chemoresistant features. Furthermore, the overexpression of circulating EVs-derived MMP1 was found to be associated with reduced overall and progression-free survival in women with OC. In conclusion, the proteomic profile of circulating EVs appears as a promising field for future developments for early diagnosis and prognostic stratification of OC patients.

6.4 Future Perspectives: A Focus on microRNAs

Quantitative proteomic profiling techniques extended the horizon of proteomics by assessing several other biomarkers beyond proteins such as miRNAs. Deregulation of mi-RNAs expression has been shown to be associated with malignant development of OC. Therefore, quantitative proteomic assessment of miRNAs expression patterns represents a further approach to improve early detection of OC. Previously, Taylor et al. reported that eight circulating exosomal miRNAs (miR-21, miR-141, miR-200a, miR-200b, miR-200c, miR-203, miR-205, and miR-214) are overexpressed in OC patients compared to benign controls (Taylor and Gercel-Taylor 2008). Similarly, another report showed that the expression levels of four serum miRNAs (miR-182, miR-200a, miRR-200b, and miR-200c) were significantly elevated in women with high-grade serous OC as compared with healthy controls (Kan et al. 2012). Moreover, serum levels of miR-25 and miR-93 were found downregulated, while miR-7 and miR-429 were found upregulated in OC patients compared with healthy women (Meng et al. 2015). This suggests that the differential expression of some selected miRNAs can be used as biomarkers.

The role of miRNAs isolated from serum, tissue, and ascites was analyzed by Chung et al. and identified five miRNAs (miR-132, miR-26a, let-7b, miR-145, and miR-143) as the most significantly downregulated miRNAs in the sera of OC patients (Chung et al. 2013). Moreover, Zhou et al. investigated the diagnostic value of urinary miRNAs in OC patients and identified a significant upregulation of mir-30a-5p in the urine samples of women with OC when compared to healthy controls (Zhou et al. 2015). The miRNA signatures from exosomes were concordant to those from the originating tumor cells, indicating that circulating miRNAs profiles accurately reflect the tumor profile. Furthermore, Zheng et al. evaluated plasma samples of 360 OC patients and 200 healthy controls, and they found a higher expression of plasma miR-205 and lower expression of let 7-f in OC patients (Zheng et al. 2013). The authors were able to propose a combination of mir-205 and let-7f to provide high diagnostic accuracy (Nakamura et al. 2016; Zheng et al. 2013). Similarly, Zuberi et al. showed that miR-200a was significantly upregulated in mucinous adenocarcinoma when compared with histotypes in 70 OC patients (Zuberi et al. 2015). Another interesting experience has been recently published evaluating the differences in terms of circulating EVs derived miRNAs between OC patients and healthy controls (Chi Pan et al. 2018). A specific panel of miRNAs (miR-23a, miR-92a, miR-21, miR-100, and miR-200b, miR-320, miR-16, miR-93, miR-126, and miR-223) was identified as potentially useful diagnostic biomarkers, but the overall discriminating performance was indecisive being below 85%, thus not allowing a further clinical validation. Very interesting results have been reported in 2017 by Yokoi et al., which demonstrated that a combination of eight circulating serum miRNAs (miR-142-3p, miR-26a-5p, let7d-5p, miR-374a-5p, miR-766-3p, miR-200a-3p, miR-328-3p, and miR-130b-3p) was able to successfully discriminate OC patients from healthy controls with remarkable diagnostic performances at ROC analysis (AUC 0.97; sensitivity 0.92 and specificity 0.91) (Yokoi et al. 2017a, b). The eight miRNAs classification model had a different AUC, sensitivity, and specificity for the different histological types of OC, thus emphasizing the need to identify histology-based diagnostic models (Yokoi et al. 2017a, b). In addition, in the same study, the authors developed a predictive algorithm able to differentiate early-stage OC from benign tumor using seven mi-RNAs (miR-200a-3p, miR-766-3p, miR-26a-5p, miR-142-3p, let-7d-5p, miR-130b-3p, and miR-328-3p) (Yokoi et al. 2017a, b). In this model, the diagnostic performance appeared promising with an AUC of 0.92, but the sensitivity and specificity were lower being 0.861, and 0.833, respectively (Yokoi et al. 2017a, b). Similarly, Yoshimura et al. identified circulating EVs embedded miR-99a-5p as a potentially useful diagnostic tool for early detection of OC patients (Yoshimura et al. 2018). Furthermore, a quantitative proteomic approach detected a relevant reduction of circulating miR-99a-5p after cytoreductive surgery, thus suggesting that this biomarker may be used for disease monitoring. Unfortunately, the diagnostic performances were always below 85% with relevant differences according to tumor histotypes, and specificity for detecting clear cell and mucinous OC above 90%. It should be acknowledged that the results of this study do not support the use of this miRNA in clinical setting; however, this is the first well-conducted experimental approach that stratified prognostic and diagnostic performances of specific proteomic profiles according to tumor histology (Yoshimura et al. 2018), which certainly support this approach to be furtherly developed. In case of endometriosis-associated OC, Suryawanshi et al. found that three plasma miRNAs (miR-16, miR-191, and miR-195) are overexpressed in peritoneal endometriotic lesions and discriminated between healthy subjects and patients with deep infiltrating endometriosis (sensitivity and specificity of 88% and 60%, respectively) (Suryawanshi et al. 2013). Kobayashi et al. showed that serum miR-1290 is significantly increased in patients with high-grade serous OC, and it can be used to early identify these patients (Kobayashi et al. 2018). In particular, this study demonstrated that CA-125 retains a better performance to early identify the OC patients as compared with miR-1290 serum levels. However, the assessment of miR-1290 serum levels showed better performance as compared to CA-125 in discriminating high-grade serous OC patients from women with non-serous ovarian malignancies. Furthermore, the authors compared the levels of miR-1290 before and after the primary debulking surgery and suggested that serum miR-1290 reflects tumor burden, which may help disease monitoring (Kobayashi et al. 2018). Similarly, in a cohort of 56 high-grade serous OC patients, Shah et al. showed that the combination of miR-375 and CA-125 was the strongest discriminator of healthy versus high-grade serous OC patients, and that the combination of miR-34a-5p and CA-125 was the strongest predictor of complete surgical debulking (Shah et al. 2018). In addition, the role of the EVs derived miRNAs have been studied also in terms of prognosis because of their implication in the development of drug resistance in OC patients. In particular, increased circulating levels of annexin A3 (Yin et al. 2012) together with a panel of miRNAs including miR-181a, miR-1908, miR-21, miR-486, and miR-223 were identified as markers of platinum-resistance in women with OC, thus suggesting a potential clinically relevant role for these biomarkers (Kuhlmann et al. 2019). To date, this approach using microRNAs and other liquid biopsy components is under investigation in several human studies but the current evidence is not mature yet for clinical use.

6.5 Conclusion

In the last decade, quantitative proteomic approaches have been used as a promising tool to be used in clinical practice. In particular, compelling evidence seems to support the role of a panel of proteins and circulating microRNAs as reliable biomarkers to achieve early diagnosis and accurate prognostic stratification of OC patients. On the other hand, despite a plethora of experimental data suggesting potential diagnostic and prognostic proteomic profiles, only a few reports have entered clinical evaluation, with contrasting results, thus producing an impressive gap between preclinical evidences, and clinical findings. Therefore, there is an urgent need to design clinically focused studies with an immediate reliable translation into clinical practice. The combination of proteomic profiles, serum CA-125 levels, *BRCA* gene status, and ultrasound examination appears as the most promising strategy. For further reading, see Box 6.1.

Box 6.1 Overview of recommended articles providing relevant scientific insights on this specific issue

Recommended reading of particular interest	DOI
Macklin A, et al. **Recent advances in mass spectrometry based clinical proteomics: applications to cancer research.** Clin Proteomics. 2020;17:17.	https://doi.org/10.1186/s12014-020-09283-w
Sobsey CA, et al. **Targeted and Untargeted Proteomics Approaches in Biomarker Development.** Proteomics. 2020;20(9):e1900029.	https://doi.org/10.1002/pmic.201900029
Bonifácio VDB. **Ovarian Cancer Biomarkers: Moving Forward in Early Detection.** Adv Exp Med Biol. 2020;1219:355–363.	https://doi.org/10.1007/978-3-030-34025-4_18
He Y, et al. **Oncoproteomics: Current status and future opportunities.** Clin Chim Acta. 2019;495:611–624.	https://doi.org/10.1016/j.cca.2019.06.006
Srivastava A, Creek DJ. **Discovery and Validation of Clinical Biomarkers of Cancer: A Review Combining Metabolomics and Proteomics.** Proteomics. 2019;19(10):e1700448.	https://doi.org/10.1002/pmic.201700448
Carvalho VP, et al. **The contribution and perspectives of proteomics to uncover ovarian cancer tumor markers.** Transl Res. 2019;206:71–90.	https://doi.org/10.1016/j.trsl.2018.11.001
Forshed J. **Experimental Design in Clinical 'Omics Biomarker Discovery.** J Proteome Res. 2017;16(11):3954–3960.	https://doi.org/10.1021/acs.jproteome.7b00418
Huang Y, Zhu H. **Protein Array-based Approaches for Biomarker Discovery in Cancer.** Genomics Proteomics Bioinformatics. 2017;15(2):73–81.	https://doi.org/10.1016/j.gpb.2017.03.001
Bonifácio VDB. **Ovarian Cancer Biomarkers: Moving Forward in Early Detection.** Adv Exp Med Biol. 2020;1219:355–363.	https://doi.org/10.1007/978-3-030-34025-4_18
Labrie M, et al. **Proteomics advances for precision therapy in ovarian cancer.** Expert Rev Proteomics. 2019;16(10):841–850.	https://doi.org/10.1080/14789450.2019.1666004
El Bairi K, et al. **Prediction of therapy response in ovarian cancer: Where are we now?** Crit Rev Clin Lab Sci. 2017;54(4):233–266.	https://doi.org/10.1080/10408363.2017.1313190

Acknowledgment and Conflicts of Interest The authors declare they have no conflict of interest. The final draft was reviewed and approved by all the authors. The contents of the chapter reflect the authors' perspectives and not of their institutions of affiliation.

Authors' Contributions MP, CR, DC, MD wrote the chapter. SD supervised the writing process.

References

Agarwal R, Kaye SB (2003) Ovarian cancer: strategies for overcoming resistance to chemotherapy. Nat Rev Cancer 3(7):502–516. https://doi.org/10.1038/nrc1123

Amintas S, Vendrely V, Dupin C, Buscail L, Laurent C, Bournet B, Merlio JP, Bedel A, Moreau-Gaudry F, Boutin J, Dabernat S, Buscail E (2021) Next-generation cancer biomarkers: extracellular vesicle DNA as a circulating surrogate of tumor DNA. Front Cell Dev Biol 8:622048. https://doi.org/10.3389/fcell.2020.622048

An HJ, Kim DS, Park YK et al (2006) Comparative proteomics of ovarian epithelial tumors. J Proteome Res 5(5):1082–1090. https://doi.org/10.1021/pr050461p

Barnabas G, Bahar-Shany K, Sapoznik S et al (2019) Microvesicle proteomic profiling of uterine liquid biopsy for ovarian cancer early detection. Mol Cell Proteomics 18(5):865–875. https://doi.org/10.1074/mcp.RA119.001362

Carvalho VP, Grassi ML, Palma CS, Carrara HHA, Faça VM, Candido Dos Reis FJ (2019) Poersch a. the contribution and perspectives of proteomics to uncover ovarian cancer tumor markers. Transl Res 206:71–90. https://doi.org/10.1016/j.trsl.2018.11.001

Chappell NP, Teng P, Hood BL et al (2012) Mitochondrial proteomic analysis of cisplatin resistance in ovarian cancer. J Proteome Res 11(9):4605–4614. https://doi.org/10.1021/pr300403d

Chen X, Wei S, Ma Y et al (2014) Quantitative proteomics analysis identifies mitochondria as therapeutic targets of multidrug-resistance in ovarian cancer. Theranostic 4(12):1164–1175. https://doi.org/10.7150/thno.8502.eCollection.2014

Chung YW, Bae HS, Song JY et al (2013) Detection of microRNA as novel biomarkers of epithelial ovarian cancer from the serum of ovarian cancer patients. Int J Gynecol Cancer 23(4):673–679. https://doi.org/10.1097/IGC.0b013e31828c166d

Davidson B, Espina V, Steinberg SM et al (2006) Proteomic analysis of malignant ovarian cancer effusions as a tool for biologic and prognostic profiling. Clin Cancer Res 12(3 Pt 1):791–799. https://doi.org/10.1158/1078-0432.CCR-05-2516

Domcke S, Sinha R, Levine DA, Sander C, Schultz N (2013) Evaluating cell lines as tumor models by comparison of genomic profiles. Nat Commun 4:2126. https://doi.org/10.1038/ncomms3126

El Bairi K, Kandhro AH, Gouri A, Mahfoud W, Louanjli N, Saadani B, Afqir S, Amrani M (2017) Emerging diagnostic, prognostic and therapeutic biomarkers for ovarian cancer. Cell Oncol (Dordr) 40(2):105–118. https://doi.org/10.1007/s13402-016-0309-1

El Bairi K, Afqir S, Amrani M (2020) Is HE4 superior over CA-125 in the follow-up of patients with epithelial ovarian cancer? Curr Drug Targets 21(10):1026–1033. https://doi.org/10.2174/1389450121666200425211732

Elewaily MI, Elsergany AR (2021) Emerging role of exosomes and exosomal microRNA in cancer: pathophysiology and clinical potential. J Cancer Res Clin Oncol 147(3):637–648. https://doi.org/10.1007/s00432-021-03534-5

Elstrand MB, Sandstad B, Oksefjell H, Davidson B, Tropé CG (2012) Prognostic significance of residual tumor in patients with epithelial ovarian cancer stage IV in a 20 year perspective. Acta Obstet Gynecol Scand 91(3):308–317. https://doi.org/10.1111/j.1600-0412.2011.01316.x

Elzek MA, Rodland KD (2015) Proteomics of ovarian cancer: functional insights and clinical applications. Cancer Metastasis Rev 34(1):83–96. https://doi.org/10.1007/s10555-014-9547-8

Faca VM, Ventura AP, Fitzgibbon MP, Pereira-Faça SR, Pitteri SJ, Green AE et al (2008) Proteomic analysis of ovarian cancer cells reveals dynamic processes of protein secretion and shedding of extra-cellular domains. PLoS One 3(6):e2425. https://doi.org/10.1371/journal.pone.0002425

Gortzak-Uzan L, Ignatchenko A, Evangelou AI, Agochiya M, Brown KA, St Onge P et al (2008) A proteome resource of ovarian cancer ascites; integrated proteomic and bioinformatic analyses to identify putative biomarkers. J Proteome Res 7(1):339–351. https://doi.org/10.1021/pr0703223

Guerra F, Paiano A, Migoni D, Girolimetti G, Perrone AM, De Iaco P et al (2019) Protein expression determines resistance to cisplatin through late endocytic pathway impairment and extracellular vesicular secretion. Cancers (Basel) 11(1):52. https://doi.org/10.3390/cancers11010052

Gunawardana CG, Kuk C, Smith CR, Batruch I, Soosaipillai A, Diamandis EP (2009) Comprehensive analysis of conditioned media from ovarian cancer cell lines identifies novel candidate markers of epithelial ovarian cancer. J Proteome Res 8(10):4705–4713. https://doi.org/10.1021/pr900411g

Kan CW, Hahn MA, Gard GB et al (2012) Elevated levels of circulating microRNA-200 family members correlate with serous epithelial ovarian cancer. BMC Cancer 12:627. https://doi.org/10.1186/1471-2407-12-627

Kobayashi M, Sawada K, Nakamura K et al (2018) Exosomal miR-1290 is a potential biomarker of high-grade serous ovarian carcinoma and can discriminate patients from those with malignancies of other histological types. J Ovarian Res 11(1):81. https://doi.org/10.1186/s13048-018-0458-0

Kuhlmann JD, Chebouti I, Kimmig R et al (2019) Extracellular vesicle-associated miRNAs in ovarian cancer-design of an integrated NGS- based workflow for the identification of blood-based biomarkers for platinum-resistance. Clin Chem Lab Med 57(7):1053–1062. https://doi.org/10.1515/cclm-2018-1048

Kuk C, Kulasingam V, Gunawardana CG, Smith CR, Batruch I, Diamandis EP (2009) Mining the ovarian cancer ascites proteome for potential ovarian cancer biomarkers. Mol Cell Proteomics 8 (4):661–669. https://doi.org/10.1074/mcp.M800313-MCP200

Leung F, Bernardini MQ, Brown MD et al (2016) Validation of a novel biomarker panel for the detection of ovarian cancer. Cancer Epidemiol Biomark Prev 25(9):1333–1340. https://doi.org/10.1158/1055-9965.EPI-15-1299

Li S-L, Ye F, Cai WJ et al (2010) Quantitative proteome analysis of multidrug resistance in human ovarian cancer cell line. J Cell Biochem 109(4):625–633. https://doi.org/10.1002/jcb.22413

Madden EC, Gorman AM, Logue SE, Samali A (2020) Tumour cell secretome in chemoresistance and tumour recurrence. Trends Cancer 6(6):489–505. https://doi.org/10.1016/j.trecan.2020.02.020

Mahdian-Shakib A, Dorostkar R, Tat M, Hashemzadeh MS, Saidi N (2016) Differential role of microRNAs in prognosis, diagnosis, and therapy of ovarian cancer. Biomed Pharmacother 84:592–600. https://doi.org/10.1016/j.biopha.2016.09.087

Meng X, Joosse SA, Müller V et al (2015) Diagnostic and prognostic potential of serum miR-7, miR-16, miR-25, miR-93, miR-182, miR-376a and miR-429 in ovarian cancer patients. Br J Cancer 113(9):1358–1366. https://doi.org/10.1038/bjc.2015.340

Montagnana M, Lippi G, Ruzzenente O et al (2009) The utility of serum human epididymis protein 4 (HE4) in patients with a pelvic mass. J Clin Lab Anal 23(5):331–335. https://doi.org/10.1002/jcla.20340

Montagnana M, Benati M, Danese E (2017) Circulating biomarkers in epithelial ovarian cancer diagnosis: from present to future perspective. Ann Transl Med 5(13):276. https://doi.org/10.21037/atm.2017.05.13

Moore RG, Brown AK, Miller MC et al (2008) The use of multiple novel tumor biomarkers for the detection of ovarian carcinoma in patients with a pelvic mass. Gynecol Oncol 108(2):402–408. https://doi.org/10.1016/j.ygyno.2007.10.017

Nakamura K, Sawada K, Yoshimura A, Kinose Y, Nakatsuka E, Kimura T (2016) Clinical relevance of circulating cell-free microRNAs in ovarian cancer. Mol Cancer 15(1):48. https://doi.org/10.1186/s12943-016-0536-0

Pan S, Chen R, Aebersold R, Brentnall TA (2011) Mass spectrometry based glycoproteomics- from a proteomics perspective. Mol Cell Proteomics 10(1):R110.003251. https://doi.org/10.1074/mcp.R110.003251

Pan C, Stevic I, Muller V et al (2018) Exosomal microRNAs as tumor markers in epithelial ovarian cancer. Mol Oncol 12(11):1935–1948. https://doi.org/10.1002/1878-0261.12371

Petrillo M, Nero C, Amadio G, Gallo D, Fagotti A, Scambia G (2016) Targeting the hallmarks of ovarian cancer: the big picture. Gynecol Oncol 142(1):176–183. https://doi.org/10.1016/j.ygyno.2016.03.037

Shah JS, Gard GB, Yang J et al (2018) Combining serum microRNA and ca-125 as prognostic indicators of preoperative surgical outcome in women with high-grade serous ovarian cancer. Gynecol Oncol 148(1):181–188. https://doi.org/10.1016/j.ygyno.2017.11.005

Srivastava A, Rathore S, Munshi A, Ramesh R (2021) Extracellular vesicles in oncology: from immune suppression to immunotherapy. AAPS J 23(2):30. https://doi.org/10.1208/s12248-021-00554-4

Sung H, Ferlay J, Siegel RL, Laversanne M, Soerjomataram I, Jemal A, Bray F (2021) Global cancer statistics 2020: GLOBOCAN estimates of incidence and mortality worldwide for 36 cancers in 185 countries. CA Cancer J Clin 71(3):209–249. https://doi.org/10.3322/caac.21660

Suryawanshi S, Huang X, Elishaev E et al (2013) Plasma microRNAs as novel biomarkers for endometriosis and endometriosis-associated ovarian cancer. Clin Cancer Res 19(5):1213–1224. https://doi.org/10.1158/1078-0432.CCR-12-2726

Taylor DD, Gercel-Taylor C (2008) MicroRNA signatures of tumor-derived exosomes as diagnostic biomarkers of ovarian cancer. Gynecol Oncol 110(1):13–21. https://doi.org/10.1016/j.ygyno.2008.04.033

Tian Y, Yao Z, Roden RB, Zhang H (2011) Identification of glycoproteins associated with different histological subtypes of ovarian tumors using quantitative glycoproteomics. Proteomics 11 (24):4677–4687. https://doi.org/10.1002/pmic.201000811

Ueland FR, Desimone CP, Seamon LG et al (2011) Effectiveness of a multivariate index assay in the preoperative assessment of ovarian tumors. Obstet Gynecol 117(6):1289–1297. https://doi.org/10.1097/AOG.0b013e31821b5118

Wegdam W, Argmann CA, Kramer G, Vissers JP, Buist MR, Kenter GG, Aerts JM, Meijer D, Moerland PD (2014) Label-free LC-MSe in tissue and serum reveals protein networks underlying differences between benign and malignant serous ovarian tumors. PLoS One 9(9):e108046. https://doi.org/10.1371/journal.pone.0108046

Wiegand KC, Hennessy BT, Leung S et al (2014) A functional proteogenomic analysis of endometrioid and clear cell carcinomas using reserve phase protein array and mutation analysis: protein expression is histotype-specific and loss of ARID1A/BAF250a is associated with AKT phosphorylation. BMC Cancer 14:120. https://doi.org/10.1186/1471-2407-14-120

Yamamoto CM, Oakes ML, Murakami T, Muto MG, Berkowitz RS, Ng SW (2018) Comparison of benign peritoneal fluid-and ovarian cancer ascites-derived extracellular vesicle RNA biomarkers. J Ovarian Res 11(1):20. https://doi.org/10.1186/s13048-018-0391-2

Yang JY, Yoshihara K, Tanaka K et al (2013) Predicting time to ovarian carcinoma recurrence using protein markers. J Clin Investig 123(9):3740–3750. https://doi.org/10.1172/JCI68509

Yin J, Yan X, Yao X et al (2012) Secretion of annexin A3 from ovarian cancer cells and its association with platinum resistance in ovarian cancer patients. J Cell Mol Med 16(2):337–348. https://doi.org/10.1111/j.1582-4934.2011.01316.x

Yokoi A, Yoshioka Y, Hirakawa A et al (2017a) A combination of circulating miRNAs for early detection of ovarian cancer. Oncotarget 8(52):89811–89823. https://doi.org/10.18632/oncotarget.20688

Yokoi A, Yoshioka Y, Yamamoto Y et al (2017b) Malignant extracellular vesicles carrying MMP1 mRNA facilitate peritoneal dissemination in ovarian cancer. Nat Commun 8:14470. https://doi.org/10.1038/ncomms14470

Yoshimura A, Sawada K, Nakamura K et al (2018) Exosomal miR-99a-5p is elevated in sera of ovarian cancer patients and promotes cancer cell invasion by increasing fibronectin and vitronectin expression in neighboring peritoneal mesothelial cells. BMC Cancer 18(1):1065. https://doi.org/10.1186/s12885-018-4974-5

Zhang Z, Bast RC Jr, Yu Y et al (2004) Three biomarkers identified from serum proteomic analysis for detection of early stage ovarian cancer. Cancer Res 64(16):5882–5890. https://doi.org/10.1158/0008-5472.CAN-04-0746

Zhao M, Ding JX, Zeng K et al (2014) Heat shock protein 27: a potential biomarker of peritoneal metastasis in epithelial ovarian cancer? Tumour Biol 35(2):1051–1056. https://doi.org/10.1007/s13277-013-1139-7

Zheng H, Zhang L, Zhao Y et al (2013) Plasma miRNAs as diagnostic and prognostic biomarkers for ovarian cancer. PLoS One 8(11):e77853. https://doi.org/10.1371/journal.pone.0077853

Zhou J, Gong G, Tan H et al (2015) Urinary microRNA-30a5p is a potential biomarker for ovarian serous adenocarcinoma. Oncol Rep 33(6):2915–2923. https://doi.org/10.3892/or.2015.3937

Zuberi M, Mir R, Das J et al (2015) Expression of serum miR-200a, miR-200b, and miR-200c as candidate biomarkers in epithelial ovarian cancer and their association with clinicopathological features. Clin Transl Oncol 17(10):779–787. https://doi.org/10.1007/s12094-015-1303-1

Cutting-Edge Technologies for Ovarian Cancer: An Overview of the Impact of Genetic Testing, Next-Generation Sequencing, and Single-Cell Analysis

7

Alia Ghoneum, Amal Tazzite, Khalid El Bairi, and Neveen Said

Abstract

Cancer genetics is increasingly becoming central in the course of patients' care. Genetic testing for pathogenic variants in ovarian cancer (OC) is becoming widely available and represents a cornerstone for cancer risk assessment, prediction of prognosis, and targeted treatments. The introduction of novel technologies for sequencing has enabled large-scale multigene panel genomic testing. In this chapter, the current genetic variants and genetic testing guidelines for OC are reviewed. We also discussed potential applications of next-generation sequencing in understanding OC genetics and its impact on patients' outcomes according to the latest research findings. We finally depict the potential of single-cell sequencing in understanding OC heterogeneity based on recent proof-of-concept studies.

A. Ghoneum
Departments of Cancer Biology, Wake Forest University School of Medicine, Winston Salem, NC, USA

A. Tazzite
Genetics and Molecular Pathology Laboratory, Medical School, Hassan II University, Casablanca, Morocco

K. El Bairi (✉)
Cancer Biomarkers Working Group, Oujda, Morocco
e-mail: k.elbairi@ump.ac.ma

N. Said (✉)
Departments of Cancer Biology, Wake Forest University School of Medicine, Winston Salem, NC, USA

Departments of Urology, Wake Forest University School of Medicine, Winston Salem, NC, USA

Comprehensive Cancer Center, Winston Salem, NC, USA
e-mail: nsaid@wakehealth.edu

K. El Bairi (ed.), *Ovarian Cancer Biomarkers*,
https://doi.org/10.1007/978-981-16-1873-4_7

Keywords

Ovarian cancer · Next-generation sequencing · Single-cell sequencing · Genetic testing

7.1 Introduction

Genetic testing in OC is currently used to identify individuals at increased disease risk as well as to predict prognosis and response to targeted therapies including platinum and poly(ADP)-ribose polymerase inhibitors (PARPi), which are currently shifting poor outcomes in this aggressive disease (Amin et al. 2020). Notably, next-generation sequencing (NGS) played a central role in delivering molecular testing for OC patients (Stoffel and Carethers 2020). These novel techniques enable massive and parallel sequencing of several clinically actionable variants simultaneously in a short period and at a lower cost as compared to the standard Sanger sequencing approach (El Bairi et al. 2020a). For these reasons, most genetics laboratories have opted for this technology for routine genetic counseling; not only for risk assessment but also for predicting prognosis and therapy response. Moreover, due to the significant tumor heterogeneity observed in OC, other technologies—principally single-cell sequencing—were applied to explore the molecular mechanisms of tumor pathogenesis, clonal evolution, and chemoresistance (Winterhoff et al. 2019). This chapter will focus on these aspects to illuminate the potential of cancer genetics to improve the management of OC in the era of precision medicine.

7.2 Overview of Guidelines and Approved Methods for Genetic Testing in Ovarian Cancer

OC is the fifth most common cancer in women and the most lethal gynecologic malignancy (Siegel et al. 2020; American Cancer Society 2020). Family history of breast cancer or OC is considered as a well-known risk factor for OC; nearly 25% of all OCs are associated with heritable genetics. Mutated *Breast Cancer type 1/2* (*BRCA*) anti-oncogenes account for almost 40% of OCs in subjects with family history, while 6% of all ovarian, fallopian tube, and peritoneal cancers are caused by germline mutated mismatch repair (MMR) genes involved in homologous recombination (HR) and those associated with the Fanconi anemia pathway (Walsh et al. 2011). Mutations in these genes have been identified as pathogenic variants (PV) or likely pathogenic variants (LPV) and they are not only limited to germline hereditary disease, but they were also identified as somatic mutations in primary and/or recurrent tumors from patients with no family history of cancer (Konstantinopoulos et al. 2020). Importantly, screening and identification of these mutations guide the clinical decision for prophylaxis, surveillance, as well as therapeutics offered to women with family history of OC, women diagnosed with OC and their blood relatives (Konstantinopoulos et al. 2020). In the last decade, multiple and simultaneous analyses of several genes associated with OC have been facilitated by the arrival of next-generation sequencing (NGS) techniques for both germline and somatic mutations in primary and/or recurrent tumors. This has enabled cost-effective screening tests, especially for patients with family history of cancer and suspected genetic syndromes (Angeli et al. 2020). However, the main challenge is defining the number of genes that must be tested for women with a genetic predisposition and risk assessment based on the penetrance of disease-causing genetic variants (Sud et al. 2017; Angeli et al. 2020). In addition to *BRCA1/2* and MMR genes, other high penetrance genes including *TP53, PTEN, STK11,* and *CDH1* have been identified and were associated with the risk of developing breast cancer and OCs. Genes including *PALB2, BRIP1, ATM, CHEK2, BARD1, NBN, NF1, RAD51C, RAD51D,* and some genes of the MMR pathway have been considered as moderate and low penetrance genes, along with other genes involved in the same pathway such as *PIK3CA* amplification and activating mutations. In this chapter, we will review the major screening markers that have been employed in genetic testing for OC, their diagnostic and prognostic value, and their significance for guiding clinical decisions.

7.2.1 Hereditary Breast and Ovarian Cancer Syndrome

Hereditary germline mutations in *BRCA1/2* genes account for approximately 20-25% of OCs leading to deficiencies in DNA repair mechanisms (Walsh et al. 2011; Arts-de Jong et al. 2016; Norquist et al. 2016a). Heterozygous carriers of germline mutations in *BRCA1/2* have a heightened risk of OC diagnosis, with 44% for *BRCA1* and 17% for *BRCA2* (Kuchenbaecker et al. 2017). *BRCA* mutations are inherited in an autosomal dominant pattern with high penetrance of cancers in individuals carrying *BRCA* mutations (Moyer 2014). Women having deleterious germline mutations, first-degree relatives have a 50% chance of carrying the same variant, while second-degree relatives have a 25% risk. Therefore, these two populations should benefit from genetic testing and appropriate surveillance protocols (Moyer 2014).

BRCA1/2 mutations are highest in the high-grade serous subtype of OC, constituting up to 20% (Ledermann et al. 2016), while constituting 10% in endometrioid and even low frequency in clear cell carcinomas (Arts-de Jong et al. 2016; Manchana et al. 2019). In addition, *BRCA1/2* genes are subject to somatic mutations in *BRCA* in 5%-7% of OC cases as well as promoter hypermethylation with subsequent downregulation/loss of their transcription (Kanakkanthara et al. 2019). Somatic *BRCA1/2* alterations have similar molecular characteristics as hereditary cancers (Faraoni and Graziani 2018). *BRCA1* and *BRCA2* confer genome stability by coordinating DNA repair via HR, a high-fidelity process responsible for repairing double-stranded breaks (DSBs). In contrast to nonhomologous DNA end joining (NHEJ), which repairs breaks merely by ligating DSB ends, HR uses a sister chromatid as a template and hence reduces errors in repair (Dziadkowiec et al. 2016; Fleury et al. 2019; Frey and Pothuri 2017).

Inactivating mutations in *BRCA1/2* lead to a deficiency in HR, forcing cells to shift to the NHEJ pathway to repair DSB with increased chromosomal instability that can be further aggravated by factors that induce DSBs, such as exposure to DNA cross-linking agents (Gorodetska et al. 2019; Mylavarapu et al. 2018). Thus, cells deficient in *BRCA1/2* are sensitive to platinum agents, which intercalate into DNA nucleotides (Mylavarapu et al. 2018), and PARP inhibitors (PARPi). PARP describes a category of enzymes that generate large branched chains of poly(ADP)ribose (PAR) from NAD+. The efficacy of PARP inhibition (PARPi) is dependent on the concept that PARP1 loss in the setting of HR dysfunction (due to *BRCA1/2* mutation) increases DNA aberrations, leading to cell death via synthetic lethality (Topatana et al. 2020; Eskander and Tewari 2014; Turk and Wisinski 2018). The synthetic lethality of PARPi–BRCA can be attributed to the fact that PARP1 contributes to the repair of single-strand breaks (SSBs), and PARP inhibition may cause destruction of replication forks, causing DSBs and hence cell death (Helleday 2011). PARP inhibitors are not only effective for EOC treatment in patients with *BRCA* dysfunction, but they have also been approved as a second-line treatment for recurrent and advanced HGSOC or endometrioid carcinoma (Mirza et al. 2016).

7.2.2 Mismatch Repair (*MMR*) Genes

Germline inactivating mutations of DNA MMR genes is the cause of Lynch syndrome (LS), also known as hereditary nonpolyposis colon cancer (HNPCC) and are inherited in an autosomal dominant manner (Carethers and Stoffel 2015). Lynch syndrome is the second most common cause of inherited OC and accounts for 10–15% of all hereditary OCs (Hampel et al. 2015). OCs associated with Lynch syndrome mainly have non-serous histology including endometrioid (19.2%), mucinous (16.9%), and clear cell (11.5%) carcinomas (Nakamura et al. 2014), and are typically diagnosed at an earlier age and stage, with a better OS (Nakamura et al. 2014). Although the incidence of MMR mutations in serous cancers has been reported to be lower than other subtypes, there is a significant between-study heterogeneity; warranting routine testing of MMR mutations in women diagnosed with other histologic types (Carethers and Stoffel 2015; Germano et al. 2018; Guillotin and Martin 2014; Konstantinopoulos et al. 2020; Zhao et al. 2018).

MMR genes, including post-meiotic segregation increased 1 and 2 (PMS1 and PMS2), mutL homolog 1 (MLH1), mutS homolog 2, 3, and 6 (MSH2, MSH3, and MSH6), as well as deletion of EPCAM gene upstream of MSH2, participate in repair during DNA replication (Carethers and Stoffel 2015; Li 2008). Inactivating mutations of MLH1 and MSH2 account for the majority of LS cases, followed by PMS2 and MSH6 mutations (Pino et al. 2009). For women with OC, the most frequent mutations were MSH2 (47%) and MLH1 (38%) (Helder-Woolderink et al. 2016). Somatic MMR gene deficiencies are detected in OC through genetic or epigenetic mechanisms and have important implications in both treatment and prognosis (Germano et al. 2018; Zhao et al. 2018). MMR proteins correct for nucleotide base mismatches, small deletions or insertions generated by DNA polymerase displacement or slippage during DNA replicative events. Typically, in LS, when there is a somatic mutation of one allele, the other allele is inactivated, and the MMR protein's normal expression is lost, leading to the accumulation of repeated nucleotide sequences and microsatellite instability with replicative errors (Moller et al. 2017; Guillotin and Martin 2014). Notably, studies of clear cell OCs with microsatellite instability revealed that these tumors are immunogenic with increased lymphocytic infiltration; thus, patients with these tumor phenotypes may benefit from immune checkpoint blockade in the setting of recurrent disease, regardless of their tissue of origin (Howitt et al. 2017). Existing clinical data do not support the recommendation of routine surveillance and screening of OC in LS patients by transvaginal ultrasound and serum CA-125 testing. However, the National Comprehensive Cancer Network (NCCN) guidelines recommend that bilateral Risk-reducing salpingo-oophorectomy (RRSO) may be considered and individualized based on patient's age (childbearing or menopausal status), comorbidities, family history, and the mutated LS gene as lifetime for OC vary by the mutated gene (NCCN Guidelines 2019).

7.2.3 DNA Repair Protein (*RAD51*)

RAD51 paralogs family proteins including X-ray repair cross-complementing proteins (*XRCC3 and XRCC2*), *RAD51D, RAD51C, and RAD51B* are involved in the DNA repair pathway (Prakash et al. 2015). Located at the human chromosome15q15.1, the RAD51 protein plays an invaluable role during HR repair by binding to DNA and initiating ATP-dependent homologous pairing and strand transfer reactions (Antony et al. 2009). When ATP is present, RAD51 self-assembles into an extended polymer on single-stranded DNA catalyzing strand exchange (Antony et al. 2009). Germline variants in several *RAD51* paralogs have been detected in ovarian and breast cancers. *RAD51C* and *RAD51D* mutations confer predisposition to OC with a lifetime risk of OC for *RAD51C* PV/LPV carriers of around 7% (Suszynska et al. 2020; Loveday et al. 2011, 2012). Risk of developing OC in case of *RAD51* variants warrants their use with *BRCA1* and *BRCA2* in routine clinical genetic screening (Song et al. 2015).

7.2.4 Tumor Protein p53 (*TP53*)

TP53 is a transcription factor, which regulates several target genes that induce DNA repair, cell cycle arrest, cell death, senescence as a response to cellular stress. *TP53* is altered in over 96% HGSOC cases (Cancer Genome Atlas 2011; Ahmed et al. 2010). Ultra-deep sequencing revealed low-frequency *TP53* mutations in ascitic fluid and blood samples from chemotherapy-naïve patients, including control samples without tumor. *TP53* mutations were detected in DNA samples derived from tumor cells present in the vagina of women with high-grade serous OC (HGSOC) and were also detected in 60% of patients with HGSOC without a prior tubal ligation (Erickson et al. 2014). Pathogenic variants of *TP53* mutations were also detected in 64% of vaginal smears (Papanicolaou tests) withdrawn six years before OC diagnosis with tumor-matching PV, strongly suggesting that noninvasive early molecular detection of HGSOC is possible based on identification of *TP53* clonal variants (Paracchini et al. 2020). There are several advantages of using *TP53* mutations as prognostic indicators for OC as the first genetic events of HGSOC formation are*TP53* mutations detected in Fallopian tubes' serous tubal intraepithelial carcinoma "STIC" lesions (Chien et al. 2015; Soong et al. 2019; Kuhn et al. 2012). However, high-accuracy NGS revealed the presence of low-frequency *TP53* mutations in several healthy tissues, regardless of age, and becoming increasingly abundant with age in all tissues investigated. Hence, it is essential to differentiate between tumor-derived versus age-associated *TP53* alterations in high-sensitivity DNA sequencing studies (Cancer Genome Atlas 2011; Vang et al. 2016).

7.2.5 *BRCA1* Interacting Protein C-Terminal Helicase 1 (BRIP1)

BRIP1 is required for DNA inter-strand cross-link (ICL) repair and is important to genome stability. Hence, germline deletions in *BRIP1* have been associated with a higher risk of breast and OC. A recent study conducted by Moyer et al., investigated NGS of germline DNA in 1199 patients with OC and 2160 patients with early-onset breast cancer, and found that approximately 2% of patients carried a missense mutation in *BRIP1* (Moyer et al. 2020). Surprisingly, this percentage was threefold higher than the frequency of *BRIP1* variant alleles seen in individuals of the general population. Inactivating mutations in the helicase domain of *BRIP1* were identified in 75% of the PV of *BRIP1* suggesting that BRIP1 is a susceptibility gene for breast and OC (Moyer et al. 2020). Deletion of *BRIP1* was also found to result in a higher risk of OC in familial index patients, and in patients with late-onset OC. Interestingly, the minority of deleterious missense variants were significantly more widespread in OC patients than in breast cancer patients (Weber-Lassalle et al. 2018; Balmana and Domchek 2015).

7.2.6 Checkpoint Kinase 2 (*CHEK2*)

CHEK2 encodes for a tumor suppressor serine-threonine kinase that is responsible for DNA repair, cell cycle arrest, and apoptosis (Zoppoli et al. 2012). Somatic missense mutation is associated with low-grade invasive cancers, borderline ovarian tumors, and ovarian cystadenomas but not with HGSOC (Zoppoli et al. 2012). Recent NGS studies identified *CHEK2* PV and PVL as the third most frequently altered susceptibility gene among OC patients, though with moderate or low penetrance (Carter et al. 2018; Kurian et al. 2019). However, the clinical implications in surveillance, prophylaxis, treatment, and prognosis are not strong (Konstantinopoulos et al. 2020).

7.2.7 Cyclin-Dependent Kinases (CDKs) and CDK Inhibitors

Loss of function (LOF) splice variant of the *CDK12* gene was found to be strongly associated with hereditary OC (Bogdanova et al. 2019; Sokol et al. 2019). *CDK12* mutation or deficiency was reported to sensitize cells to agents that target cell cycle checkpoints, including *CHK1* inhibitors (Chou et al. 2020; Zhu et al. 2020). Hence, *CDK12* not only serves as a prognostic biomarker, but can enhance the antiproliferative effects of CHK1 inhibitors (Paculova et al. 2017). In OC, the Cyclin-Dependent Kinase (CDK) inhibitor *p16* gene exhibits a somatic mutation rate of 15–30% (Wang et al. 2017), as well as promoter methylation and homozygous deletions (Ruan et al. 2018). The expression of p16 protein was significantly reduced in OC compared to normal ovarian tissue, and negatively correlated with patient prognosis (Wang et al. 2017). Sallum et al. demonstrated that the IHC of p53/p16 index was a reliable marker for differentiation of low-grade serous OC (LGSOC) from HGSOC (Sallum et al. 2018).

7.2.8 Cyclin E1 (*CCNE1*)

Cyclin E1 is encoded by *CCNE1* gene, which is amplified in approximately 30% of HGSOC cases (Petersen et al. 2020; Gorski et al. 2020). Tumors amplified by *CCNE1* are characterized by abnormal replication, replicative stress, and genomic instability (Kuhn et al. 2016). Thus, intact *BRCA1* is integral for the survival of tumors with amplified *CCNE1* as they are deemed HR proficient (Patch et al. 2015). Accordingly, a degree of synthetic lethality exists as chromosomal instability generated by HR pathway mutations and *CCNE1* amplification cannot coexist within the same cell (Etemadmoghadam et al. 2013; Kawahara et al. 2017). The amplification of *CCNE1* is associated with poor prognosis in tubo-ovarian high-grade serous carcinomas particularly in primary or refractory chemoresistant disease (Au-Yeung et al. 2017; da Costa et al. 2019; Chan et al. 2020; Gorski et al. 2020).

7.2.9 Phosphatase and Tensin Homologue (*PTEN*)

The tumor suppressor *PTEN* is commonly known as a potent inhibitor of the phosphoinositide-3 kinase (PI3K) pathway, and is seminal in the regulation of cellular proliferation, metastasis, cellular survival, genomic stability, and metabolic homeostasis (Carracedo and Pandolfi 2008). The lifetime risk of germline *PTEN* PV/LPVs carriers is approximately 25–85% for breast cancer, while the risk of OC is low or none, ranking *PTEN* as a low penetrance gene in OC (Angeli et al. 2020). Alterations in *PTEN* are mainly somatic in ovarian tumors with 6% of HGSOC showing homozygous loss of *PTEN* (Cancer Genome Atlas 2011; Martins et al. 2014), whereas in STIC lesions, *PTEN* loss was observed in 33% of patients (Roh et al. 2010).

7.2.10 Serine/Threonine Kinase 11 (*STK11*)

The serine/threonine kinase 11 (*STK11*) gene is located on chromosome 19p13.3 and encodes for a tumor suppressor that regulates cell polarity and apoptosis (Xu et al. 2013; Li et al. 2018; Zhao and Xu 2014). Commonly serving as an upstream kinase for AMP-activated protein kinase (AMPK), *STK11* is essential in regulating cell metabolism and homeostasis (Faubert et al. 2014). Germline inactivating mutations of *STK11* has historically been linked to Peutz-Jeghers syndrome, an autosomal dominant disorder with distinct clinical manifestations including melanocytic macules in lips, buccal mucosa, and digits, with multiple hamartomatous polyps in the gastrointestinal tract, and importantly a heightened risk of sporadic tumor formation (Hemminki et al. 1998; Beggs et al. 2010). In the case of *STK11* variants, the lifetime risk of breast and gynecological cancer development is 32–54%, and 13%, respectively (Lim et al. 2004; Syngal et al. 2015; George et al. 2016; Angeli et al. 2020).

7.2.11 Clinical Implications of Genetic Screening on Decision-Making

The National Comprehensive Cancer Network (NCCN) (NCCN Guidelines 2019) and the American Association of Clinical Oncology (ASCO) (Konstantinopoulos et al. 2020) published recommendations and guidelines for the management of hereditary OC (Fig. 7.1):

1. *"Germline genetic testing for BRCA1/2 and other susceptibility genes of OC should be offered to all women diagnosed with epithelial OC, irrespective of their clinical features or family history. Women who do not carry germline alterations, somatic tumor testing for BRCA1 and BRCA2 PV or LPV should be performed. Therapeutically, PARP inhibitors, that act through the mechanism of synthetic lethality, can be offered to OC patients with germline or somatic BRCA1/2 variants* (Lord and Ashworth 2017). *Importantly, the decision of sequencing germline DNA based on mutations found in tumor tissues is not recommended because of reduced sensitivity. 5% of germline mutations could be missed if tumor somatic variants are used to determine germline mutations. Missing a germline mutation could provide false reassurance for family members who may be at risk* (Konstantinopoulos et al. 2020)*."*
2. *"First-, and second-degree blood relatives of patients with germline BRCA1/2 PV or LPV, should be offered genetic testing for BRCA1 and BRCA2 PV or LPV. Surveillance protocols, including annual transvaginal ultrasound combined with serum CA-125 (although of uncertain benefit), beginning as early as 30–35 years of age) should be followed. RRSO should be considered typically between 35 and 40 years of age, and/or upon completion of childbearing* (Konstantinopoulos et al. 2020)*."*

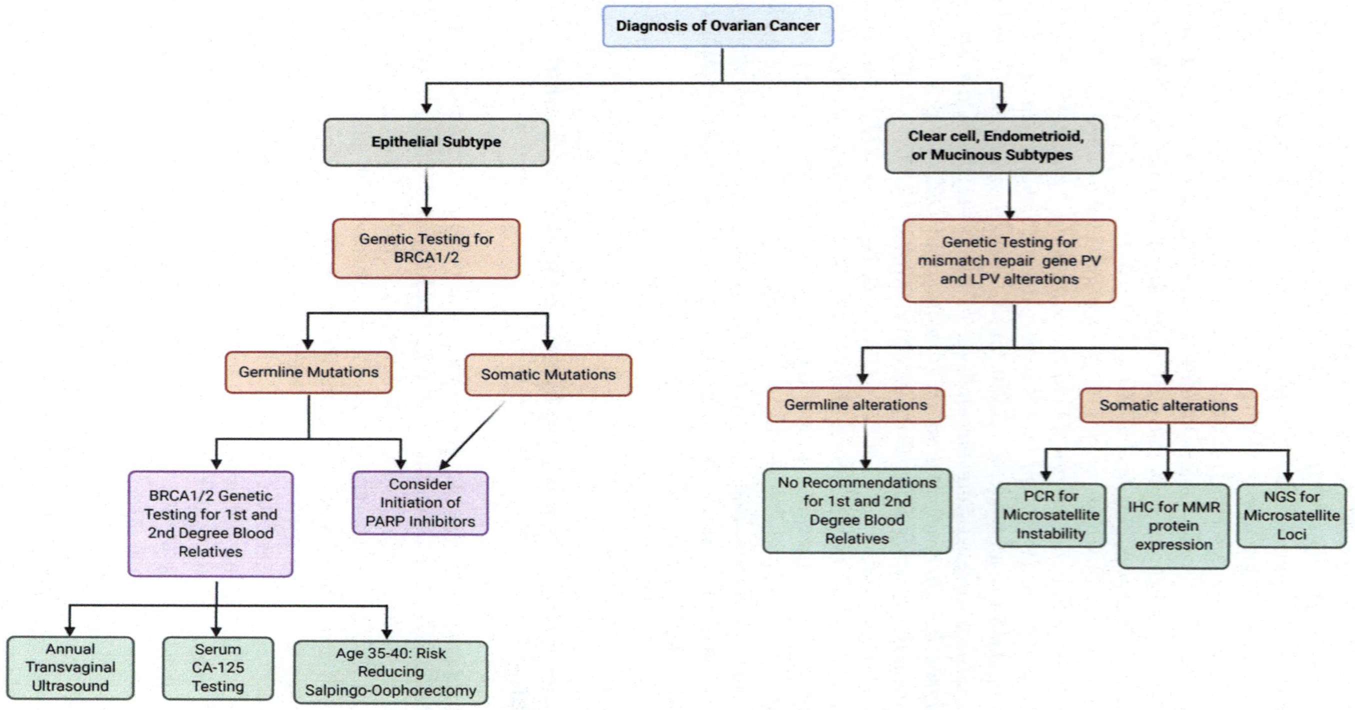

Fig. 7.1 Summary of genetic testing in ovarian cancer. Abbreviations: *BRCA* breast cancer gene, *CA-125* cancer antigen 125, *IHC* immunohistochemistry, *LPV* likely pathogenic variants, *MMR* mismatch repair, *NGS* next-generation sequencing, *PARP* poly(ADP)-ribose polymerase, *PCR* polymerase chain reaction, *PV* pathogenic variants

3. *"In case of other OC histotypes including clear cell, endometrioid, or mucinous carcinomas, patients should be offered somatic tumor testing for MMR gene PV and LPV alterations. These MMR genes can be evaluated using several available tests including polymerase chain reaction (PCR) for microsatellite instability assessment and immunohistochemistry (IHC) for the evaluation of expression status of the key MMR proteins* (McConechy et al. 2015). *Targeted NGS panels of known microsatellite loci or microsatellite regions are also valuable. However, these lack the sensitivity and the specificity for diagnostic and prognostic purposes* (Konstantinopoulos et al. 2019)."
4. *"Clinical decisions based on variants of uncertain significance (VUS) is not recommended as clinical and preclinical research and assessment of whether a variant is deleterious or benign is still underway and hence reclassification of VUS is anticipated* (Barbosa et al. 2020). *In this respect, many preclinical and clinical trials are investigating targeted agents and other innovative synthetic lethal approaches for various somatic alterations in OC subtypes, including activating or inactivating mutations of BRAF, KRAS, ARID1A, PIK3CA, and PTEN, and amplification of CCNE1, CCND1, CCND2, and MYC, as well as deletion of RB and CDKN2A genes. However, it should be appreciated that the association between specific variants and drug response to therapy may be contextual and impacted by specific tumor site, type, histology, as well as concomitant mutational landscape and molecular alterations in the tumor* (Song et al. 2015; Giri et al. 2019; Alexandrova et al. 2020; Kobayashi et al. 2018; Caumanns et al. 2018)."

7.2.12 Challenges in Developing Effective Genetic Screening Methods

Several factors pose challenges to the development of an effective and consistent screening method (NCCN Guidelines 2019; Alexandrova et al. 2020; Bowtell et al. 2015; Carter et al. 2018; Patni 2019; Soletormos et al. 2016). One factor is the low prevalence of OC in the US population. Hence, studies with large prospective cohorts, which are necessary to determine the screening accuracy of a plausible test, are difficult to conduct. Second, the inherent lack of sensitivity and specificity of putative screening markers increase the overall risk of false-negative and false-positive test results. Third, the accrued cost of testing a panel of markers poses a challenge as insurance companies are not likely to cover them (Angeli et al. 2020). Fourth, there is a lack of patient and provider education regarding the importance of genetic information which may lead to increased uncertainty and unwarranted anxiety in patient populations (Konstantinopoulos et al. 2020). Fifth, there is limited availability of genetic counselors and access to facilities that offer genetic testing. Finally, the majority of OC biomarkers are derived from advanced stages and hence are less useful for early diagnostic/screening modalities (Rauh-Hain et al. 2011).

7.3 Exploring the Impact of Next-Generation Sequencing in Ovarian Cancer Management

NGS has led to the discovery of diverse genomic alterations in epithelial OC that impacts drug resistance and survival outcomes (Gorringe and Campbell 2009; Stoffel and Carethers 2020). Unfortunately, a majority of OC patients relapse or develop resistance although the high initial response rate to standard chemotherapy. Based on both clinicopathologic and molecular features of tumors, epithelial OC is categorized into two subtypes. Type I OC is characterized by a high rate of mutations in *KRAS*, *BRAF*, *PIK3CA*, *PTEN*, and *ERBB2* genes and includes low-grade serous, mucinous, endometrioid, and clear cell tumors (Terada et al. 2016). Type II has a high frequency of *TP53* mutations and comprises high-grade serous, undifferentiated carcinomas and carcinosarcomas (Koshiyama et al. 2014; Kurman and Shih 2016). Genomic profiling studies using NGS have confirmed this genetic heterogeneity, especially in serous and endometrioid tumors. Accordingly, genetic variants and gene expression profiles can be used to better stratify patients for optimizing treatment responses. Based on a cancer panel covering the most frequently mutated genomic regions, a significant association has been found between tumor heterogeneity and OS in OC patients (Oh et al. 2019). A large proportion of high-grade epithelial OC cases have shown deficiencies in HR, in particular high-grade serous carcinoma that is the most common and the aggressive subtype (da Cunha Colombo Bonadio et al. 2018). Additionally, genomic profiling revealed that *TP53* and *BRCA1/2* are the most frequently mutated genes (Ross et al. 2013; Norquist et al. 2016b; Maru et al. 2017; Zhang et al. 2019). Approximately all tubo-ovarian high-grade serous carcinomas present *TP53* mutations (The Cancer Genome Atlas Research Network. 2011). However, *TP53* wild-type tumors show distinct morphological characteristics (The Cancer Genome Atlas Research Network. 2011). In a large cohort of sequenced tubo-ovarian high-grade serous carcinomas, the histomorphological, immunophenotypical, and molecular characteristics have been compared between *TP53* mutant and wild-type patients (Chui et al. 2020). The study confirmed that 40% of *TP53* wild-type tumors exhibit similar genetic and phenotypic characteristics as low and high-grade serous cancers while the remaining share common morphological features with *TP53* mutant high-grade serous carcinomas (Chui et al. 2020). In addition, Mandilaras et al. performed an immunohistochemical and molecular analysis of HGSOC and observed that the six studied *TP53* mutation classification schemes did not affect the patients' platinum-free interval and OS (Mandilaras et al. 2019). Remarkably, four distinct transcriptomic types of high-grade serous carcinomas have been identified; namely mesenchymal, immunoreactive, differentiated, and proliferative (Cancer Genome Atlas Research Network 2011; Bowtell 2010). Survival analyses showed that immunoreactive tumors had better outcomes than proliferative and mesenchymal subtypes (Verhaak et al. 2013; Konecny et al. 2014). Also, copy number alterations of genes involved in HR were detected in high-grade serous (63%) and clear cell carcinomas (30%) (Saotome et al. 2020). Furthermore, a significant association was observed between increased copy number alteration count ratio and advanced stages of the disease ($p = 0.0187$) (Saotome et al. 2020).

Both genes *BRCA1* and *BRCA2* are involved in many cellular pathways including DNA double-strand breaks repair by HR mechanism, transcriptional and posttranscriptional regulation of gene expression, and protein ubiquitination (Wang et al. 2000). Deficiency in HR repair pathways (Roy et al. 2011) may enhance tumor response to some targeted therapies based on platinum salts or PARPi. The large "Cancer Genome Atlas" project revealed that almost half of HGSOC are HR deficient, 20% of which are due to somatic or germline *BRCA1/2* mutations and 11% presented *BRCA1* promoter hypermethylation (The Cancer Genome Atlas Research Network 2011). Various studies that used NGS platforms have identified other genes related to this cancer type beyond the classical *BRCA* (Alsop et al. 2012; The Cancer Genome Atlas Research Network. 2011; Pennington et al. 2014; Cunningham et al. 2014; Harter et al. 2017; Norquist et al. 2016b; Yates et al. 2017; Hahnen et al. 2016). Lynch syndrome genes, especially *MHL1* and *MSH2*, involved in the human MMR system seem to play an important role in OC predisposition (Bonadona et al. 2011; Engel et al. 2012). The lifetime OC risk is estimated to be 20% and 24% for women with *MLH1* and *MSH2* mutations respectively by the age of 70 (Nielsen et al. 2016). Subsequent studies have shown that HR deficiency may be due to other genes involved in this pathway as well. DNA sequencing of 1195 women with advanced OC recruited as part of GOG218 randomized phase III trial revealed that 25% of patients have germline mutations on genes involved in HR repair pathway (Norquist et al. 2018). Nearly 12.4% of mutations have been reported in the *BRCA1* gene, 6.5% in *BRCA2*, and 6.8% in other genes including *ATM, ATR, BARD1, BLM, BRIP1, CHEK2, MRE11A, NBN, PALB2, RAD51C, RAD51D, RBBP8, SLX4*, and *XRCC2* (Norquist et al. 2018). Somatic mutations have also been found in 9.9% of patients with respective frequencies of 5.2%, 2.2%, and 2.5% (Norquist et al. 2018). Similarly, Zhao et al. performed NGS of 31 HR genes in 50 Chinese women with confirmed epithelial OC and germline mutations were found in 36% patients (Zhao et al. 2017). Somatic mutations have also been found in 10% of patients and the most frequent alterations identified were in *RAD50, ATR,* and *CHEK2* genes (41.7%) (Zhao et al. 2017).

BRCA1/2 mutational status is considered as an accurate predictive and prognostic biomarker for platinum-based treatments. This is mainly due to HR deficiency that characterizes such tumors. Indeed, cancers associated with pathogenic *BRCA1/2* variants are unable to repair DNA double-strand breaks induced by platinum compounds. It has been found that OC patients harboring *BRCA1/2* germline mutation and treated with platinum have better survival. High platinum sensitivity and increased remission rates have been observed in epithelial OC patients with germline or somatic mutations in *BRCA1/2* (Zhao et al. 2017). In a cohort of 353 OC patients, the investigators observed that women with mutations in the RAD51-binding domain of *BRCA* have a significantly prolonged platinum-free interval (29.7 vs. 83 15.5 months; $p = 0.011$) and superior progression-free survival (PFS) at 5 years (HR: 0.36; 95% CI: 0.20-0.64; $p = 0.001$) as compared with patients with non-*BRCA* carriers (Labidi-Galy et al. 2018).

Germline and somatic mutations in *BRCA1/2* genes have also been considered as potential biomarkers of tumor response to PARPi therapy (*see previous chapters for details*). PARP is a key enzyme in the base excision repair pathway. It mediates the recruitment of many other proteins to DNA damage sites, to trigger the repair process. Inhibition of these enzymes blocks the base excision repair system leading to the conversion of single-strand breaks to double-strand breaks during replication (Dedes et al. 2011; Ledermann 2016). Consequently, the use of PARPi would be more effective when HR pathway is dysfunctional, such as in tumors with *BRCA1/2* mutations particularly OC (Bryant et al. 2005; Donawho et al. 2007; Ashworth 2008). Several clinical trials have assessed the benefit of PARPi in OC patients with germline *BRCA1/2* mutations (*see Chap. 3 for details*). Various PARPi such as olaparib, rucaparib, and niraparib are currently approved and used for OC treatment (Boussios et al. 2020; Balasubramaniam et al. 2017). Olaparib was the first PARPi approved for use as maintenance therapy for patients with platinum-sensitive relapsed OC and *BRCA1/2* mutations. This was mainly based on the promising results of randomized phase III trials such as SOLO-1 (Moore et al. 2018) and ARIEL-related studies (Kristeleit et al. 2017, 2019; Swisher et al. 2017; Coleman et al. 2017). In addition, investigation of HR pathway in OC treated with rucaparib showed that patients with *BRCA* mutations and those with high loss of heterozygosity (LOH) had longer PFS and better median duration of response than patients with low LOH tumors (Swisher et al. 2017). Simultaneously, the approval of these PARPi authorized a tumor tissue-based NGS assay called FoundationFocus™ CDxBRCA LOH able to detect somatic and germline *BRCA1/2* mutations as well as the percentage of LOH for patient's selection. Furthermore, mutational screening of *BRCA1/2* mutations in formalin-fixed and paraffin-embedded (FFPE) tumors using NGS has been found to be valid and reliable (Ellison et al. 2015; Mafficini et al. 2016; Weren et al. 2017). An international round-robin has approved *BRCA1/2* NGS screening in FFPE tumors of patients with high-grade serous carcinoma with an overall success rate of 81% (Endris et al. 2016).

In order to identify predictive biomarkers of chemotherapy resistance, NGS was used in other OC studies that focused on additional genes and pathways beyond BRCA such as *ARID1A* and *c-MYC*. Aurora kinases (AURK) play an important role in OC development (Pérez-Fidalgo et al. 2020) and are involved in cell division, cell cycle control, and DNA repair defects. Experimental data showed that OC cells overexpress AURK proteins, especially AURKA and AURKB (Lassmann et al. 2007; Chen et al. 2009). These kinases influence response to chemotherapy (Yang et al. 2006; Sun et al. 2007, 2020). In this perspective, a phase II study of ENMD-2076—a selective AURK inhibitor—in patients with recurrent ovarian clear cell carcinoma found that 6-month PFS was better in patients with loss of AT-rich interactive domain 1A (ARID1A) expression than those with normal *ARID1A* (33% vs. 12%, $p = 0.023$) (Lheureux et al. 2018). In contrast, no significant difference was observed in median PFS by sequencing *ARID1A* gene, thus suggesting the existence of an alternative mechanism of loss of expression (Lheureux et al. 2018). *ARID1A* gene encodes for a subunit of the human SWI/SNF chromatin remodelling complex, which plays a role in epigenetic regulatory mechanisms. Mutations in this gene appear to be more common in clear cell and low-grade endometrioid tumors (Wiegand et al. 2010; Jones et al. 2010). These findings suggest that *ARID1A* gene expression could be considered as a predictive biomarker to guide patients' selection for treatment with AURKA inhibitors. On the other hand, *c-MYC* gene amplification has been previously described in OC and is implicated in drug resistance. *C-MYC* is a proto-oncogene involved in the regulation of cell growth, proliferation, metabolism, and apoptosis (Kalkat et al. 2017). Moreover, high levels of c-MYC expression in patients with HGSOS have been found to be significantly associated with decreased PFS ($p = 0.0277$) and OS ($p = 0.0058$) (Reyes-González et al. 2015). More importantly, inactivation of bromodomain and extra-terminal motif (BET) protein can downregulate *c-MYC* gene transcription (Delmore et al. 2011). Therefore, BET inhibitors may represent a potential therapy for ovarian tumors overexpressing c-MYC. Recently, a whole-exome sequencing study showed that *c-MYC* amplifications occur in 74% of primary ovarian tumors, 78% of metastatic tumors, and 82% of recurrent OCs (Li et al. 2019). Moreover, preclinical analyses performed in xenografts and patient-derived xenografts models using ovarian resistant cell lines demonstrated that increased sensitivity to BET inhibitors (GS-626510 and JQ1) is associated with *c-MYC* amplification (Li et al. 2019).

Genomics has also the potential to examine the actionable information in circulating tumor cells (CTC), cell-free DNA (cfDNA), and circulating tumor DNA (ctDNA) derived from fragmented tumor cells released in body fluids (El Bairi et al. 2020b). The implementation of liquid biopsy approaches provided information on disease screening, progression, relapse, and treatment response. Furthermore, ctDNA methylation analyses enabled precise evaluation of tissue of origin, fragmentation size, structures, and release mechanisms. In OC, *BRCA1* and *TP53* mutations are also present in cfDNA suggesting its possible role as a potential biomarker (Giannopoulou et al. 2018). A number of studies have used high-throughput sequencing to assess genetic alterations in liquid biopsy samples from OC patients. Recently, a report of 20 HGSOC patients confirmed that digital PCR or NGS technologies were able to detect *TP53* mutations in serum cfDNA (Vitale et al. 2020). *TP53* missense mutations were present in tumor tissues and serum cfDNA in 53% of patients at diagnosis. Interestingly, these mutations disappeared with treatment and reappeared at tumor progression which makes this strategy promising for monitoring therapy and follow-up. Vanderstichele et al. compared the chromosome instability in cfDNA and tumor samples in OC patients with adnexal masses and found that somatic copy number variations in cfDNA were similar to those detected in tumors (Vanderstichele et al. 2017). In terms of accuracy, *TP53* and *BRCA1* mutations in both ctDNA and tumor tissues of drug resistant recurrent OCs seem to be highly consistent with tumor bulky data (Du et al. 2018). *BRCA1* and *BRCA2* somatic mutations have been detected in cfDNA of OC patients harboring germline *BRCA* mutations and resistant to platinum-based chemotherapy and PARPi. *BRCA1/2* reversion somatic mutations in cfDNA of patients with recurrent high-grade serous OC can be explored using NGS which may be used for monitoring response to PARPi (Christie and Bowtell 2017). In agreement with these findings, a large cohort of HGSOC recently explored *BRCA* reversion mutations after earlier treatment with platinum-based chemotherapy and their ability to predict response to PARPi (Li et al. 2019). NGS of plasma cfDNA collected from patients with germline or somatic *BRCA* mutations revealed that the presence of *BRCA* reversion mutations of platinum-resistant or refractory HGSOC were correlated with reduced benefits from rucaparib treatment (Li et al. 2019). Therefore, the combination of NGS and liquid biopsy approaches, especially circulating DNA may be used in the future for this purpose if mature findings from large interventional trials support the current evidence (*see Chap. 5 for further reading on this topic*).

7.4 Single-Cell Sequencing Technology to Depict Ovarian Cancer Heterogeneity

The advent of NGS and single-cell sequencing (SCS) has transformed the current understanding of the cancer contexture (Lawson et al. 2018; Suvà and Tirosh 2019; Bagger and Probst 2020). SCS enables high throughput sequencing of cancer cells one at a time, which allows for better assessment of tumor cellular heterogeneity, clonal evolution, and mechanisms of drug resistance (El Bairi et al. 2020b). A number of recent translational studies have illuminated the single-cell landscape of ovarian tumors and its considerable association with clinical outcomes (Winterhoff et al. 2019). Previously, Winterhoff et al. investigated the levels of heterogeneity in HGSOC based on single-cell RNA sequencing of tumor and stromal cells (Winterhoff et al. 2017). The investigators were able to demonstrate two major clones of cells. In the epithelial group, genes related to proliferative properties such as MYC were markedly noticed. In addition, high expression of genes associated with extracellular matrix and epithelial-to-mesenchymal transition was observed in the stromal subpopulation. Notably, these identified cells and their signatures were not found to be correlated with chemoresistant phenotypes. However, these markers were associated with cancer cell stemness (Winterhoff et al. 2017) which is a well-known hallmark that confers drug resistance (reviewed elsewhere: Chen et al. 2021; Marzagalli et al. 2021). Soon after, two other teams confirmed that this technology is also applicable for identifying the cell of origin of OC (Vuong et al. 2018; Shih et al. 2018). In a preclinical study, cells of the ovarian surface epithelium were treated with estradiol and were characterized by single-cell RNA sequencing to decipher their transcriptional dynamics (Vuong et al. 2018). These dysplastic cells were distinguished by their upregulation of genes related to proliferation, metabolism, and survival signaling. Moreover, the study findings also showed that the *Greb1* gene is expressed in an estrogen-driven precancerous state of these cells and is a potential biomarker for the transition from dysplasia to cancer (Vuong et al. 2018). Of note, OCs commonly express GREB1 which is an estrogen receptor-regulated tumor promoter (Hodgkinson et al. 2018) and involved in ovarian tumor progression (Laviolette et al. 2014). In another study using human OC samples, sixteen different cancer cell subpopulations were identified and were associated with various OC histotypes and benign tumors (Shih et al. 2018).

Notably, the proportion of these cells changed noticeably between the primary and metastatic sites (Shih et al. 2018). To date, the origins of OC including fallopian tubes and ovarian surface epithelia and the related mechanisms of tumor progression are still debated and the arrival of SCS may provide additional discoveries for this unresolved mystery. More recently, Hu et al. showed that nongenetic heterogeneity in serous OC can be precisely assessed when guided by the molecular profiling of normal fallopian tube cells, which are believed to drive ovarian tumorigenesis (Hu et al. 2020). Analysis of 6000 fallopian tube cells identified 6 cell subpopulations and substantial intra-tumor nongenetic heterogeneity was noticed, which was associated with survival outcomes in this setting (Hu et al. 2020). The single-cell RNA sequencing of 11,000 cells in the ascites of OC patients demonstrated an important inter-patient variability of ascites cells including fibroblasts with immunomodulatory properties and macrophages (Izar et al. 2020). In addition, the findings of this report confirmed the previous subclassification of HGSOC into immunoreactive and mesenchymal types with abundant immune infiltrates and fibroblasts. This highlights the notable place of tumor microenvironment in this novel classification. Genetically, this variability was associated with heterogeneous copy number alterations and activation of cancer stemness. Based on OC patient-derived xenografts, the authors showed that the expressed JAK/STAT signaling in cancer cells and cancer-associated fibroblasts is potentially targetable for drug discovery (Izar et al. 2020). The chronology of HGSOC subtype clonal evolution was investigated in another recent study using data from The Cancer Genome Atlas and SCS of ovarian tumors (Geistlinger et al. 2020). A marked difference between OC subtypes in terms of subclonality, ploidy, and tumor purity was noticed. Furthermore, genomic alterations in these subtypes diverged at later stages of tumor evolution and were typically subclonal. In proliferative tumors, this subclonality was characterized by prominent genomic instability and absence of immune infiltrates. On the contrary, differentiated tumors had undamaged genome integrity and high immune infiltrates. SCS of 42,000 tumor cells also demonstrated prevalent heterogeneity in the composition of ovarian tumors regarding tumor cell types (Geistlinger et al. 2020). Therapeutically, SCS also presents a good opportunity for improved comprehension of the mechanisms of resistance to the emerging PARPi. In this perspective, Färkkilä et al. generated single-cell clones of resistant tumor cells to PARPi based on CRISPR/Cas9 technology and showed various mechanisms of resistance (Färkkilä et al. 2021). In some studied clones, multiple mechanisms of resistance at the same time were observed. Clonal selection of resistant cells occurred in a heterogeneous sensitive cell population with pre-existent drug tolerance. The analysis of tumor specimens from a patient with mutated *BRCA1* and having resistance to PARPi showed a clonal and spatial heterogeneity. Remarkably, the study also showed that these clones have different responses to targeted agents and therefore, demonstrating that resistant cells to PARPi need additional therapies to bypass PARPi resistance (Färkkilä et al. 2021). The utility of SCS in depicting the global picture of OC heterogeneity was supported by these proof-of-concept studies. Additional research using this technology is needed to determine molecular features that influence outcomes in this aggressive cancer.

7.5 Conclusion

The genetics of OC is becoming actionable especially with the emergence of targeted therapeutics that require predictive biomarkers for patients' selection as well as cancer risk assessment. NGS enables multiple and simultaneous OC genetic testing of relevant genes with a rapid turnaround time. Moreover, SCS provides a window of opportunities to better characterize OC heterogeneity. Further studies of OC genetics particularly in the context of clinical trials are awaited. For additional reading, see Box 7.1.

Box 7.1 Recommended reading of particular interest

	DOI
McAlarnen L, et al. **Challenges of Genomic Testing for Hereditary Breast and Ovarian Cancers**. Appl Clin Genet. 2021 14;14:1-9.	https://doi.org/10.2147/TACG.S245021
Pujol P, et al. **Clinical practice guidelines for BRCA1 and BRCA2 genetic testing**. Eur J Cancer. 2021;146:30-47.	https://doi.org/10.1016/j.ejca.2020.12.023
Koldehoff A, et al. **Cost-Effectiveness of Targeted Genetic Testing for Breast and Ovarian Cancer: A Systematic Review**. Value Health. 2021;24(2):303-312.	https://doi.org/10.1016/j.jval.2020.09.016
Bonadio RC, et al. **Ovarian cancer risk assessment in the era of next-generation sequencing**. Ann Transl Med. 2020;8(24):1704.	https://doi.org/10.21037/atm-20-1582
Ponzone R. **BRCA1/2 status and chemotherapy response score to tailor ovarian cancer surgery**. Crit Rev Oncol Hematol. 2021;157:103128.	https://doi.org/10.1016/j.critrevonc.2020.103128
Haunschild CE, Tewari KS. **The current landscape of molecular profiling in the treatment of epithelial ovarian cancer**. Gynecol Oncol. 2021;160(1):333-345.	https://doi.org/10.1016/j.ygyno.2020.09.043
Shih IM, et al. **The Origin of Ovarian Cancer Species and Precancerous Landscape**. Am J Pathol. 2021;191(1):26-39.	https://doi.org/10.1016/j.ajpath.2020.09.006
Pietragalla A, et al. **Ovarian cancer predisposition beyond BRCA1 and BRCA2 genes**. Int J Gynecol Cancer. 2020;30(11):1803-1810.	https://doi.org/10.1136/ijgc-2020-001556
Yoshida R. **Hereditary breast and ovarian cancer (HBOC): review of its molecular characteristics, screening, treatment, and prognosis**. Breast Cancer. 2020.	https://doi.org/10.1007/s12282-020-01148-2

Acknowledgment and Conflicts of Interest KE is an editor in Springer Nature Journals and a previous editor for a Springer Book (https://link.springer.com/book/10.1007/978-3-030-53821-7). AG and NS are supported by T32 GM127261 R01-CA193437 grants respectively.

Authors' Contribution AG and NS wrote Sect. 7.2. AT and KE wrote Sects. 7.3 and 7.4, respectively. KE coordinated the development of the chapter idea and shared a preliminary content discussion. The final draft was reviewed and approved by all the authors. The contents of the chapter reflect the authors' perspectives and not of their institutions of affiliation.

References

Ahmed AA et al (2010) Driver mutations in TP53 are ubiquitous in high grade serous carcinoma of the ovary. J Pathol 221(1):49–56

Alexandrova E et al (2020) An overview of candidate therapeutic target genes in ovarian cancer. Cancers 12(6):1470

Alsop K, Fereday S, Meldrum C, de Fazio A, Emmanuel C, George J, Dobrovic A, Birrer MJ, Webb PM, Stewart C, Friedlander M, Fox S, Bowtell D, Mitchell G (2012) BRCA mutation frequency and patterns of treatment response in BRCA mutation-positive women with ovarian cancer: a report from the Australian Ovarian Cancer Study Group. J Clin Oncol 30 (21):2654–2663. https://doi.org/10.1200/JCO.2011.39.8545

American Cancer Society (2020) Key statistics for ovarian cancer. Accessed 12/2020

Amin N, Chaabouni N, George A (2020) Genetic testing for epithelial ovarian cancer. Best Pract Res Clin Obstet Gynaecol 65:125–138. https://doi.org/10.1016/j.bpobgyn.2020.01.005

Angeli D, Salvi S, Tedaldi G (2020) Genetic predisposition to breast and ovarian cancers: how many and which genes to test? Int J Mol Sci 21(3):1128

Antony E et al (2009) Srs2 disassembles Rad51 filaments by a protein-protein interaction triggering ATP turnover and dissociation of Rad51 from DNA. Mol Cell 35(1):105–115

Arts-de Jong M et al (2016) Germline BRCA1/2 mutation testing is indicated in every patient with epithelial ovarian cancer: a systematic review. Eur J Cancer 61:137–145

Ashworth A (2008) Drug resistance caused by reversion mutation. Cancer Res 68 (24):10021–10023. https://doi.org/10.1158/0008-5472.CAN-08-2287

Au-Yeung G et al (2017) Selective targeting of cyclin E1-amplified high-grade serous ovarian Cancer by cyclin-dependent kinase 2 and AKT inhibition. Clin Cancer Res 23(7):1862–1874

Bagger FO, Probst V (2020) Single cell sequencing in cancer diagnostics. Adv Exp Med Biol 1255:175–193. https://doi.org/10.1007/978-981-15-4494-1_15

Balasubramaniam S, Beaver JA, Horton S et al (2017) FDA approval summary: Rucaparib for the treatment of patients with deleterious BRCA mutation-associated advanced ovarian cancer. Clin Cancer Res 23(23):7165–7170. https://doi.org/10.1158/1078-0432.CCR-17-1337

Balmana J, Domchek SM (2015) BRIP1 as an ovarian cancer susceptibility gene: ready for the clinic? J Natl Cancer Inst 107(11):djv262

Barbosa A et al (2020) Gene panel tumor testing in ovarian cancer patients significantly increases the yield of clinically actionable germline variants beyond BRCA1/BRCA2. Cancers 12 (10):2834

Beggs AD et al (2010) Peutz-Jeghers syndrome: a systematic review and recommendations for management. Gut 59(7):975–986

Bogdanova NV et al (2019) A splice site variant of CDK12 and breast cancer in three Eurasian populations. Front Oncol 9:493

Bonadona V, Bonaïti B, Olschwang S, Grandjouan S, Huiart L, Longy M, Guimbaud R, Buecher B, Bignon YJ, Caron O, Colas C, Noguès C, Lejeune-Dumoulin S, Olivier-Faivre L, Polycarpe-Osaer F, Nguyen TD, Desseigne F, Saurin JC, Berthet P, Leroux D, Duffour J, Manouvrier S, Frébourg T, Sobol H, Lasset C, Bonaïti-Pellié C, French Cancer Genetics Network (2011) Cancer risks associated with germline mutations in MLH1, MSH2, and MSH6 genes in lynch syndrome. JAMA 305(22):2304–2310. https://doi.org/10.1001/jama.2011.743

Boussios S, Karihtala P, Moschetta M, Abson C, Karathanasi A, Zakynthinakis-Kyriakou N, Ryan JE, Sheriff M, Rassy E, Pavlidis N (2020) Veliparib in ovarian cancer: a new synthetically lethal therapeutic approach. Investig New Drugs 38(1):181–193. https://doi.org/10.1007/s10637-019-00867-4

Bowtell DD (2010) The genesis and evolution of high-grade serous ovarian cancer. Nat Rev Cancer 10(11):803–808. https://doi.org/10.1038/nrc2946

Bowtell DD et al (2015) Rethinking ovarian cancer II: reducing mortality from high-grade serous ovarian cancer. Nat Rev Cancer 15(11):668–679

Bryant H, Schultz N, Thomas H et al (2005) Specific killing of BRCA2-deficient tumours with inhibitors of poly (ADP-ribose) polymerase. Nature 434:913–917. https://doi.org/10.1038/nature03443

Cancer Genome Atlas Research Network (2011) Integrated genomic analyses of ovarian carcinoma. Nature 474(7353):609–615. https://doi.org/10.1038/nature10166. Erratum in: Nature. 2012; 490 (7419): 298

Carethers JM, Stoffel EM (2015) Lynch syndrome and lynch syndrome mimics: the growing complex landscape of hereditary colon cancer. World J Gastroenterol 21(31):9253–9261

Carracedo A, Pandolfi PP (2008) The PTEN-PI3K pathway: of feedbacks and cross-talks. Oncogene 27(41):5527–5541

Carter NJ, Marshall ML, Susswein LR, Zorn KK, Hiraki S, Arvai KJ, Torene RI, McGill AK, Yackowski L, Murphy PD, Xu Z, Solomon BD, Klein RT, Hruska KS (2018) Germline pathogenic variants identified in women with ovarian tumors. Gynecol Oncol 151 (3):481–488. https://doi.org/10.1016/j.ygyno.2018.09.030

Caumanns JJ et al (2018) ARID1A mutant ovarian clear cell carcinoma: a clear target for synthetic lethal strategies. Biochim Biophys Acta Rev Cancer 1870(2):176–184

Chan AM et al (2020) Combined CCNE1 high-level amplification and overexpression is associated with unfavourable outcome in tubo-ovarian high-grade serous carcinoma. J Pathol Clin Res 6 (4):252–262

Chen YJ, Chen CM, Twu NF, Yen MS, Lai CR, Wu HH, Wang PH, Yuan CC (2009) Overexpression of Aurora B is associated with poor prognosis in epithelial ovarian cancer patients. Virchows Arch 455(5):431–440. https://doi.org/10.1007/s00428-009-0838-3

Chen P, Hsu WH, Han J, Xia Y, DePinho RA (2021) Cancer stemness meets immunity: from mechanism to therapy. Cell Rep 34(1):108597. https://doi.org/10.1016/j.celrep.2020.108597

Chien J et al (2015) TP53 mutations, tetraploidy and homologous recombination repair defects in early stage high-grade serous ovarian cancer. Nucleic Acids Res 43(14):6945–6958

Chou J et al (2020) Transcription-associated cyclin-dependent kinases as targets and biomarkers for cancer therapy. Cancer Discov 10(3):351–370

Christie EL, Bowtell DDL (2017) Acquired chemotherapy resistance in ovarian cancer. Ann Oncol 28(suppl_8):viii13–viii15. https://doi.org/10.1093/annonc/mdx446

Chui MH, Momeni Boroujeni A, Mandelker D, Ladanyi M, Soslow RA (2020) Characterization of TP53-wildtype tubo-ovarian high-grade serous carcinomas: rare exceptions to the binary classification of ovarian serous carcinoma. Mod Pathol 34:490–501. https://doi.org/10.1038/s41379-020-00648-y

Coleman RL, Oza AM, Lorusso D et al (2017) Rucaparib maintenance treatment for recurrent ovarian carcinoma after response to platinum therapy (ARIEL3): a randomised, double-blind, placebo-controlled, phase 3 trial. Lancet 390(10106):1949–1961. https://doi.org/10.1016/S0140-6736(17)32440-6

Cunningham JM, Cicek MS, Larson NB, Davila J, Wang C, Larson MC, Song H, Dicks EM, Harrington P, Wick M, Winterhoff BJ, Hamidi H, Konecny GE, Chien J, Bibikova M, Fan JB, Kalli KR, Lindor NM, Fridley BL, Pharoah PP, Goode EL (2014) Clinical characteristics of ovarian cancer classified by BRCA1, BRCA2, and RAD51C status. Sci Rep 4:4026. https://doi.org/10.1038/srep04026

da Costa A et al (2019) Genomic profiling in ovarian cancer retreated with platinum based chemotherapy presented homologous recombination deficiency and copy number imbalances of CCNE1 and RB1 genes. BMC Cancer 19(1):422

da Cunha Colombo Bonadio RR, Fogace RN, Miranda VC, MDPE D (2018) Homologous recombination deficiency in ovarian cancer: a review of its epidemiology and management. Clinics (Sao Paulo) 73(suppl 1):e450s. https://doi.org/10.6061/clinics/2018/e450s

Dedes KJ, Wilkerson PM, Wetterskog D, Weigelt B, Ashworth A, Reis-Filho JS (2011) Synthetic lethality of PARP inhibition in cancers lacking BRCA1 and BRCA2 mutations. Cell Cycle 10 (8):1192–1199. https://doi.org/10.4161/cc.10.8.15273

Delmore JE, Issa GC, Lemieux ME, Rahl PB, Shi J, Jacobs HM, Kastritis E, Gilpatrick T, Paranal RM, Qi J, Chesi M, Schinzel AC, McKeown MR, Heffernan TP, Vakoc CR, Bergsagel PL, Ghobrial IM, Richardson PG, Young RA, Hahn WC, Anderson KC, Kung AL, Bradner JE, Mitsiades CS (2011) BET bromodomain inhibition as a therapeutic strategy to target c-Myc. Cell 146(6):904–917. https://doi.org/10.1016/j.cell.2011.08.017

Donawho CK, Luo Y, Luo Y et al (2007) ABT-888, an orally active poly (ADP-ribose) polymerase inhibitor that potentiates DNA-damaging agents in preclinical tumor models. Clin Cancer Res 13(9):2728–2737. https://doi.org/10.1158/1078-0432.CCR-06-3039

Du ZH, Bi FF, Wang L, Yang Q (2018) Next-generation sequencing unravels extensive genetic alteration in recurrent ovarian cancer and unique genetic changes in drug-resistant recurrent ovarian cancer. Mol Genet Genomic Med 6(4):638–647. https://doi.org/10.1002/mgg3.414

Dziadkowiec KN et al (2016) PARP inhibitors: review of mechanisms of action and BRCA1/2 mutation targeting. Prz Menopauzalny 15(4):215–219

El Bairi K, Azzam F, Amrani M (2020a) The arrival of next-generation sequencing: an overview of current technologies. In: El Bairi K (ed) Illuminating colorectal cancer genomics by next-generation sequencing. Springer, Cham. https://doi.org/10.1007/978-3-030-53821-7_3

El Bairi K, Trapani D, Amrani M (2020b) The revolution of liquid biopsy and single-cell sequencing in the management of colorectal cancer. In: El Bairi K (ed) Illuminating colorectal cancer genomics by next-generation sequencing. Springer, Cham. https://doi.org/10.1007/978-3-030-53821-7_6

Ellison G, Huang S, Carr H, Wallace A, Ahdesmaki M, Bhaskar S, Mills J (2015) A reliable method for the detection of BRCA1 and BRCA2 mutations in fixed tumour tissue utilising multiplex PCR-based targeted next generation sequencing. BMC Clin Pathol 15:5. https://doi.org/10.1186/s12907-015-0004-6

Endris V, Stenzinger A, Pfarr N et al (2016) NGS-based BRCA1/2 mutation testing of high-grade serous ovarian cancer tissue: results and conclusions of the first international round robin trial. Virchows Arch 468(6):697–705. https://doi.org/10.1007/s00428-016-1919-8

Engel C, Loeffler M, Steinke V, Rahner N, Holinski-Feder E, Dietmaier W, Schackert HK, Goergens H, von Knebel Doeberitz M, Goecke TO, Schmiegel W, Buettner R, Moeslein G, Letteboer TG, Gómez García E, Hes FJ, Hoogerbrugge N, Menko FH, van Os TA, Sijmons RH, Wagner A, Kluijt I, Propping P, Vasen HF (2012) Risks of less common cancers in proven mutation carriers with lynch syndrome. J Clin Oncol 30(35):4409–4415. https://doi.org/10.1200/JCO.2012.43.2278

Erickson BK et al (2014) Detection of somatic TP53 mutations in tampons of patients with high-grade serous ovarian cancer. Obstet Gynecol 124(5):881–885

Eskander RN, Tewari KS (2014) PARP inhibition and synthetic lethality in ovarian cancer. Expert Rev Clin Pharmacol 7(5):613–622

Etemadmoghadam D et al (2013) Synthetic lethality between CCNE1 amplification and loss of BRCA1. Proc Natl Acad Sci U S A 110(48):19489–19494

Faraoni I, Graziani G (2018) Role of BRCA mutations in cancer treatment with poly (ADP-ribose) polymerase (PARP) inhibitors. Cancers 10(12):487

Färkkilä A, Rodríguez A, Oikkonen J, Gulhan DC, Nguyen H, Domínguez J, Ramos S, Mills CE, Perez-Villatoro F, Lazaro JB, Zhou J, Clairmont CS, Moreau LA, Park PJ, Sorger PK, Hautaniemi S, Frias S, D'Andrea AD (2021) Heterogeneity and clonal evolution of acquired PARP inhibitor resistance in TP53- and BRCA1-deficient cells. Cancer Res 81(10):2774–2787. canres.2912.2020. https://doi.org/10.1158/0008-5472.CAN-20-2912

Faubert B et al (2014) Loss of the tumor suppressor LKB1 promotes metabolic reprogramming of cancer cells via HIF-1alpha. Proc Natl Acad Sci U S A 111(7):2554–2559

Fleury H et al (2019) Exploiting interconnected synthetic lethal interactions between PARP inhibition and cancer cell reversible senescence. Nat Commun 10(1):2556

Frey MK, Pothuri B (2017) Homologous recombination deficiency (HRD) testing in ovarian cancer clinical practice: a review of the literature. Gynecol Oncol Res Pract 4:4

Geistlinger L, Oh S, Ramos M, Schiffer L, LaRue RS, Henzler CM, Munro SA, Daughters C, Nelson AC, Winterhoff BJ, Chang Z, Talukdar S, Shetty M, Mullany SA, Morgan M, Parmigiani G, Birrer MJ, Qin LX, Riester M, Starr TK, Waldron L (2020) Multiomic analysis of subtype evolution and heterogeneity in high-grade serous ovarian carcinoma. Cancer Res 80 (20):4335–4345. https://doi.org/10.1158/0008-5472.CAN-20-0521

George SH et al (2016) Loss of LKB1 and p53 synergizes to alter fallopian tube epithelial phenotype and high-grade serous tumorigenesis. Oncogene 35(1):59–68

Germano G, Amirouchene-Angelozzi N, Rospo G, Bardelli A (2018) The clinical impact of the genomic landscape of mismatch repair-deficient cancers. Cancer Discov 8(12):1518–1528. https://doi.org/10.1158/2159-8290.CD-18-0150

Giannopoulou L, Kasimir-Bauer S, Lianidou ES (2018) Liquid biopsy in ovarian cancer: recent advances on circulating tumor cells and circulating tumor DNA. Clin Chem Lab Med 56 (2):186–197. https://doi.org/10.1515/cclm-2017-0019

Giri VN, Hyatt C, Gomella LG (2019) Germline testing for men with prostate cancer: navigating an expanding New World of genetic evaluation for precision therapy and precision management. J Clin Oncol 37(17):1455–1459

Gorodetska I, Kozeretska I, Dubrovska A (2019) BRCA genes: the role in genome stability, cancer stemness and therapy resistance. J Cancer 10(9):2109–2127

Gorringe KL, Campbell IG (2009) Large-scale genomic analysis of ovarian carcinomas. Mol Oncol 3(2):157–164. https://doi.org/10.1016/j.molonc.2008.12.005

Gorski JW, Ueland FR, Kolesar JM (2020) CCNE1 amplification as a predictive biomarker of chemotherapy resistance in epithelial ovarian cancer. Diagnostics (Basel) 10(5):279

Guillotin D, Martin SA (2014) Exploiting DNA mismatch repair deficiency as a therapeutic strategy. Exp Cell Res 329(1):110–115

Hahnen E, Baumann KH, Heimbach A et al (2016) Prevalence of somatic mutations in risk genes including BRCA1/2 in consecutive ovarian cancer patients (AGO-TR-1 study). J Clin Oncol 34 (15_suppl):5544–5544. https://doi.org/10.1200/JCO.2016.34.15_suppl.5544

Hampel H et al (2015) A practice guideline from the American College of Medical Genetics and Genomics and the National Society of genetic counselors: referral indications for cancer predisposition assessment. Genet Med 17(1):70–87

Harter P, Hauke J, Heitz F et al (2017) Prevalence of deleterious germline variants in risk genes including BRCA1/2 in consecutive ovarian cancer patients (AGO-TR-1). PLoS One 12(10): e0186043. https://doi.org/10.1371/journal.pone.0186043

Helder-Woolderink JM et al (2016) Ovarian cancer in lynch syndrome; a systematic review. Eur J Cancer 55:65–73

Helleday T (2011) The underlying mechanism for the PARP and BRCA synthetic lethality: clearing up the misunderstandings. Mol Oncol 5(4):387–393

Hemminki A et al (1998) A serine/threonine kinase gene defective in Peutz-Jeghers syndrome. Nature 391(6663):184–187

Hodgkinson K, Forrest LA, Vuong N, Garson K, Djordjevic B, Vanderhyden BC (2018) GREB1 is an estrogen receptor-regulated tumour promoter that is frequently expressed in ovarian cancer. Oncogene 37(44):5873–5886. https://doi.org/10.1038/s41388-018-0377-y

Howitt BE et al (2017) Clear cell ovarian cancers with microsatellite instability: a unique subset of ovarian cancers with increased tumor-infiltrating lymphocytes and PD-1/PD-L1 expression. Onco Targets Ther 6(2):e1277308

Hu Z, Artibani M, Alsaadi A, Wietek N, Morotti M, Shi T, Zhong Z, Santana Gonzalez L, El-Sahhar S, Karami Nejad Ranjbar M, Mallett G, Feng Y, Masuda K, Zheng Y, Chong K,

Damato S, Dhar S, Campo L, Garruto Campanile R, Soleymani Majd H, Rai V, Maldonado-Perez D, Jones S, Cerundolo V, Sauka-Spengler T, Yau C, Ahmed AA (2020) The repertoire of serous ovarian cancer non-genetic heterogeneity revealed by single-cell sequencing of normal fallopian tube epithelial cells. Cancer Cell 37(2):226–242.e7. https://doi.org/10.1016/j.ccell.2020.01.003

Izar B, Tirosh I, Stover EH, Wakiro I, Cuoco MS, Alter I, Rodman C, Leeson R, Su MJ, Shah P, Iwanicki M, Walker SR, Kanodia A, Melms JC, Mei S, Lin JR, Porter CBM, Slyper M, Waldman J, Jerby-Arnon L, Ashenberg O, Brinker TJ, Mills C, Rogava M, Vigneau S, Sorger PK, Garraway LA, Konstantinopoulos PA, Liu JF, Matulonis U, Johnson BE, Rozenblatt-Rosen O, Rotem A, Regev A (2020) A single-cell landscape of high-grade serous ovarian cancer. Nat Med 26(8):1271–1279. https://doi.org/10.1038/s41591-020-0926-0

Jones S, Wang TL, IeM S, Mao TL, Nakayama K, Roden R, Glas R, Slamon D, Diaz LA Jr, Vogelstein B, Kinzler KW, Velculescu VE, Papadopoulos N (2010) Frequent mutations of chromatin remodeling gene ARID1A in ovarian clear cell carcinoma. Science 330 (6001):228–231. https://doi.org/10.1126/science.1196333

Kalkat M, De Melo J, Hickman KA, Lourenco C, Redel C, Resetca D, Tamachi A, Tu WB, Penn LZ (2017) MYC deregulation in primary human cancers. Genes (Basel) 8(6):151. https://doi.org/10.3390/genes8060151

Kanakkanthara A et al (2019) BRCA1 deficiency upregulates NNMT, which reprograms metabolism and sensitizes ovarian cancer cells to mitochondrial metabolic targeting agents. Cancer Res 79(23):5920–5929

Kawahara N et al (2017) Candidate synthetic lethality partners to PARP inhibitors in the treatment of ovarian clear cell cancer. Biomed Rep 7(5):391–399

Kobayashi H et al (2018) Conceptual frameworks of synthetic lethality in clear cell carcinoma of the ovary. Biomed Rep 9(2):112–118

Konecny GE, Wang C, Hamidi H, Winterhoff B, Kalli KR, Dering J, Ginther C, Chen HW, Dowdy S, Cliby W, Gostout B, Podratz KC, Keeney G, Wang HJ, Hartmann LC, Slamon DJ, Goode EL (2014) Prognostic and therapeutic relevance of molecular subtypes in high-grade serous ovarian cancer. J Natl Cancer Inst 106(10):dju 249. https://doi.org/10.1093/jnci/dju249

Konstantinopoulos PA et al (2019) Phase II study of Avelumab in patients with mismatch repair deficient and mismatch repair proficient recurrent/persistent endometrial cancer. J Clin Oncol 37 (30):2786–2794

Konstantinopoulos PA et al (2020) Germline and somatic tumor testing in epithelial ovarian cancer: ASCO guideline. J Clin Oncol 38(11):1222–1245

Koshiyama M, Matsumura N, Konishi I (2014) Recent concepts of ovarian carcinogenesis: type I and type II. Biomed Res Int 2014:934261. https://doi.org/10.1155/2014/934261

Kristeleit R, Shapiro GI, Burris HA, Oza AM, LoRusso P, Patel MR, Domchek SM, Balmaña J, Drew Y, Chen LM, Safra T, Montes A, Giordano H, Maloney L, Goble S, Isaacson J, Xiao J, Borrow J, Rolfe L, Shapira-Frommer R (2017) A phase I-II study of the oral PARP inhibitor Rucaparib in patients with germline BRCA1/2-mutated ovarian carcinoma or other solid tumors. Clin Cancer Res 23(15):4095–4106. https://doi.org/10.1158/1078-0432.CCR-16-2796

Kristeleit RS, Oaknin A, Ray-Coquard I, Leary A, Balmaña J, Drew Y, Oza AM, Shapira-Frommer R, Domchek SM, Cameron T, Maloney L, Goble S, Lorusso D, Ledermann JA, McNeish IA (2019) Antitumor activity of the poly(ADP-ribose) polymerase inhibitor rucaparib as monotherapy in patients with platinum-sensitive, relapsed, BRCA-mutated, high-grade ovarian cancer, and an update on safety. Int J Gynecol Cancer 29(9):1396–1404. https://doi.org/10.1136/ijgc-2019-000623

Kuchenbaecker KB et al (2017) Risks of breast, ovarian, and contralateral breast cancer for BRCA1 and BRCA2 mutation carriers. JAMA 317(23):2402–2416

Kuhn E et al (2012) TP53 mutations in serous tubal intraepithelial carcinoma and concurrent pelvic high-grade serous carcinoma--evidence supporting the clonal relationship of the two lesions. J Pathol 226(3):421–426

Kuhn E et al (2016) CCNE1 amplification and centrosome number abnormality in serous tubal intraepithelial carcinoma: further evidence supporting its role as a precursor of ovarian high-grade serous carcinoma. Mod Pathol 29(10):1254–1261

Kurian AW et al (2019) Genetic testing and results in a population-based cohort of breast cancer patients and ovarian cancer patients. J Clin Oncol 37(15):1305–1315

Kurman RJ, Shih IM (2016) The dualistic model of ovarian carcinogenesis: revisited, revised, and expanded. Am J Pathol 186(4):733–747. https://doi.org/10.1016/j.ajpath.2015.11.011

Labidi-Galy SI, Olivier T, Rodrigues M, Ferraioli D, Derbel O, Bodmer A, Petignat P, Rak B, Chopin N, Tredan O, Heudel PE, Stuckelberger S, Meeus P, Meraldi P, Viassolo V, Ayme A, Chappuis PO, Stern MH, Houdayer C, Stoppa-Lyonnet D, Buisson A, Golmard L, Bonadona V, Ray-Coquard I (2018) Location of mutation in BRCA2 gene and survival in patients with ovarian cancer. Clin Cancer Res 24(2):326–333. https://doi.org/10.1158/1078-0432.CCR-17-2136

Lassmann S, Shen Y, Jütting U, Wiehle P, Walch A, Gitsch G, Hasenburg A, Werner M (2007) Predictive value of Aurora-a/STK15 expression for late stage epithelial ovarian cancer patients treated by adjuvant chemotherapy. Clin Cancer Res 13(14):4083–4091. https://doi.org/10.1158/1078-0432.CCR-06-2775

Laviolette LA, Hodgkinson KM, Minhas N, Perez-Iratxeta C, Vanderhyden BC (2014) 17-β-estradiol upregulates GREB1 and accelerates ovarian tumor progression in vivo. Int J Cancer 135(5):1072–1084. https://doi.org/10.1002/ijc.28741

Lawson DA, Kessenbrock K, Davis RT, Pervolarakis N, Werb Z (2018) Tumour heterogeneity and metastasis at single-cell resolution. Nat Cell Biol 20(12):1349–1360. https://doi.org/10.1038/s41556-018-0236-7

Ledermann JA (2016) PARP inhibitors in ovarian cancer. Ann Oncol 27(Suppl 1):i40–i44. https://doi.org/10.1093/annonc/mdw094

Ledermann JA, Drew Y, Kristeleit RS (2016) Homologous recombination deficiency and ovarian cancer. Eur J Cancer 60:49–58

Lheureux S, Tinker A, Clarke B et al (2018) A clinical and molecular phase II trial of Oral ENMD-2076 in ovarian clear cell carcinoma (OCCC): a study of the Princess Margaret phase II consortium. Clin Cancer Res 24(24):6168–6174. https://doi.org/10.1158/1078-0432.CCR-18-1244

Li GM (2008) Mechanisms and functions of DNA mismatch repair. Cell Res 18(1):85–98

Li R et al (2018) Two novel STK11 missense mutations induce phosphorylation of S6K and promote cell proliferation in Peutz-Jeghers syndrome. Oncol Lett 15(1):717–726

Li C, Bonazzoli E, Bellone S et al (2019) Mutational landscape of primary, metastatic, and recurrent ovarian cancer reveals c-MYC gains as potential target for BET inhibitors. Proc Natl Acad Sci U S A 116(2):619–624. https://doi.org/10.1073/pnas.1814027116. Epub 2018 Dec 24. Erratum in: Proc Natl Acad Sci U S A. 2019; 116 (12): 5829

Lim W et al (2004) Relative frequency and morphology of cancers in STK11 mutation carriers. Gastroenterology 126(7):1788–1794

Lord CJ, Ashworth A (2017) PARP inhibitors: synthetic lethality in the clinic. Science (New York, NY) 355(6330):1152–1158

Loveday C, Turnbull C, Ramsay E et al (2011) Germline mutations in RAD51D confer susceptibility to ovarian cancer. Nat Genet 43(9):879–882. https://doi.org/10.1038/ng.893

Loveday C et al (2012) Germline RAD51C mutations confer susceptibility to ovarian cancer. Nat Genet 44(5):475–476. author reply 476

Mafficini A, Simbolo M, Parisi A, Rusev B, Luchini C, Cataldo I, Piazzola E, Sperandio N, Turri G, Franchi M, Tortora G, Bovo C, Lawlor RT, Scarpa A (2016) BRCA somatic and germline mutation detection in paraffin embedded ovarian cancers by next-generation sequencing. Oncotarget 7(2):1076–1083. https://doi.org/10.18632/oncotarget.6834

Manchana T, Phoolcharoen N, Tantbirojn P (2019) BRCA mutation in high grade epithelial ovarian cancers. Gynecol Oncol Rep 29:102–105

Mandilaras V, Garg S, Cabanero M, Tan Q, Pastrello C, Burnier J, Karakasis K, Wang L, Dhani NC, Butler MO, Bedard PL, Siu LL, Clarke B, Shaw PA, Stockley T, Jurisica I, Oza AM, Lheureux S (2019) TP53 mutations in high grade serous ovarian cancer and impact on clinical outcomes: a comparison of next generation sequencing and bioinformatics analyses. Int J Gynecol Cancer 29(2):346–352. ijgc-2018-000087. https://doi.org/10.1136/ijgc-2018-000087

Martins FC et al (2014) Combined image and genomic analysis of high-grade serous ovarian cancer reveals PTEN loss as a common driver event and prognostic classifier. Genome Biol 15(12):526

Maru Y, Tanaka N, Ohira M, Itami M, Hippo Y, Nagase H (2017) Identification of novel mutations in Japanese ovarian clear cell carcinoma patients using optimized targeted NGS for clinical diagnosis. Gynecol Oncol 144(2):377–383. https://doi.org/10.1016/j.ygyno.2016.11.045

Marzagalli M, Fontana F, Raimondi M, Limonta P (2021) Cancer stem cells-key players in tumor relapse. Cancers (Basel) 13(3):E376. https://doi.org/10.3390/cancers13030376

McConechy MK et al (2015) Detection of DNA mismatch repair (MMR) deficiencies by immunohistochemistry can effectively diagnose the microsatellite instability (MSI) phenotype in endometrial carcinomas. Gynecol Oncol 137(2):306–310

Mirza MR et al (2016) Niraparib maintenance therapy in platinum-sensitive, recurrent ovarian cancer. N Engl J Med 375(22):2154–2164

Moller P et al (2017) Cancer incidence and survival in lynch syndrome patients receiving colonoscopic and gynaecological surveillance: first report from the prospective lynch syndrome database. Gut 66(3):464–472

Moore K, Colombo N, Scambia G, Kim BG, Oaknin A, Friedlander M, Lisyanskaya A, Floquet A, Leary A, Sonke GS, Gourley C, Banerjee S, Oza A, González-Martín A, Aghajanian C, Bradley W, Mathews C, Liu J, Lowe ES, Bloomfield R, DiSilvestro P (2018) Maintenance Olaparib in patients with newly diagnosed advanced ovarian cancer. N Engl J Med 379 (26):2495–2505. https://doi.org/10.1056/NEJMoa1810858

Moyer VA (2014) Risk assessment, genetic counseling, and genetic testing for BRCA-related cancer in women: U.S. Preventive Services Task Force recommendation statement. Ann Intern Med 160(4):271–281

Moyer CL et al (2020) Rare BRIP1 missense alleles confer risk for ovarian and breast cancer. Cancer Res 80(4):857–867

Mylavarapu S, Das A, Roy M (2018) Role of BRCA mutations in the modulation of response to platinum therapy. Front Oncol 8:16

Nakamura K et al (2014) Features of ovarian cancer in lynch syndrome (review). Mol Clin Oncol 2 (6):909–916

NCCN Guiedelines (2019) National Comprehensive Cancer Network: ovarian cancer including fallopian tube cancer and primary peritoneal cancer, version 1. Available from https://www.nccn.org/physician_gls/pdf/ovarian.pdf

Nielsen FC, van Overeem HT, Sørensen CS (2016) Hereditary breast and ovarian cancer: new genes in confined pathways. Nat Rev Cancer 16(9):599–612. https://doi.org/10.1038/nrc.2016.72

Norquist BM, Harrell MI, Brady MF, Walsh T, Lee MK, Gulsuner S, Bernards SS, Casadei S, Yi Q, Burger RA, Chan JK, Davidson SA, Mannel RS, DiSilvestro PA, Lankes HA, Ramirez NC, King MC, Swisher EM, Birrer MJ (2016a) Inherited mutations in women with ovarian carcinoma. JAMA Oncol 2(4):482–490. https://doi.org/10.1001/jamaoncol.2015.5495

Norquist BS, Brady MF, Harrell MI, Walsh T, Lee MK, Gulsuner SI et al (2016b) Mutations in homologous recombination genes and response to treatment in GOG 218: an NRG oncology study. Gynecol Oncol 141:2. https://doi.org/10.1016/j.ygyno.2016.04.033

Norquist BM, Brady MF, Harrell MI, Walsh T, Lee MK, Gulsuner S, Bernards SS, Casadei S, Burger RA, Tewari KS, Backes F, Mannel RS, Glaser G, Bailey C, Rubin S, Soper J, Lankes HA, Ramirez NC, King MC, Birrer MJ, Swisher EM (2018) Mutations in homologous recombination genes and outcomes in ovarian carcinoma patients in GOG 218: an NRG oncology/gynecologic oncology group study. Clin Cancer Res 24(4):777–783. https://doi.org/10.1158/1078-0432.CCR-17-1327

Oh BY, Shin HT, Yun JW, Kim KT, Kim J, Bae JS, Cho YB, Lee WY, Yun SH, Park YA, Park YH, Im YH, Lee J, Joung JG, Kim HC, Park WY (2019) Intratumor heterogeneity inferred from targeted deep sequencing as a prognostic indicator. Sci Rep 9(1):4542. https://doi.org/10.1038/s41598-019-41098-0

Paculova H et al (2017) BRCA1 or CDK12 loss sensitizes cells to CHK1 inhibitors. Tumour Biol 39(10):1010428317727479. https://doi.org/10.1177/1010428317727479

Paracchini L et al (2020) Detection of TP53 clonal variants in Papanicolaou test samples collected up to 6 years prior to high-grade serous epithelial ovarian cancer diagnosis. JAMA Netw Open 3 (7):e207566

Patch AM et al (2015) Whole-genome characterization of chemoresistant ovarian cancer. Nature 521(7553):489–494

Patni R (2019) Screening for ovarian cancer: an update. J Midlife Health 10(1):3–5

Pennington KP, Walsh T, Harrell MI, Lee MK, Pennil CC, Rendi MH, Thornton A, Norquist BM, Casadei S, Nord AS, Agnew KJ, Pritchard CC, Scroggins S, Garcia RL, King MC, Swisher EM (2014) Germline and somatic mutations in homologous recombination genes predict platinum response and survival in ovarian, fallopian tube, and peritoneal carcinomas. Clin Cancer Res 20 (3):764–775. https://doi.org/10.1158/1078-0432.CCR-13-2287

Pérez-Fidalgo JA, Gambardella V, Pineda B, Burgues O, Piñero O, Cervantes A (2020) Aurora kinases in ovarian cancer. ESMO Open 5(5):e000718. https://doi.org/10.1136/esmoopen-2020-000718

Petersen S et al (2020) CCNE1 and BRD4 co-amplification in high-grade serous ovarian cancer is associated with poor clinical outcomes. Gynecol Oncol 157(2):405–410

Pino MS et al (2009) Deficient DNA mismatch repair is common in lynch syndrome-associated colorectal adenomas. J Mol Diagn 11(3):238–247

Prakash R et al (2015) Homologous recombination and human health: the roles of BRCA1, BRCA2, and associated proteins. Cold Spring Harb Perspect Biol 7(4):a016600

Rauh-Hain JA et al (2011) Ovarian cancer screening and early detection in the general population. Rev Obstet Gynecol 4(1):15–21

Reyes-González JM, Armaiz-Peña GN, Mangala LS, Valiyeva F, Ivan C, Pradeep S, Echevarría-Vargas IM, Rivera-Reyes A, Sood AK, Vivas-Mejía PE (2015) Targeting c-MYC in platinum-resistant ovarian cancer. Mol Cancer Ther 14(10):2260–2269. https://doi.org/10.1158/1535-7163.MCT-14-0801

Roh MH et al (2010) High-grade fimbrial-ovarian carcinomas are unified by altered p53, PTEN and PAX2 expression. Mod Pathol 23(10):1316–1324

Ross JS, Ali SM, Wang K, Palmer G, Yelensky R, Lipson D, Miller VA, Zajchowski D, Shawver LK, Stephens PJ (2013) Comprehensive genomic profiling of epithelial ovarian cancer by next generation sequencing-based diagnostic assay reveals new routes to targeted therapies. Gynecol Oncol 130(3):554–559. https://doi.org/10.1016/j.ygyno.2013.06.019

Roy R, Chun J, Powell SN (2011) BRCA1 and BRCA2: different roles in a common pathway of genome protection. Nat Rev Cancer 12(1):68–78. https://doi.org/10.1038/nrc3181

Ruan J et al (2018) Quantitative assessment of aberrant P16(INK4a) methylation in ovarian cancer: a meta-analysis based on literature and TCGA datasets. Cancer Manag Res 10:3033–3046

Sallum LF et al (2018) WT1, p53 and p16 expression in the diagnosis of low- and high-grade serous ovarian carcinomas and their relation to prognosis. Oncotarget 9(22):15818–15827

Saotome K, Chiyoda T, Aimono E, Nakamura K, Tanishima S, Nohara S, Okada C, Hayashi H, Kuroda Y, Nomura H, Susumu N, Iwata T, Yamagami W, Kataoka F, Nishihara H, Aoki D (2020) Clinical implications of next-generation sequencing-based panel tests for malignant ovarian tumors. Cancer Med 9(20):7407–7417. https://doi.org/10.1002/cam4.3383

Shih AJ, Menzin A, Whyte J, Lovecchio J, Liew A, Khalili H, Bhuiya T, Gregersen PK, Lee AT (2018) Identification of grade and origin specific cell populations in serous epithelial ovarian cancer by single cell RNA-seq. PLoS One 13(11):e0206785. https://doi.org/10.1371/journal.pone.0206785. Erratum in: PLoS One. 2018 Dec 4; 13 (12): e0208778

Siegel RL, Miller KD, Jemal A (2020) Cancer statistics, 2020. CA Cancer J Clin 70(1):7–30

Sokol ES et al (2019) Pan-Cancer analysis of CDK12 loss-of-function alterations and their association with the focal tandem-duplicator phenotype. Oncologist 24(12):1526–1533

Soletormos G et al (2016) Clinical use of Cancer biomarkers in epithelial ovarian cancer: updated guidelines from the European group on tumor markers. Int J Gynecol Cancer 26(1):43–51

Song H, Dicks E, Ramus SJ et al (2015) Contribution of germline mutations in the RAD51B, RAD51C, and RAD51D genes to ovarian cancer in the population. J Clin Oncol 33 (26):2901–2907. https://doi.org/10.1200/JCO.2015.61.2408

Soong TR et al (2019) The fallopian tube, "precursor escape" and narrowing the knowledge gap to the origins of high-grade serous carcinoma. Gynecol Oncol 152(2):426–433

Stoffel EM, Carethers JM (2020) Current approaches to germline cancer genetic testing. Annu Rev Med 71:85–102. https://doi.org/10.1146/annurev-med-052318-101009

Sud A, Kinnersley B, Houlston RS (2017) Genome-wide association studies of cancer: current insights and future perspectives. Nat Rev Cancer 17(11):692–704

Sun C, Chan F, Briassouli P, Linardopoulos S (2007) Aurora kinase inhibition downregulates NF-kappaB and sensitises tumour cells to chemotherapeutic agents. Biochem Biophys Res Commun 352(1):220–225. https://doi.org/10.1016/j.bbrc.2006.11.004

Sun H, Wang H, Wang X, Aoki Y, Wang X, Yang Y, Cheng X, Wang Z, Wang X (2020) Aurora-A/SOX8/FOXK1 signaling axis promotes chemoresistance via suppression of cell senescence and induction of glucose metabolism in ovarian cancer organoids and cells. Theranostics 10 (15):6928–6945. https://doi.org/10.7150/thno.43811

Suszynska M, Ratajska M, Kozlowski P (2020) BRIP1, RAD51C, and RAD51D mutations are associated with high susceptibility to ovarian cancer: mutation prevalence and precise risk estimates based on a pooled analysis of ~30,000 cases. J Ovarian Res 13(1):50

Suvà ML, Tirosh I (2019) Single-cell RNA sequencing in cancer: lessons learned and emerging challenges. Mol Cell 75(1):7–12. https://doi.org/10.1016/j.molcel.2019.05.003

Swisher EM, Lin KK, Oza AM et al (2017) Rucaparib in relapsed, platinum-sensitive high-grade ovarian carcinoma (ARIEL2 part 1): an international, multicentre, open-label, phase 2 trial. Lancet Oncol 18(1):75–87. https://doi.org/10.1016/S1470-2045(16)30559-9

Syngal S et al (2015) ACG clinical guideline: genetic testing and management of hereditary gastrointestinal cancer syndromes. Am J Gastroenterol 110(2):223–262. quiz 263

Terada KY, Ahn HJ, Kessel B (2016) Differences in risk for type 1 and type 2 ovarian cancer in a large cancer screening trial. J Gynecol Oncol 27(3):e25. https://doi.org/10.3802/jgo.2016.27.e25

Topatana W et al (2020) Advances in synthetic lethality for cancer therapy: cellular mechanism and clinical translation. J Hematol Oncol 13(1):118

Turk AA, Wisinski KB (2018) PARP inhibitors in breast cancer: bringing synthetic lethality to the bedside. Cancer 124(12):2498–2506

Vanderstichele A, Busschaert P, Olbrecht S, Lambrechts D, Vergote I (2017) Genomic signatures as predictive biomarkers of homologous recombination deficiency in ovarian cancer. Eur J Cancer 86:5–14. https://doi.org/10.1016/j.ejca.2017.08.029

Vang R et al (2016) Molecular alterations of TP53 are a defining feature of ovarian high-grade serous carcinoma: a rereview of cases lacking TP53 mutations in the cancer genome atlas ovarian study. Int J Gynecol Pathol 35(1):48–55

Verhaak RG, Tamayo P, Yang JY et al (2013) Prognostically relevant gene signatures of high-grade serous ovarian carcinoma. J Clin Invest 123(1):517–525. https://doi.org/10.1172/JCI65833

Vitale SR, Groenendijk FH, van Marion R, Beaufort CM, Helmijr JC, Dubbink HJ, Dinjens WNM, Ewing-Graham PC, Smolders R, van Doorn HC, Boere IA, Berns EMJJ, Helleman J, Jansen MPHM (2020) TP53 mutations in serum circulating cell-free tumor DNA as longitudinal biomarker for high-grade serous ovarian cancer. Biomol Ther 10(3):415. https://doi.org/10.3390/biom10030415

Vuong NH, Cook DP, Forrest LA, Carter LE, Robineau-Charette P, Kofsky JM, Hodgkinson KM, Vanderhyden BC (2018) Single-cell RNA-sequencing reveals transcriptional dynamics of estrogen-induced dysplasia in the ovarian surface epithelium. PLoS Genet 14(11):e1007788. https://doi.org/10.1371/journal.pgen.1007788

Walsh T et al (2011) Mutations in 12 genes for inherited ovarian, fallopian tube, and peritoneal carcinoma identified by massively parallel sequencing. Proc Natl Acad Sci U S A 108 (44):18032–18037

Wang Y, Cortez D, Yazdi P, Neff N, Elledge SJ, Qin J (2000) BASC, a super complex of BRCA1-associated proteins involved in the recognition and repair of aberrant DNA structures. Genes Dev 14(8):927–939

Wang H et al (2017) Expression of the tumor suppressor gene p16, and lymph node metastasis in patients with ovarian cancer. Oncol Lett 14(4):4689–4693

Weber-Lassalle N et al (2018) BRIP1 loss-of-function mutations confer high risk for familial ovarian cancer, but not familial breast cancer. Breast Cancer Res 20(1):7

Weren RD, Mensenkamp AR, Simons M, Eijkelenboom A, Sie AS, Ouchene H, van Asseldonk M, Gomez-Garcia EB, Blok MJ, de Hullu JA, Nelen MR, Hoischen A, Bulten J, Tops BB, Hoogerbrugge N, Ligtenberg MJ (2017) Novel BRCA1 and BRCA2 tumor test as basis for treatment decisions and referral for genetic counselling of patients with ovarian carcinomas. Hum Mutat 38:226–235. https://doi.org/10.1002/humu.23137

Wiegand KC, Shah SP, Al-Agha OM et al (2010) ARID1A mutations in endometriosis-associated ovarian carcinomas. N Engl J Med 363(16):1532–1543. https://doi.org/10.1056/NEJMoa1008433

Winterhoff BJ, Maile M, Mitra AK, Sebe A, Bazzaro M, Geller MA, Abrahante JE, Klein M, Hellweg R, Mullany SA, Beckman K, Daniel J, Starr TK (2017) Single cell sequencing reveals heterogeneity within ovarian cancer epithelium and cancer associated stromal cells. Gynecol Oncol 144(3):598–606. https://doi.org/10.1016/j.ygyno.2017.01.015. Erratum in: Gynecol Oncol. 2018 Oct; 151(1): 182–186

Winterhoff B, Talukdar S, Chang Z, Wang J, Starr TK (2019) Single-cell sequencing in ovarian cancer: a new frontier in precision medicine. Curr Opin Obstet Gynecol 31(1):49–55. https://doi.org/10.1097/GCO.0000000000000516

Xu X et al (2013) LKB1 controls human bronchial epithelial morphogenesis through p114RhoGEF-dependent RhoA activation. Mol Cell Biol 33(14):2671–2682

Yang H, He L, Kruk P et al (2006) Aurora-A induces cell survival and chemoresistance by activation of Akt through a p53-dependent manner in ovarian cancer cells. Int J Cancer 119:2304–2312. https://doi.org/10.1002/ijc.22154

Yates MS, Timms K, Daniels MS, Oakley HD, Munsell MF, Lanchbury JS et al (2017) Evaluation of BRCA1/2 and homologous recombination defects in ovarian cancer and impact on clinical outcomes. J Clin Oncol 35(15 Suppl):5511. https://doi.org/10.1200/JCO.2017.35.15_suppl.5511

Zhang L, Luo M, Yang H, Zhu S, Cheng X, Qing C (2019) Next-generation sequencing-based genomic profiling analysis reveals novel mutations for clinical diagnosis in Chinese primary epithelial ovarian cancer patients. J Ovarian Res 12(1):19. https://doi.org/10.1186/s13048-019-0494-4

Zhao RX, Xu ZX (2014) Targeting the LKB1 tumor suppressor. Curr Drug Targets 15(1):32–52

Zhao Q, Yang J, Li L, Cao D, Yu M, Shen K, BGI Group (2017) Germline and somatic mutations in homologous recombination genes among Chinese ovarian cancer patients detected using next-generation sequencing. J Gynecol Oncol 28(4):e39. https://doi.org/10.3802/jgo.2017.28.e39

Zhao C, Li S, Zhao M, Zhu H, Zhu X (2018) Prognostic values of DNA mismatch repair genes in ovarian cancer patients treated with platinum-based chemotherapy. Arch Gynecol Obstet 297 (1):153–159. https://doi.org/10.1007/s00404-017-4563-x

Zhu H et al (2020) Harnessing DNA replication stress for novel cancer therapy. Genes (Basel) 11 (9):990

Zoppoli G et al (2012) CHEK2 genomic and proteomic analyses reveal genetic inactivation or endogenous activation across the 60 cell lines of the US National Cancer Institute. Oncogene 31 (4):403–418

Printed by Printforce, the Netherlands